SHELF-LIFE
SURGERY

SHELF-LIFE SURGERY

Editor

Stanley Zaslau, MD
Professor and Chief, Urology Residency
 Program Director
Associate Chair, Education and Research,
 Department of Surgery
Department of Surgery/Division of Urology
West Virginia University
Morgantown, West Virginia

Series Editors

Veeral Sudhakar Sheth, MD, FACS
Director, Scientific Affairs
University Retina and Macula Associates
Clinical Assistant Professor
University of Illinois at Chicago
Chicago, Illinois

Stanley Zaslau, MD, MBA, FACS
Professor and Chief
Urology Residency Program Director
Department of Surgery/Division
 of Urology
West Virginia University
Morgantown, West Virginia

Robert Casanova, MD
Assistant Dean of Clinical Sciences
 Curriculum
Associate Professor Obstetrics and
 Gynecology
Texas Tech University Health Sciences
 Center
Lubbock, Texas

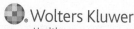
. Wolters Kluwer

Health

Philadelphia • Baltimore • New York • London
Buenos Aires • Hong Kong • Sydney • Tokyo

Acquisitions Editor: Susan Rhyner
Product Manager: Catherine Noonan
Marketing Manager: Joy Fisher-Williams
Designer: Stephen Druding
Compositor: Integra Software Services Pvt. Ltd.

9 8 7 6 5 4 3 2 1

Library of Congress Cataloging-in-Publication Data
Shelf-life surgery / editor Stanley Zaslau.
   p. ; cm.
  Includes index.
  ISBN 978-1-4511-9147-9
  I. Zaslau, Stanley, editor.
  [DNLM: 1. Surgical Procedures, Operative—Problems and Exercises. WO 18.2]
  RD37.2
  617.0076—dc23
             2013049598

DISCLAIMER

    Care has been taken to confirm the accuracy of the information present and to describe
generally accepted practices. However, the authors, editors, and publisher are not responsible for
errors or omissions or for any consequences from application of the information in this book and
make no warranty, expressed or implied, with respect to the currency, completeness, or accuracy
of the contents of the publication. Application of this information in a particular situation remains
the professional responsibility of the practitioner; the clinical treatments described and recommended may not be considered absolute and universal recommendations.

    The authors, editors, and publisher have exerted every effort to ensure that drug selection
and dosage set forth in this text are in accordance with the current recommendations and practice
at the time of publication. However, in view of ongoing research, changes in government regula-
tions, and the constant flow of information relating to drug therapy and drug reactions, the reader
is urged to check the package insert for each drug for any change in indications and dosage and
for added warnings and precautions. This is particularly important when the recommended agent
is a new or infrequently employed drug.

    Some drugs and medical devices presented in this publication have Food and Drug Admin-
istration (FDA) clearance for limited use in restricted research settings. It is the responsibility of
the health care provider to ascertain the FDA status of each drug or device planned for use in their
clinical practice.

To purchase additional copies of this book, call our customer service department at **(800)
638-3030** or fax orders to **(301) 223-2320**. International customers should call **(301) 223-2300**.

Visit Lippincott Williams & Wilkins on the Internet: http://www.lww.com. Lippincott Williams &
Wilkins customer service representatives are available from 8:30 am to 6:00 pm, EST.

Contributors

John Bozek, MD
Resident, Department of Anesthesiology
West Virginia University
Morgantown, West Virginia

David Greenwald, MD
Resident, Department of Surgery
Stanford University
Palo Alto, California

Morris Jessop, MD
Resident, Division of Urology,
    Department of Surgery
West Virginia University
Morgantown, West Virginia

Jared Manwaring, MD
Resident, Department of Urology
SUNY Syracuse Health Science Center
Syracuse, New York

Chad Morley, MD
Resident, Division of Urology/Department
    of Surgery
West Virginia University
Morgantown, West Virginia

Introduction to the Shelf-Life Series

The Shelf-Life series is an entirely new concept. The books have been designed from the ground up with student input. With academic faculty helping guide the production of these books, the Shelf-Life series is meant to help supplement the student's educational experience while on clinical rotation as well as prepare the student for the end-of-rotation shelf exam. We feel you will find these question books challenging but an irreplaceable part of the clinical rotation. With high quality, up-to-date content and hundreds of images and tables, this resource will be something you will continue to refer to even after you have completed your rotation.

The series editors would like to thank Susan Rhyner for supporting this concept from its inception. We would like to express our appreciation to Catherine Noonan, Laura Blyton, Amanda Ingold, Ashley Fischer, and Stacey Sebring, all of whom have been integral parts of the publishing team; their project management has been invaluable.

Veeral S. Sheth, MD, FACS
Stanley Zaslau, MD, MBA, FACS
Robert Casanova, MD

Acknowledgments

To Susan Rhyner and Catherine Noonan whose continued inspiration and well-wishes made this journey possible. To Veeral Sheeth and Bob Casanova, thanks for your support, timely feedback and enthusiasm for this great collaborative efforts in creating this series. To all of our current, future and former students of surgery, thank you for having the passion to be students of surgery which fuels my passion to be the best educator possible.

Contents

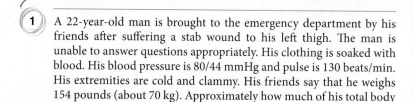

CHAPTER

1

Surgical Physiology

1 A 22-year-old man is brought to the emergency department by his friends after suffering a stab wound to his left thigh. The man is unable to answer questions appropriately. His clothing is soaked with blood. His blood pressure is 80/44 mmHg and pulse is 130 beats/min. His extremities are cold and clammy. His friends say that he weighs 154 pounds (about 70 kg). Approximately how much of his total body weight is composed of his intravascular fluid volume?

(A) 5 kg
(B) 16 kg
(C) 30 kg
(D) 42 kg
(E) 55 kg

The answer is A: 5 kg. A large amount of variation exists between patients and from time to time within the same patient in the proportion of body weight due to the fluid compartments, but a close approximation can be made with the two-thirds rule. This rule states that approximately two-thirds of body weight is made up of total body water. Two-thirds of the total body water is intracellular and one-third extracellular. Of the extracellular fluid, two-thirds are interstitial and one-third is intravascular. Using this rule, 2/3 × 70 kg = 47 kg (total body water). 2/3 × 47 kg = 31 kg (intracellular fluid) so the rest (16 kg) is extracellular fluid. 2/3 × 16 kg = 11 kg in the interstitial compartment so the rest (about 5 kg) is intravascular.

(B) Using the two-thirds rule, 2/3 × 70 kg = 47 kg (total body water). 2/3 × 47 kg = 31 kg (intracellular fluid) so the rest (16 kg) is extracellular fluid. 2/3 × 16 kg = 11 kg in the interstitial compartment so the rest (about 5 kg) is intravascular. (C) Using the two-thirds rule, 2/3 × 70 kg = 47 kg (total body water). 2/3 × 47 kg = 31 kg (intracellular fluid) so the rest (16 kg) is extracellular fluid. 2/3 × 16 kg = 11 kg in the interstitial compartment so the rest (about 5 kg) is intravascular. (D) Using the two-thirds rule, 2/3 × 70 kg = 47 kg (total body water). 2/3 × 47 kg = 31 kg (intracellular fluid) so the rest (16 kg) is extracellular fluid. 2/3 × 16 kg = 11 kg in the interstitial compartment so the rest (about 5 kg) is intravascular. (E) Using the two-thirds rule, 2/3 × 70 kg = 47 kg (total body water). 2/3 × 47 kg = 31 kg (intracellular fluid) so the rest (16 kg) is extra-cellular fluid. 2/3 × 16 kg = 11 kg in the interstitial compartment so the rest (about 5 kg) is intravascular.

---

2   A 45-year-old 70-kg man is hospitalized following a right direct ingui-nal hernia repair. The surgery was without complications. His blood pressure is 132/80 mmHg and pulse is 76 beats/min. About how much IV fluid should he be receiving per hour?

(A) 50 mL/h
(B) 75 mL/h
(C) 110 mL/h
(D) 125 mL/h
(E) 150 mL/h

The answer is C: 110 mL/h. There are two formulas for calculating main-tenance fluid doses. The 100/50/20 rule gives the amount of fluid a patient should receive in 24 hours: for the first 10 kg give 100 mL/kg, for the next 10 kg give 50 mL/kg, then for each kg above 20 kg give 20 mL/kg. For our 70-kg patient, this would be (10 kg × 100 mL/kg) + (10 kg × 50 mL/kg) + (50 kg × 20 mL/kg) = 2,500 mL in 24 hours, or about 104 mL per hour. An alternative is the 4/2/1 rule, which is similar but gives the rate per hour instead of per day. This rule counsels 4 mL/kg for the first 10 kg, 2 mL/kg for the next 10 kg, then 1 mL/kg for all above 20 kg. For our 70-kg patient, this would be (10 kg × 4 mL/kg) + (10 kg × 2 mL/kg) + (50 kg × 1 mL/kg) = 100 mL/h, very close to the 104 mL/h estimate given by the 100/50/20 rule.

(A) The 4/2/1 rule estimates 110 mL/h for a 70-kg man. The 100/50/20 rule (which gives a 24-hour fluid estimate) is close, with an hourly estimate of 104 mL/kg. (B) The 4/2/1 rule estimates 110 mL/h for a 70-kg man. The 100/50/20 rule (which gives a 24-hour fluid estimate) is close, with an hourly estimate of 104 mL/kg. (D) The 4/2/1 rule estimates 110 mL/h for a 70-kg man. The 100/50/20 rule (which gives a 24-hour fluid estimate) is close, with an hourly estimate of 104 mL/kg. (E) The 4/2/1 rule estimates 110 mL/h for a 70-kg man. The 100/50/20 rule (which gives a 24-hour fluid estimate) is close, with an hourly estimate of 104 mL/kg.

---

3   A 27-year-old woman presents to the emergency department with 6 hours of abdominal pain and vomiting. The pain started around her umbilicus at 4/10 but is now localized to her right lower quadrant and is 8/10. Her blood pressure is 130/82 mmHg, pulse is 90 beats/min, respirations are 18 breaths/min, and temperature is 38.5°C. She under-goes an uneventful emergency appendectomy. Her pre-op sodium was

145 mEq/L and is now 152 mEq/L. Her current fractional excretion of sodium (FE$_{Na}$) is <1%. Which of the following is the most likely cause of her hypernatremia?

(A) Acute tubular necrosis (ATN)
(B) High salt diet
(C) Iatrogenic
(D) Syndrome of inappropriate antidiuretic hormone secretion (SIADH)
(E) Vomiting

The answer is E: **Vomiting.** Most cases of hypernatremia are due to excessive free water loss. This can occur in any fluid deficit state in which hypotonic fluid is lost as in vomiting or diarrhea as well as the insensible losses from burns, mechanical ventilation, and fever. The polyuric phase of ATN can also result in hypernatremia. The cause is usually easy to identify. In cases of hypovolemia, resuscitation with isotonic fluids should be the first step. This can be switched to 1/2 normal saline or D5W once volume has been restored. In cases of hypervolemia, the first step would be to decrease sodium administration (via IV fluids). Diuretics may be useful as well.

(A) ATN can result in hypotonic fluid loss and hypernatremia, but it is characterized by a FE$_{Na}$ of >3% signifying a failure of the kidneys to retain sodium in the face of a volume deficit (caused by her vomiting). (B) Ingestion of excess sodium in a patient with intact renal function would not result in hypernatremia because of autoregulatory mechanisms that maintain serum sodium within a narrow range. (C) Iatrogenic hypernatremia is rare. It is due to infusion of too much saline. (D) SIADH is often the result of small cell lung cancers that produce antidiuretic hormone (ADH) with no negative feedback mechanism to inhibit its secretion. The excess ADH causes the kidneys to retain free water resulting in hyponatremia.

---

 4 A 65-year-old man who underwent surgery for a perforated gastric ulcer and has a nasogastric tube in place. His serum potassium is found to be 2.8 mEq/L. About how many mEq of potassium will be required to raise his serum potassium to 3.5 mEq/L?

(A) 20 mEq
(B) 35 mEq
(C) 50 mEq
(D) 70 mEq
(E) 105 mEq

The answer is D: **70 mEq.** Replacing potassium in hypokalemic patients reverses the weakness and ileus that accompanies hypokalemia (K$^+$ <3.5 mEq/L) and potentially prevents the cardiac arrhythmias it can cause. Replacing potassium by

IV infusion is advisable in patients with severe symptoms in the setting of hypoka-lemia, and replacement in these patients should continue until symptoms resolve. Replacing at a rate of 20 mEq/h is standard, and may increase up to 40 mEq/h in a closely monitored patient. Each 10 mEq of infused is expected to raise serum potassium by 0.1 mEq. By this estimation, about 70 mEq of potassium would be needed to bring this patient's level to 3.5 mEq/L.

(A) Each 10 mEq of infused is expected to raise serum potassium by 0.1 mEq. By this estimation, about 70 mEq of potassium would be needed to bring this patient's level to 3.5 mEq/L. (B) Each 10 mEq of infused is expected to raise serum potassium by 0.1 mEq. By this estimation, about 70 mEq of potassium would be needed to bring this patient's level to 3.5 mEq/L. (C) Each 10 mEq of infused is expected to raise serum potassium by 0.1 mEq. By this estimation, about 70 mEq of potassium would be needed to bring this patient's level to 3.5 mEq/L. (E) Each 10 mEq of infused is expected to raise serum potassium by 0.1 mEq. By this estimation, about 70 mEq of potassium would be needed to bring this patient's level to 3.5 mEq/L.

5 An 18-year-old male high school football player is tackled when he is rammed in the left abdomen by another player's head during practice. He complains of diffuse abdominal pain. He reports having a sore throat and fatigue for the past 10 days or so. On arrival, his blood pressure was 90/52 and pulse is 128. Focused assessment with sonography for trauma (FAST) examination shows a large intraperitoneal fluid collection. He is given normal saline for fluid resuscitation. The next day his sodium is 142, potassium 3.8, chloride 118, and bicarbonate 23. What is the most likely cause of his electrolyte abnormality?

(A) Adverse effect of paralytic used in surgery
(B) Free water retention
(C) Iatrogenic
(D) Massive tissue necrosis
(E) Vomiting

The answer is C: Iatrogenic. This patient has suffered a splenic laceration due to blunt abdominal trauma. His sore throat and fatigue should raise suspicion for mononucleosis, which increases the risk of splenic injury due to the spleno-megaly that often accompanies mononucleosis. The first step in answering this question is to determine which electrolyte value is abnormal. All except chloride are within the normal ranges. Any serum chloride value over 110 mEq/L is con-sidered high, so this patient has hyperchloremia. The most common cause of hyperchloremia in surgical patients is due to excessive use of normal saline for hydration. Normal saline has a much higher chloride content (154 mEq/L) than serum (100 to 110 mEq/L). Lactated Ringer solution or normal saline with an ampule of sodium bicarbonate or sodium acetate can provide the same amount of isotonic fluid for resuscitation while avoiding the infusion excess chloride.

(A) The depolarizing paralytic succinylcholine that is often used in surgery can cause or exacerbate hyperkalemia. This occurs because the depolarization of muscle cells involves potassium leaving the cells and entering the serum. Chloride abnormalities are not seen with succinylcholine. (B) Free water retention can cause hyponatremia as the sodium concentration is diluted and sodium is excreted as the body attempts to maintain euvolemia, but this patient's electrolyte abnormality is hyperchloremia. Hyperchloremia in surgical patients is most commonly caused by infusion of too much chloride. (D) Massive tissue necrosis can cause hyperkalemia as the large amount of intracellular potassium is released into the serum. This patient's hyperchloremia is more likely a result of infusion of too much chloride. (E) Vomiting can lead to hypochloremia, but this patient's chloride is above the normal range at 118 mEq/L. Normal values for serum chloride range from 100 to 110 mEq/L.

 6 A 47-year-old alcoholic woman presents to the emergency department with 2 hours of hematemesis. This is the second time in 2 months she has presented with hematemesis. She reports feeling short of breath and appears anxious and pale. Her blood pressure is 84/30 mmHg and pulse is 126 beats/min. Her hemoglobin is 7.2 g/dL. She is transfused with 6 units of packed red cells and her hemoglobin increases to 11.8 g/dL. Her next comprehensive metabolic panel shows a calcium level of 7.4 mg/dL. What is the most likely cause of her hypocalcemia?

(A) Blood loss
(B) Citrate chelation
(C) Malnutrition
(D) Parathyroid infarct
(E) Volume contraction

The answer is B: Citrate chelation. Serum calcium is maintained within a narrow range as are other electrolytes in order to support normal physiology. There are a number of regulatory hormones that adjust calcium levels including parathyroid hormone, vitamin D, and calcitonin. Hypocalcemia can be caused by failure of any of these hormones or by some extrinsic factor. Other causes of hypocalcemia include medication side effects, buildup of lactate, and citrate from blood transfusions. In a patient such as this woman who has recently received a large transfusion, the most likely cause is binding up of serum calcium by the citrate added to blood products to inhibit coagulation.

(A) Blood loss itself on the scale presented in this patient would not be expected to lead to hypocalcemia because even though total body calcium may be low the ionized portion would be relatively constant from the release of calcium bound to albumin. (C) Malnutrition could lead to hypocalcemia by leading to a decrease either in vitamin D or in the amount of albumin available to bind calcium. However, given the fact that this patient recently received a relatively large transfusion, citrate chelation of serum calcium is a more likely explanation. (D) Parathyroid infarct is not a common cause of hypocalcemia as the parathyroids receive a rich blood supply. Damage to the parathyroids during thyroid surgery can lead to hypocalcemia, but this patient underwent no such procedure. (E) Volume contraction would not be expected to cause significant variations in serum calcium. The most likely explanation for this patient's hypocalcemia is chelation by the citrate found in the blood products she received.

---

7 A 37-year-old woman undergoes a laparoscopic hysterectomy for leiomyomata. In the postanesthesia care unit (PACU), she appears somnolent. Blood pressure is 118/86 mmHg, pulse is 74 beats/min, respirations are 10 breaths/min, and temperature is 37°C. Her lungs are clear to auscultation. An arterial blood gas (ABG) drawn showed the following values: pH is 7.3, $PaCO_2$ is 50 mmHg, PaO_2 is 75 mmHg, and bicarbonate is 24 mEq/L. What is the most likely cause of her acid–base disorder?

(A) Excessive lactate production
(B) Hyperventilation
(C) Medication side effect
(D) Pneumonia
(E) Her values are within the normal range

The answer is C: Medication side effect. The first ABG value to check is the pH as this will determine whether the disorder is an acidosis or an alkalosis. In this patient, the pH of 7.3 is below normal (7.35 to 7.45) so the disorder is an acidosis. Metabolic acidosis is characterized by a low bicarbonate level, but this patient's bicarbonate is normal. Physiologically, respiratory acidosis is caused by hypoventilation leading to buildup of carbon dioxide in the blood. More carbon dioxide = more carbonic acid, so if a patient has a respiratory acidosis the $PaCO_2$ must be elevated. The low pH, high $PaCO_2$, low PaO_2, and normal bicarbonate level in this patient suggest respiratory acidosis. A patient in the PACU with respiratory acidosis may well be under the influence of narcotics (either those used during surgery or afterward or both). This is further supported by the findings of somnolence and decreased respirations.

(A) Excessive lactate production from poor tissue perfusion results in a metabolic acidosis. Metabolic acidosis is characterized by a low bicarbonate level, but this patient's bicarbonate is normal. The low pH, high $PaCO_2$, low PaO_2, and normal bicarbonate level in this patient suggest respiratory acidosis. (B) Hyperventilation would cause respiratory alkalosis, with a pH above 7.45 and a $PaCO_2$ less than 40 mmHg. This patient's respirations of 10 are also not consistent with respiratory alkalosis. (D) Pneumonia has been observed to be associated with slight hyperventilation, but not usually significant enough to cause an acid–base imbalance. Furthermore, pneumonia is unlikely in a patient only a few hours post-op with a clear chest to auscultation. (E) In this patient, the pH of 7.3 is below normal (7.35 to 7.45). Her low PaO_2 and elevated $PaCO_2$ are also abnormal and consistent with respiratory acidosis, likely due to the influence of narcotics.

8 A 24-year-old man suffers a liver laceration in a motor vehicle accident. He was hypotensive for a prolonged period of time. An ABG is drawn which shows a pH of 7.26, $PaCO_2$ of 33 mmHg, PaO_2 of 100 mmHg, and a bicarbonate of 14 mEq/L. Which of the following would be best to manage his acid–base imbalance?

(A) 100% oxygen
(B) Bicarbonate
(C) Fluid resuscitation
(D) Hemodialysis
(E) Insulin with D5W

The answer is C: Fluid resuscitation. The first ABG value to check is the pH as this will determine whether the disorder is an acidosis or an alkalosis. In this patient, the pH of 7.26 is below normal (7.35 to 7.45) so the disorder is an acidosis. Metabolic acidosis is characterized by a low bicarbonate level as seen in this patient. His low $PaCO_2$ is a compensatory response by the respiratory system to blow off more CO_2 in order to bring the pH toward normal. Treatment for metabolic acidosis involves correcting the underlying cause of the acidosis. This patient likely has lactic acidosis secondary to poor perfusion (tissues undergo anaerobic metabolism) and would best benefit from fluid resuscitation and possibly blood transfusion.

(A) This patient's blood oxygenation is within normal limits; he is suffering from hypoxia from poor perfusion but is not suffering hypoxemia. Fluid resuscitation would most rapidly restore perfusion and reverse the underlying lactic acidosis. (B) Bicarbonate has not been shown to be beneficial in treating acidosis of this degree. Treatment of metabolic acidosis should be targeted to the underlying cause rather than the acidosis itself. Bicarbonate may be therapeutic more severe cases of acidosis (pH <7.2), but in this case the next best step would be volume expansion. (D) Hemodialysis is only indicated in patients with acidosis who are refractory to other simpler treatment or have some contraindication. In this case, the next best step would be volume expansion to correct the poor perfusion leading to the acidosis. (E) Insulin and glucose can be used to treat diabetic ketoacidosis (a type of metabolic acidosis), but this patient's history is more consistent with lactic acidosis due to poor tissue perfusion. In this case, the next best step would be volume expansion.

9 A 34-year-old woman undergoes a cholecystectomy for an episode of cholecystitis. While recovering from the operation, she complains of feeling lightheaded. She appears uncomfortable. An ABG showed a pH of 7.48, $PaCO_2$ of 24 mmHg, PaO_2 of 106 mmHg, and bicarbonate of 24 mEq/L. Which of the following would be the best treatment?

(A) Administer bicarbonate
(B) Administer fentanyl
(C) Administer imipenem
(D) Administer oral lemon juice
(E) No intervention is necessary

The answer is B: **Administer fentanyl.** The first ABG value to check is the pH as this will determine whether the disorder is an acidosis or an alkalosis. In this patient, the pH of 7.48 is above normal (7.35 to 7.45) so the disorder is an alkalosis. The next step is to determine whether the alkalosis is primarily metabolic or respiratory. Metabolic alkalosis is characterized by a high pH and a high bicarbonate level. Respiratory alkalosis is characterized by a high pH and a low $PaCO_2$. This patient has both high pH and a low $PaCO_2$, consistent with respiratory alkalosis. Respiratory alkalosis is ultimately caused by hyperventilation; perhaps the patient in the question stem is hyperventilating in response to pain from her operation. The best choice under these circumstances would be to see if treating her pain would correct her acid–base imbalance.

(A) Treating the acidosis or alkalosis in a patient with an acid–base imbalance is ineffective because it does not correct the underlying cause of the imbalance. Regardless of this principle, this patient already has an alkalosis so adding bicarbonate would only worsen her condition. (C) Imipenem is a broad-spectrum antibiotic and may be useful in a patient with systemic inflammatory response syndrome (SIRS) or sepsis of unknown cause. Such serious infections may result in metabolic acidosis, not respiratory alkalosis (as seen in this patient). (D) Treating the acidosis or alkalosis in a patient with an acid–base imbalance is ineffective because it does not correct the underlying cause of the imbalance. (E) This patient's high pH and low $PaCO_2$ suggest respiratory alkalosis. Anxiety and pain can cause this so a trial of a pain reliever would be wise considering her recent operation.

---

 10 A 2-year-old boy suffers a traumatic amputation of his right index finger when a glass bowl fell and shattered on his hand while he was pulling on a tablecloth. What is the first step in hemostasis following the trauma?

(A) Factor X activation
(B) Formation of fibrin split products
(C) Gamma-glutamate carboxylation
(D) Platelet activation
(E) Platelet adherence

The answer is E: **Platelet adherence.** The question stem refers to the mechanisms of hemostasis. There are many steps in and factors contributing to hemostasis. The first step of hemostasis consists of platelet adherence to the basement membrane of the injured vessel. Next, platelets are activated and produce vasoconstrictors and adhere to each other. Clot formation also begins soon after the basement membrane of the damaged vessel is exposed. The intrinsic and extrinsic pathways converge by activating factor X which in turn activates thrombin which turns soluble fibrinogen into insoluble fibrin strands. Clot breakdown occurs as plasmin degrades the fibrin strands producing fibrin split products (d-dimers).

(A) Factor X activation is not the first step in hemostasis. Factor X activation occurs only after the extrinsic and/or intrinsic pathways have been activated. The first step in hemostasis is platelet adherence to the basement membrane of the damaged vessel. (B) Formation of fibrin split products occurs as plasmin breaks down the clot to restore normal circulation. The first step in hemostasis is platelet adherence to the basement membrane of the damaged vessel. (C) Gamma-glutamate carboxylation is a step preceding hemostasis during which vitamin K serves as a cofactor in the final step of factors II, VII, IX, and X to prepare them for their future role in coagulation. The first step in hemostasis is platelet adherence to the basement membrane of the damaged vessel. (D) Platelet activation occurs after platelets adhere to damaged vessels. The first step in hemostasis is platelet adherence to the basement membrane of the damaged vessel.

11 A 62-year-old alcoholic man presents to the emergency department with abdominal pain. He notes that his gums have been bleeding when he has been brushing his teeth over the past few days. He has no family history of bleeding disorders. A complete blood count (CBC) shows a white cell count of 8,000/mm³, hemoglobin of 14 g/dL, a hematocrit of 44%, and a platelet count of 210,000/mm³. His prothrombin time (PT) is 13 seconds and partial thromboplastin time (PTT) is 24 seconds. His sodium is 138 mEq/L, potassium 4.0 mEq/L, chloride 102 mEq/L, bicarbonate 23 mEq/L, blood urea nitrogen (BUN) 47 mg/dL, and creatinine 2.1 mg/dL. A CT scan shows a 3.3 cm × 3.1 cm × 2.8 cm renal mass with characteristics suggestive of renal cell carcinoma in the upper pole of his left kidney. A partial nephrectomy is recommended. Which of the following is the next best step in the management of this patient?

(A) Dialysis
(B) Fresh frozen plasma administration
(C) Platelet transfusion
(D) Proceed with partial nephrectomy
(E) Vitamin K administration

The answer is A: Dialysis. This patient's coagulopathy in the presence of a normal platelet count, normal PT, and normal PTT suggests platelet dysfunction is to blame. As an alcoholic, this patient is at increased risk for uremia as suggested by his elevated BUN. Uremia impairs platelet function so a patient with uremia may have a normal platelet count (as in this case), but has nonfunctional platelets. Dialysis is the definitive treatment for uremia.

(B) Fresh frozen plasma is given to correct clotting factor deficiencies but would not correct the uremia that is causing his platelet dysfunction. A clotting factor deficiency is not the cause of this man's coagulopathy as can be seen from his normal PT and PTT. (C) Transfused platelets would be deactivated by the uremia in the same manner as his native platelets have been. This man has a sufficient number of platelets but they are impaired because of his uremia. (D) A major surgery of this kind would likely result in a large, unnecessary, and potentially life-threatening blood loss in a patient with a coagulopathy such as this man. His coagulopathy will likely be reversed with dialysis to correct the uremia. (E) Vitamin K is necessary for the production of clotting factors II, VII, IX, and X. These factors are not deficient in this patient as seen by his normal PT and PTT. In any case, vitamin K will not result in acute reversal of any coagulopathy because these factors take days to synthesize.

 12 A 67-year-old man undergoes a right knee arthroplasty for osteoarthitis. He is otherwise healthy. Which of the following would be the most appropriate method of thromboembolism chemoprophylaxis in this patient?

(A) Aspirin
(B) IVC filter
(C) Low-molecular-weight heparin
(D) Warfarin
(E) None needed

The answer is C: Low-molecular-weight heparin. Many surgical patients are at risk for thromboembolism. Additional risk factors include smoking, immobilization, obesity, and cancer. Thromboembolic prophylaxis is an easy method for preventing major complications due to thromboembolic events such as deep vein thrombosis (DVT) and pulmonary emboli. Unfractionated heparin at a dose of 5,000 units subcutaneously every 8 hours or low-molecular-weight heparin 30 mg subcutaneously twice daily or 40 mg subcutaneously daily is an effective means of thromboembolic prophylaxis. Low-molecular-weight heparin is appealing because of its relative ease of use even though it is harder to reverse than unfractionated heparin.

(A) Aspirin is used as an antiplatelet drug in patients at risk for stroke and myocardial infarction. It is not useful in preventing thromboembolism. (B) An inferior vena cava filter may be used in patients with contraindications to chemoprophylaxis such as a patient with an intracranial bleed. Placing a filter is much more costly and invasive than simple chemoprophylaxis and is not done on a routine basis. (D) Warfarin is effective for long-term anticoagulation such as in patients with atrial fibrillation when it is used to prevent mural thrombi. It has a slow onset of action and is not useful it prevent thromboembolism in the acute setting. (E) Thromboembolic events are potentially devastating and easily preventable; all surgical patients should be assessed for thromboembolic prophylaxis.

13 A 58-year-old man undergoing radical prostatectomy for Gleason 9 prostate cancer loses 1,800 mL of blood during the operation and in transfused with 5 units of packed red cells. One week later, he develops a fever. His hematocrit upon discharge was 34% but is now 26%. What is the most likely etiology of his fever?

(A) ABO incompatibility
(B) Hepatitis B infection
(C) Hepatitis C infection
(D) Leukocytes present in the donor blood
(E) Minor antigen incompatibility

The answer is E: Minor antigen incompatibility. The delayed nature of this fever following this patient's transfusion suggests a minor antibody incompatibility such as Rh incompatibility. This reaction is known as a delayed hemolytic reaction as opposed to the acute hemolysis that occurs in ABO incompatibility. Treatment is supportive and this condition can usually be prevented by properly matching blood types.

(A) ABO incompatibility also causes hemolysis, but this reaction occurs within seconds to minutes of the start of transfusion. This type of reaction is entirely preventable. (B) Hepatitis B infection is rarely the result of a blood transfusion (1 in 220,000) and would not cause hemolysis. The most likely etiology in this case is a delayed hemolytic reaction from minor antigen incompatibility. (C) Hepatitis C infection is rarely the result of a blood transfusion (1 in 600,000) and would not cause hemolysis. The most likely etiology in this case is a delayed hemolytic reaction from minor antigen incompatibility. (D) Leukocytes present in the donor blood can cause a febrile reaction, but one that occurs on the order of minutes rather than days after the transfusion. There would be no hemolysis with this type of reaction.

14 A 58-year-old woman complains of progressively worsening left lower quadrant pain with blood in her stool. Her temperature is 39°C. An abdominal CT scan is suggestive of diverticulitis with a perforated viscus. She undergoes a partial colon resection. Which term would best classify this wound type?

(A) Clean
(B) Clean-contaminated
(C) Contaminated
(D) Dirty
(E) None of the above

The answer is D: Dirty. Surgical wounds are classified as clean, clean-contaminated, contaminated, or dirty/infected. This classification scheme takes into account how the wound was made and the expected rate of infection in order to determine whether the wound should be closed or left open to heal by secondary intent. Clean wounds are those made under sterile conditions and do not compromise any epithelial lining other than prepped skin. Clean-contaminated wounds are those made under sterile conditions but that do traverse a potentially contaminated epithelial lining such as bowel, GU tract, or respiratory tract but without gross contamination evident. A contaminated wound is similar to clean-contaminated wound except that gross contamination is present (as spillage of stool from the colon). This category also includes traumatic wounds. Dirty and infected wounds are those in which an infection is established before a cut is made in the skin, such as an abscess or perforated viscus following infection (as in this patient). Contaminated and dirty wounds are often left open to heal.

(A) A clean wound is one made under sterile conditions. This patient's wound would be classified as dirty because of the preexisting infection and perforated viscus. (B) This patient's wound would be considered clean-contaminated if her bowel was transected but no infection was present. The presence of a preexisting infection and perforated viscus would make her wound a dirty wound. (C) A contaminated wound is one in which there is gross spillage of stool from and uninfected bowel or the compromise of an infected respiratory or GU tract. (E) This patient's bowel infection (diverticulitis) with a perforated viscus fit the criteria for a dirty wound.

---

 15 A 64-year-old man with hydronephrosis secondary ureteral obstruction following radiation therapy for prostate cancer undergoes an operation in which a segment of small bowel is resected and attached to the renal pelvis and bladder to create a new ureter. Which term would best classify this wound?

(A) Clean
(B) Clean-contaminated
(C) Contaminated
(D) Dirty
(E) None of the above

The answer is B: Clean-contaminated. Surgical wounds are classified as clean, clean-contaminated, contaminated, or dirty/infected. This classification scheme takes into account how the wound was made and the expected rate of infection in order to determine whether the wound should be closed or left open to heal by secondary intent. Clean wounds are those made under sterile conditions and do not compromise any epithelial lining other than prepped skin. Clean-contaminated wounds are those made under sterile conditions but that do traverse a potentially contaminated epithelial lining such as bowel, GU tract, or respiratory tract but without gross contamination evident. A contaminated wound is similar to clean-contaminated wound except that gross contamination is present (as spillage of stool from the colon). This category also includes traumatic wounds. Dirty and infected wounds are those in which an infection is established before a cut is made in the skin, such as an abscess being drained. Contaminated and dirty wounds are often left open to heal.

(A) Any time an uninfected bowel mucosa is compromised during surgery, the wound is classified as clean-contaminated at best. If gross stool is spilled, the wound would be classified as contaminated (which did not occur in this case). (C) A contaminated wound is one in which gross contamination is present (spilled stool, infected GI, or respiratory tract that is transected). The act of transecting healthy, uninfected bowel in this case would be best classified as a clean-contaminated wound. (D) A dirty wound is one in which gross infection is present before the skin is cut. The act of transecting healthy, uninfected bowel in this case would be best classified as a clean-contaminated wound. (E) The act of transecting healthy, uninfected bowel in this case would be best classified as a clean-contaminated wound.

16 A 28-year-old woman with Crohn disease undergoes a partial colectomy through an abdominal incision. On post-op day 5, the wound is closed but is slightly erythematous. Her temperature is 37.1°C, pulse is 74 mmHg, blood pressure is 122/82 beats/min, and respirations are 16 breaths/min. No pus or other discharge is present at the incision. What is the most likely status of this wound?

(A) Infected
(B) Normal healing—coagulative phase
(C) Normal healing—inflammatory phase
(D) Normal healing—proliferative phase
(E) Normal healing—wound remodeling

The answer is C: Normal healing—inflammatory phase. Normal wound healing occurs through a series of phases by which a large measure of the original tensile strength of a tissue returns. First is the coagulation phase in which platelets and coagulation factors combine to stem bleeding and bring about hemostasis. Next comes the inflammatory phase, which lasts about 1 week. During this phase, polymorphonuclear leucocytes (PMNs) and macrophages invade to clean the area while epithelial cells form a barrier. Angiogenesis also occurs and contributes to the erythema and edema associated with this phase. This patient's wound is in the inflammatory phase. Then the proliferative phase begins in which fibroblasts invade and haphazardly lay down collagen, lasting about 3 weeks. The final phase is wound remodeling in which more collagen is laid down and reinforced along stress lines while excess collagen is degraded. Disruptions such as infections and hematomas can delay wound healing and may result in a chronic, nonhealing wound.

(A) The slight redness present around this woman's incision is most likely due to angiogenesis and associated edema that occurs during the inflammatory phase of wound healing. This is supported by the absence of fever and purulent drainage. (B) The coagulative phase occurs during the first minutes to hours following an insult. This patient's timing (5 days after her operation) suggests that her wound is going through the inflammatory phase. (D) The proliferative phase begins about 1 week after the original insult and corresponds to the end of the inflammatory phase. This patient's timing (5 days after her operation) and the finding of slight erythema suggest that her wound is going through the inflammatory phase. (E) Wound remodeling is the final phase in healing and occurs approximately 3 weeks after the injury. This patient's timing (5 days after her operation) and the finding of slight erythema suggest that her wound is going through the inflammatory phase.

 17 An 82-year-old man with metastatic prostate cancer has refused to eat anything for the past 18 hours. Which bodily nutrition source is utilized first during starvation?

(A) Glycogen
(B) Protein from collagen
(C) Protein from skeletal muscle
(D) Subcutaneous fat
(E) Visceral fat

The answer is A: Glycogen. Protein is one of the last energy sources used because proteins serve so many additional functions. Proteins can be broken down to amino acids which are converted to glucose by the liver, but the body preferentially uses glycogen stores and then fat stores as much as possible to spare proteins. The first fuel source during starvation is glycogen. It is easily and quickly broken down to glucose for use by any body cell but stores last only about 24 hours. The brain, which has a high metabolic need, can use ketones from fat breakdown once glycogen has been depleted so proteins can be conserved. After all glycogen and fat stores have been depleted, protein is metabolized rapidly until protein levels drop to half of baseline when death occurs.

(B) Protein from any source is spared by the body until glycogen and fat stores are depleted. At 18 hours, this man would still be using glucose from glycogen as his primary energy source. (C) Protein from any source is spared by the body until glycogen and fat stores are depleted. At 18 hours, this man would still be using glucose from glycogen as his primary energy source. (D) Fat stores are tapped only as glycogen becomes scarce. At 18 hours, this man would still be using glucose from glycogen as his primary energy source. (E) Fat stores are tapped only as glycogen becomes scarce. At 18 hours, this man would still be using glucose from glycogen as his primary energy source.

 18 A 42-year-old diabetic obese woman presents with a 4 × 6 cm² festering wound on her left lower extremity. The bulk of the necrotic tissue was successfully debrided surgically. Following her operation, which dressing would be best?

(A) Betadine-impregnated gauze
(B) Petrolatum-impregnated gauze
(C) Wet-to-dry
(D) Wet-to-wet
(E) No dressing

The answer is C: Wet-to-dry. The basic purposes of a dressing are to protect the underlying tissue until the epithelial covering reforms to seal the wound (about 48 hours) and wick away moisture and drainage so bacteria are not able to accumulate. Above this, certain types of dressings provide added benefit. For example, a wet-to-dry dressing involves a layer of saline-moistened gauze covered by a layer of dry gauze. As the underlying wet layer dries, necrotic tissue adheres and is easily pulled away when the dressing is changed to allow healthy tissue to grow.

(A) Betadine kills bacteria but would also destroy the body's leukocytes and fibroblasts that have migrated to the area to repair the wound. Betadine is for external use and would delay wound healing if applied directly. (B) Petrolatum-impregnated gauze would be more useful in dermal wounds such as abrasions and skin grafts. The nonpermeable gauze layer promotes more rapid epithelialization. A wound with necrotic tissue would be better served with a wet-to-dry dressing. (D) A wet-to-wet dressing would confer no benefit and may delay healing by providing a warm, moist area for bacteria to grow. A wet-to-dry dressing would be best for this woman's wound. (E) As mentioned in the explanation, dressings provide protection to allow rapid epithelialization and keep the wound dry to prevent bacterial buildup. A wet-to-dry dressing would be the best option in this case.

 A 72-year-old man undergoes partial colon resection for stage II colorectal cancer. The operation goes smoothly and he is transferred to the floor after recovering in the PACU. Later that night, he becomes hypotensive and requires vasopressors to maintain a mean arterial pressure (MAP) above 60 mmHg. Which of the following is an appropriate step in his management?

(A) Administer 100% oxygen
(B) Administer nitroprusside
(C) Administer total parenteral nutrition (TPN)
(D) Intubate
(E) Transfer to ICU

The answer is E: Transfer to ICU. The intensive care unit (ICU) is well prepared and equipped to handle critically ill patients. The care received in the ICU is much more than what is generally available in other areas of the hospital. Some reasons to place a patient in the ICU include intubation and ventilation, vasopressor requirement, invasive monitors (such as arterial lines), and any other condition demanding more intensive care. An appropriate next step in the management of this patient who has just been placed on vasopressors would be a transfer to the ICU.

(A) Administration of 100% oxygen would do nothing for this patient's hypotension. Oxygen therapy may be valuable to him overall, but a better step would be a transfer to the ICU. (B) Nitroprusside is a vasodilator and would only worsen his condition. Patients requiring vasopressors are better cared for in an ICU setting. (C) There is no obvious reason to give this man total parenteral nutrition. The fact that he requires vasopressors suggests that he would be better served in the ICU. (D) There is no reason to intubate this patient; his problem is hypotension requiring vasopressors. This requirement is a reason enough to transfer him to the ICU.

---

20   A 24-year-old 60-kg woman is severely injured in an automobile accident. She suffers a blunt closed head injury and requires intubation and ventilatory support. After being on the ventilator for an hour, an ABG shows pH 7.32, $PaCO_2$ is 48 mmHg, PaO_2 190 mmHg, and bicarbonate 18 mEq/L. Current ventilator settings are 10 bpm, tidal volume is 600 mL, positive end expiratory pressure (PEEP) 5 mmHg, and FiO_2 0.4. Which setting should increase?

(A) Breaths per minute (bpm)
(B) FiO_2
(C) PEEP
(D) Tidal volume
(E) No changes are necessary

The answer is A: Breaths per minute (bpm). The ventilator addresses two different issues the lungs normally handle: ventilation (ridding the body of CO_2) and oxygenation. Depending on the patient's underlying problem, the ventilator may be correcting one aspect more than the other. The variety of settings on the ventilator allows the physician to modify oxygenation and ventilation independently of each other. In this case, the patient's ABG shows an appropriate response to her FiO_2—the normal ratio of PaO_2 (normally ~100) to FiO_2 (~0.2 for room air) is 500. A ratio less than 200 defines ARDS. Her oxygenation needs no change, but her $PaCO_2$ is slightly high and her pH is slightly low suggesting ventilation is inadequate. To increase ventilation, tidal volume or breaths per minute (bpm) or both can be increased. 600 mL is a large volume for this size patient (values between 8 and 10 mL/kg are appropriate). Increasing her tidal volume further will likely result in lung damage (volutrauma). The best way to safely increase this patient's ventilation is to increase her breathing rate. 12 to 15 breaths/min would likely correct her mild respiratory acidosis.

(B) This woman's oxygenation is appropriate (PaO_2 to FiO_2 ratio is 475). Her low pH and elevated $PaCO_2$ suggest instead that she is not being sufficiently ventilated. (C) A PEEP of 5 mmHg is appropriate for this patient. Increasing the

PEEP may compensate for some degree of hypoxia but high PEEP decreases venous return to the heart and can lead to hypotension and poor perfusion. (D) Appropriate tidal volume for a patient on a ventilator can be calculated by estimated between 8 and 10 mL/kg. At 60 kg this patient would tolerate at most 600 mL per breath, so increasing the tidal volume any more would likely lead to lung injury. (E) This patient's $PaCO_2$ is high and her pH is low suggesting ventilation is inadequate. To increase ventilation, tidal volume or breaths per minute (bpm) or both can be increased.

---

 21 A 66-year-old man undergoes a four-vessel coronary artery bypass graft. In order to monitor his cardiac output, a pulmonary artery catheter is inserted. The PCWP on the catheter reads 10 mmHg. With which value does this measurement most closely correlate?

(A) Inferior vena cava pressure
(B) Left atrial pressure
(C) Right atrial pressure
(D) Right ventricular pressure during diastole
(E) Right ventricular pressure during systole

The answer is B: Left atrial pressure. A pulmonary artery catheter consists of a long tube with a balloon at one end which is inserted usually through a subclavian or jugular vein into the right ventricle. The balloon allows the catheter to be floated through the heart along with normal blood flow into one of the pulmonary arteries. The balloon follows the flow until it becomes lodged in a pulmonary artery too small to let it pass. A port on the distal end of the balloon allows accurate measurement of venous pressure from the left side of the heart. The catheter's pulmonary capillary wedge pressure (PCWP) is a close approximation of left atrial and left diastolic ventricular pressures.

(A) The pressure in the inferior vena cava or any other central vein would not be measured by a pulmonary artery catheter. Additionally, central venous pressure is normally between 3 and 8 mmHg. (C) Right atrial pressure would not be measured with a pulmonary artery catheter. Right atrial pressure is normally between 3 and 8 mmHg. (D) Right ventricular pressure during diastole would be essentially the same as central venous pressure or right atrial pressure. These pressures are not measured by pulmonary artery catheterization and are normally between 3 and 8 mmHg. (E) Right ventricular systolic pressure is normally between 15 and 30 mmHg. A pulmonary artery catheter would not measure this pressure because the balloon at the catheter's tip ensures that the distal port is in contact only with left cardiac venous blood.

---

 22 A 74-year-old woman undergoes a left partial nephrectomy for a 3 cm lower pole renal mass. The surgical procedure is uneventful. During her first postoperative night, the nurse calls to say her blood pressure is 88/40 mmHg, pulse is 110 beats/min, and she appears to be in distress.

Physical examination reveals normal heart sounds, normal breath sounds, cold, clammy skin, and distended neck veins. Which of the following types of shock is this patient experiencing?

(A) Cardiogenic
(B) Hypovolemic
(C) Neurogenic
(D) Obstructive
(E) Septic

The answer is A: Cardiogenic. Shock refers to any situation in which the cardiovascular system is unable to maintain adequate tissue perfusion. This can be due to inappropriate systemic vasodilation (as occurs in septic and neurogenic shock), inability of the heart to pump with sufficient contractility (cardiogenic shock), insufficient intravascular volume (hypovolemic shock), or some obstruction causing decreased cardiac output (obstructive shock). This woman's findings of cold, clammy skin suggest systemic vasoconstriction (ruling out septic and neurogenic shock). Her distended neck veins suggest congestion (ruling out hypovolemic shock). The otherwise normal pulmonary and cardiac examinations make cardiogenic shock the most likely of the remaining two choices. Examples of obstructive shock include cardiac tamponade and tension pneumothorax, and would likely have some abnormality on physical examination.

(B) Hypovolemic shock is due to insufficient circulating volume (such as following a major bleed). The finding of distended neck veins effectively rules out this possibility. (C) Neurogenic shock is characterized by a decrease in autonomic tone of the vasculature resulting in warm, well-perfused skin. Cold, clammy skin is characteristic of hypovolemic and cardiogenic shock. (D) Obstructive shock occurs when cardiac output is impaired by some physical obstruction such as a tension pneumothorax or cardiac tamponade. (E) Septic shock would present with a similar appearance to neurogenic shock—warm, well-perfused skin.

---

23 A 33-year-old morbidly obese man presents to the emergency department with 8 hours of worsening fever and chills following 5 days of a red, swollen, left lower extremity. He had tripped and cut his knee on a brick staircase outside his home and has not yet seen a doctor. Past medical history is significant for poorly controlled type II diabetes. His blood pressure is 86/42 mmHg and pulse is 122 beats/min. His skin is warm and flushed. From which type of shock is he most likely suffering?

(A) Cardiogenic
(B) Hypovolemic
(C) Neurogenic
(D) Obstructive
(E) Septic

The answer is E: Septic. Shock refers to any situation in which the cardiovascular system is unable to maintain adequate tissue perfusion. This can be due to inappropriate systemic vasodilation (as occurs in septic and neurogenic shock), inability of the heart to pump with sufficient contractility (cardiogenic shock), insufficient intravascular volume (hypovolemic shock), or some obstruction causing decreased cardiac output (obstructive shock). This man's findings of warm, flushed skin suggest systemic vasodilation (ruling out cardiogenic and hypovolemic shock). His history of a dirty wound with a background of diabetes is concerning for infection and sepsis, making septic shock more likely than neurogenic shock.

(A) Cardiogenic shock occurs when some injury to the heart (such as in an MI) impairs the heart's contractility, leading to poor perfusion. The skin of the extremities will be cold and clammy from the vasoconstrictive response to decreased cardiac output. (B) Hypovolemic shock is due to insufficient circulating volume (such as following a major bleed). The skin of the extremities will be cold and clammy from the vasoconstrictive response to decreased cardiac output. (C) Neurogenic shock is characterized by a decrease in autonomic tone of the vasculature resulting in warm, well-perfused skin. The history of a dirty wound in a patient with diabetes, fever, and chills makes septic shock more likely. (D) Obstructive shock occurs when cardiac output is impaired by some physical obstruction such as a tension pneumothorax or cardiac tamponade.

24 A 65-year-old 60-kg woman undergoes a hemicolectomy for diverticulitis. Postoperatively she exhibits poor respiratory drive and must remain intubated. Crackles are heard bilaterally. An arterial blood gas shows that pH is 7.41, $PaCO_2$ 41 mmHg, PaO_2 110 mmHg, and bicarbonate 24 mEq/L. Current ventilator settings are 14 bpm, tidal volume is 500 mL, PEEP 5 mmHg, and FiO_2 0.5. Which ventilator setting should be increased?

(A) Breathing rate
(B) FiO_2
(C) PEEP
(D) Tidal volume
(E) No changes are necessary

The answer is B: FiO_2. The ventilator addresses two different issues the lungs normally handle: ventilation (ridding the body of CO_2) and oxygenation. Depending on the patient's underlying problem, the ventilator may be correcting one aspect more than the other. The variety of settings on the ventilator allows the physician to modify oxygenation and ventilation independently of each other. In this case, the patient's ABG shows a "normal" PaO_2 of 90 mmHg; this represents an inappropriate response to her FiO_2 of 40%. The normal ratio of PaO_2 (normally ~100) to FiO_2 (~0.2 for room air) is 500. A ratio less than 200 defines ARDS. Her ratio is 90/0.4 = 225, suggesting respiratory distress

and close to the diagnostic level for ARDS. An increase in her FiO_2 would be prudent. Her pH, $PaCO_2$, and bicarbonate levels are within normal limits so no changes in ventilation are necessary at this time.
(A) Breathing rate affects ventilation more than oxygenation. She requires better oxygenation while her pH, $PaCO_2$, and bicarbonate levels are within normal limits so no changes in ventilation are necessary at this time. (C) A PEEP of 6 mmHg is appropriate for this patient. Increasing the PEEP may compensate for some degree of hypoxia but high PEEP decreases venous return to the heart and can lead to hypotension and poor perfusion. Her relative hypoxia would best be corrected by increasing the FiO_2. (D) Appropriate tidal volume for a patient on a ventilator can be calculated by estimated between 8 and 10 mL/kg (500 mL is appropriate for this patient). Increasing the tidal volume affects ventilation more than oxygenation. She requires better oxygenation while her pH, $PaCO_2$, and bicarbonate levels are within normal limits so no changes in ventilation are necessary at this time. (E) This patient's relative hypoxia suggests oxygenation is inadequate. To increase oxygenation, PEEP can be increased (already is above 5 mmHg for her) or FiO_2 can be increased.

---

 25 A 48-year-old morbidly obese man undergoes a panectomy for intractable cellulitis. His weight was decreased by 23 kg and is placed on a low-calorie diabetic diet. What is the best way to measure adequate protein intake in this patient?

(A) Calculate protein content of food
(B) Daily weights
(C) Hemoglobin level
(D) Prealbumin level
(E) Urinary urea nitrogen level

The answer is D: Prealbumin level. Adequate protein intake for a normal adult is approximately 0.8 g/kg/d, but this can increase to 2 g/kg/d during times of illness and stress. A number of indicators can be used to evaluate adequate protein intake. These include measuring nitrogen output (urine plus stool) vs. nitrogen intake (grams of protein/6.25) to maintain a positive balance, monitoring weight gain (though this is the least reliable), and measuring visceral protein levels (albumin, prealbumin, transferrin). Of the choices listed, measuring a prealbumin level would be the most reliable indicator in this patient.
(A) Calculating the protein content of food is only part of the steps needed to determine nitrogen balance. This amount must be compared with excreted nitrogen (urinary nitrogen and estimated stool nitrogen) to determine whether the patient has a positive or negative balance. (B) Daily weights is the least accurate method of determining protein nutrition because many other unrelated factors also affect weight. (C) Hemoglobin levels do not fluctuate

with changes in protein metabolism nearly as much as prealbumin. Albumin and transferrin levels may be used to evaluate protein nutritional status, but hemoglobin is not. (E) Calculating the excreted urinary nitrogen is only part of the steps needed to determine nitrogen balance. This amount of excreted nitrogen (urinary nitrogen and estimated stool nitrogen) must be compared to the dietary intake of nitrogen (protein grams/6.25) to determine whether the patient has a positive or negative balance.

2

Trauma and Burns

1 A 25-year-old college student arrives in the emergency department after an altercation at the bar over his girlfriend. During the fight, he was stabbed in the upper chest. He is alert, but is complaining of difficulty swallowing. His body temperature is 37.5°C, blood pressure 135/90 mmHg, pulse 110/min and respirations 20/min. On examination, there is a defect in the skin slightly off midline and directly above the sternal notch. There are crackling noises heard on expiration. Immediately lateral to the defect there is significant swelling. The skin over the swelling has a "tissue paper"-like texture. There are no other wounds visible on the rest of the body. Which of the following is the next best step in management?

(A) Cricothyrotomy
(B) Fiberoptic bronchoscopy
(C) Insert two large bore peripheral intravenous lines
(D) Orotracheal intubation
(E) Radiographs of the neck

The answer is D: **Orotracheal intubation.** This patient most likely has a penetrating injury to his trachea with possible additional injury to his esophagus or other important structures. Although he is currently not complaining of difficulty breathing, the swelling in his neck is most likely subcutaneous emphysema, which could progress to airway compression at any moment. Thus, the initial step is to secure an airway with orotracheal intubation. If unsuccessful, additional methods can be applied including intubation through the wound, fiberoptic laryngoscopy, tracheotomy, or cricothyrotomy.

(A) Cricothyrotomy (an incision through the cricothyroid membrane) is almost always performed as a last resort to secure an airway. Other methods for securing an airway should be attempted first. (B) Although fiberoptic bronchoscopy is the diagnostic modality of choice for a tracheal or bronchial injury, securing an airway is the most important initial step in this patient. (C) The airway should be secured before worrying about circulation. This patient's blood pressure is stable and there are no other signs of vascular trauma. (E) Radiographs of the neck are helpful in the diagnosis of airway injuries. They can show defects in the tracheal wall as well as subcutaneous emphysema. Although this will most likely be necessary, securing an airway is the most important initial step in this patient.

---

2 A 45-year-old white man is brought into the emergency department. He is unconscious on arrival. His oxygen saturation is 95% on 2 L, body temperature 37.3°C, blood pressure 110/65 mmHg, pulse 100/min, and respirations 20/min. He does not respond to commands. A computed tomography (CT) scan of the head shows multiple small intraparenchymal hemorrhages at the gray–white matter interface along with other focal areas of low density. Which of the following mechanisms of injury is most likely in this patient?

(A) Bleeding after a fall in a patient on warfarin
(B) Hemorrhagic stroke
(C) Restrained driver in a high-speed motor vehicle collision
(D) Temporal bone fracture from blunt injury
(E) Vascular injury to the carotid arteries

The answer is C: **Restrained driver in a high-speed motor vehicle collision.** This patient's head imaging suggests diffuse axonal injury. Diffuse axonal injury is characterized by axonal separation from severe deceleration, accelerating, or rotational forces. Although CT imaging is often initially normal, occasionally small petechial hemorrhages can be visualized at the gray–white matter junction of the cerebral cortex, the corpus collosum, or brain stem. MRI imaging is more sensitive than CT, but may also be initially normal. The injury is often more severe than realized on presentation. Motor vehicle collisions are the most common cause of diffuse axonal injury. Other less common causes include child abuse, falls, and assaults.

(A) Even minor head trauma with a patient on warfarin can result in a subdural hematoma. Patients are often immediately unconscious or may progressively deteriorate. Most subdural hematoma patients are older, with some studies citing an average age of 41. In subdural hematomas, blood forms in the subdural space following tearing of the bridging veins. CT imaging will show a hyperdense crescent-shaped collection of blood between the skull and the surface of the brain. Unlike epidural hematomas, subdural hematomas can cross suture lines. (B) CT imaging of a hemorrhagic stroke will show more often a single intraparenchymal hemorrhage. These are most common in the thalamus or basal ganglia. (D) A temporal bone fracture from a blunt injury (such as a hammer or baseball bat) is more likely to cause a laceration to the middle meningeal artery and a subsequent epidural hematoma. Patients classically present with an initial lucid interval, followed by rapid deterioration. CT imaging will classically show a biconvex homogenous density that does not cross the suture lines of the dura. (E) Vascular injury to the carotid arteries may cause diffuse cerebral hypoxia. CT imaging, although it may be unremarkable at first, would eventually show cerebral edema with obliteration of the cerebral ventricles, blurring of the gray–white matter junction and effacement of the delineation of deep gray matter structures.

3 A 26-year-old woman falls while mountain climbing and fractures her femur and tibia on her right leg. She arrives several hours later in the emergency department in severe pain. She describes it as constant and deep, with "pins and needles" in her foot. Her leg is edematous and cool to touch. Which of the following is the next best step in management?

(A) Emergent repair of fractures
(B) Fasciotomy
(C) Intravenous morphine
(D) Laboratory workup
(E) X-ray of the leg

The answer is B: Fasciotomy. This patient is presenting with symptoms of acute compartment syndrome. Acute compartment syndrome is a serious and life-threatening condition caused by increased pressure within a muscle compartment that can cause compression of the blood vessels and subsequent tissue ischemia/death. Symptoms of compartment syndrome include the 5 "Ps": pain (often out of proportion to findings and often the initial complaint), paresthesias, paralysis (often a late finding), pulse loss, and pallor. Diagnosis can be clinical or made with gauging the pressure within the compartment. Treatment is with an emergent fasciotomy to relieve pressure.

(A) Although repair of the fractures should be performed as part of this patient's treatment, the most urgent priority should be restoring blood flow to the patient's right leg. This is best accomplished with a fasciotomy. (C) Intravenous morphine is important to help control the pain, but often the pain associated with compartment syndrome is unresponsive to morphine. Urgent relief of the pressure will do the most to relieve this patient's pain. (D) Laboratory workup with acute compartment syndrome is not a first priority. Obtaining tissue reperfusion should not be delayed for laboratory studies. (E) Imaging studies are usually not helpful in the workup of acute compartment syndrome as the findings are often nonspecific and delay urgent treatment.

4 A 2-year-old boy is brought into the emergency department after being backed over by his aunt in a van. He arrives unresponsive, but the paramedics say that a few minutes ago he was complaining of abdominal pain. His blood pressure is 60/35 mmHg, pulse 144/min, and respirations symmetric and unlabored. On examination, the child's abdomen seems tense and distended and a tire mark is grossly visible. His pupils are round and reactive to light and accommodation. There are also several bruises on his shins and an obvious fracture of his left lower arm. Intravenous access is obtained and 2 L of normal saline are infused. His blood pressure increases to 65/40 mmHg. Which of the following is the next best step in management?

(A) CT scan of the head
(B) Emergent laparotomy
(C) Focused assessment with sonography for trauma (FAST) examination
(D) Peritoneal lavage
(E) Start chest compressions

The answer is B: **Emergent laparotomy.** This child is most likely bleeding within the abdomen. Since the suspicion is very high in this case, and no other injuries that could account for the drop in blood pressure are apparent, immediate laparotomy to identify the source(s) and stop the bleeding is the next best step in management.

(A) A CT scan of the head is not necessary, as there are no neurologic deficits. Furthermore, even if the head was injured it could not account for the amount of blood loss this patient has had. The most urgent problem is the intraabdominal blood loss. (C) Although a FAST would be appropriate if the site of blood loss was not obvious, the patient in this case has a distended and tense abdomen with obvious abdominal injury on the outside. (D) Performing a peritoneal lavage might be useful if the source of the bleeding was questionable, but in this case it would only serve to further delay treatment. (E) This patient is not in cardiac arrest and chest compressions are not needed.

5   An 8-year-old boy is brought into the emergency department after being pulled from a burning house. On examination, the patient has second and third-degree burns covering both of his upper extremities. The patient weighs 25 kg. An airway is secured and two large bore intravenous lines are started. Approximately how much fluid should be infused in the initial management of this patient?

(A) 800 mL over 8 hours
(B) 1,500 mL over 16 hours
(C) 1,500 mL over 8 hours
(D) 4,000 mL over 8 hours
(E) 8,500 mL over 8 hours

The answer is C: **1,500 mL over 8 hours.** The fluid requirement can be calculated for this patient using the Parkland formula along with a slightly modified "rule of 9s" for estimating body surface area (BSA) of the burn (compensating for the increased size of the head in children). Other more accurate body surface charts based on age are available, but the rule of 9s remains useful for a rough estimate in emergency situations. The initial step is to calculate BSA, which in a child can be determined as follows:

Head—18%
Each arm—9%
Abdomen and chest—18%
Back—18%
Each leg—14%

The Parkland formula for fluid in children is the same as that of adults (different numbers are used for infants). The formula is as follows:

(2 to 4 mL × %BSA × weight in kg) lactate ringers + 2,000 mL D5W.

Half of this should be given over the first 8 hours, and the other half over the subsequent 16 hours. In this patient, with a body weight of 25 kg, and with both arms burned (18% BSA), the fluid requirement is calculated as follows:

(2 to 4 mL × 18% × 25 kg) + 2,000 mL = 2,900 to 3,800 mL
2,900/2 or 3,800 mL/2 = 1,450 to 1,900 mL.

Thus, the choice of 1,500 mL is the approximate amount of fluid that should be given over the first 8 hours.
(A) This amount of fluid is too little. (B) This amount of fluid is too little. (D) This amount of fluid will result in overload. (E) This amount of fluid will result in overload.

---

6 A 5-year-old girl is out camping with her family when she accidently falls into the fire. She sustains full thickness burns of both arms up to her elbows and some minor burns on her face. She is admitted to the burn unit and does well until day 3, when she starts complaining of severe pain in her left arm. Examination shows thick, course, and leathery skin that completely encircles her left forearm. Her left radial pulse is markedly diminished when compared to her right. Which of the following is the next best step in management?

(A) Amputation of the limb
(B) Doppler ultrasound of the left radial pulse
(C) Elevation of the limb and optimization of fluids
(D) Escharotomy
(E) Intravenous morphine and serial examinations

The answer is D: Escharotomy. Following third-degree burns, full thickness tough, leathery eschars form. As the underlying tissue becomes rehydrated, tissue and blood vessels beneath the eschar can become compressed due to the inelasticity of the eschar. This can ultimately result in tissue hypoxia and limb loss if not corrected. An escharotomy is a surgical procedure used to treat the compression, which involves making an incision through the eschar to release the pressure.

(A) Amputation of the limb would be premature. An escharotomy should be performed first. If the tissue damage is already established, then amputation may be required. (B) This patient's pulse is diminished with palpation, which is an indication for emergent escharotomy. Although Doppler ultrasound of the radial pulse might be useful for monitoring pressure buildup and ensuring patency of the vessels after the escharotomy, it would only delay treatment in this patient. (C) If circumferential burns are present but adequate tissue perfusion is maintained, elevation of the limb and optimization of fluid is the best management. (E) While pain control is important for this patient, the next step is to reestablish limb perfusion before tissue death.

---

 7 A 50-year-old man is an unrestrained driver during a car accident. He had several beers prior to driving and was on his way home when he veered off the road and ran into a tree. On arrival in the emergency department, he has several contusions over his lower legs but otherwise appears stable. A chest x-ray shows a fracture of his left scapula and a widened mediastinum. Which of the following is the next best step in diagnosis?

(A) Aortic angiography
(B) Arterial blood gas
(C) CT scan of the chest, abdomen, and pelvis
(D) MRI of the chest
(E) Transthoracic echocardiogram

The answer is C: CT scan of the chest, abdomen, and pelvis. This patient appears to have only minor injuries on examination, but an x-ray shows a widened mediastinum. This finding, along with the fracture of his scapula (normally very difficult to fracture), is concerning for aortic trauma. The most rapid and effective diagnostic test for blunt aortic trauma in this case is CT imaging. It has both high sensitivity and specificity. If positive, the patient will need urgent operative repair before the aorta ruptures.

(A) Before advanced imaging, aortic angiography was the traditional method for working up a traumatic aortic injury. It is still used in facilities without CT imaging or when CT scanning is equivocal. (B) An arterial blood gas is generally not important in the acute workup of suspected aortic trauma. (D) While MRI may be useful for more chronic aortic pathology, it takes too much time to be useful for the diagnosis of acute aortic trauma. In addition, continued monitoring of the patient is important and is often difficult during MRI imaging. (E) Transthoracic echocardiography is generally not useful for imaging of blunt aortic trauma because patients with chest wall injury often have suboptimal echocardiographic findings. However, transesophageal echography can be used for diagnosis and is gaining popularity.

8 A 16-year-old boy is texting on his phone while driving when he drifts into oncoming traffic. He hits another car and is ejected. He is brought to the emergency department on a stretcher. His blood pressure is 75/40 mmHg, pulse 125/min and respirations 30/min. On examination, his trachea is deviated to the left and his breath sounds are decreased on the right side. His abdomen has no visible injury and is not tender to palpation. He has point tenderness over his left sixth rib. Chest x-ray is obtained and is shown in *Figure 2-1*.

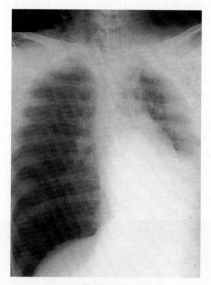

Figure 2-1

Which of the following is the next best step in management?

(A) Chest x-ray to be repeated in 30 minutes
(B) FAST
(C) Needle thoracostomy
(D) Orotracheal intubation
(E) Placement of two large bore intravenous lines

The answer is C: Needle thoracostomy. This patient is most likely suffering from a tension pneumothorax. The symptoms that indicate a tension pneumothorax in the setting of trauma include respiratory distress, tachypnea, hypotension, tracheal deviation away from affected side, and diminished breath sounds in the same side. This patient's broken rib may have caused the trauma. The most urgent next step is to place a needle into the pleural space to relieve the buildup of pressure.

(A) Although signs such as a flattened diaphragm, ipsilateral lung collapse, and mediastinal shift may be seen on chest x-ray, the diagnosis of tension pneumothorax can be made clinically and treatment should not be delayed. (B) FAST is useful for examination of possible blood loss in the abdomen. Although with this patient's hypotension it is possible that he is bleeding, proper ventilation must be secured before circulation is addressed. Additionally, further delay may worsen the patient's condition. (D) Needle thoracostomy is the first step in managing this patient's respiratory distress. Additionally orotracheal intubation may increase mediastinal pressure and worsen the symptoms. (E) Although intravenous hydration is also important in this trauma patient, the most urgent requirement is addressing the respiratory distress from the tension pneumothorax.

 9 A 45-year-old man who is hit by a car while crossing a busy highway is brought to the emergency department with multiple injuries. There is tenderness over his upper back, left pelvis, and lower mid abdomen. The patient is conscious and in pain. He also complains of difficulty voiding. A digital rectal examination shows no blood and a normal prostate. There is no blood visualized at the urethral meatus. Bloody urine is voided after insertion of a Foley catheter. Urinalysis shows many red blood cells. An x-ray shows fractures of his right third rib, left fourth rib, 1st thoracic vertebrae, pelvis, and right femur. Cystogram is obtained and is shown in *Figure 2-2*.

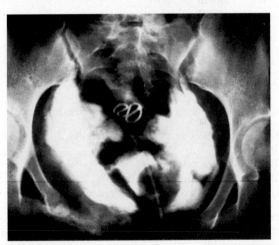

Figure 2-2

Which of the following is the most likely cause of this man's hematuria?

(A) Bladder injury

(B) Bowel injury

(C) Femur fracture
(D) Renal injury
(E) Urethral injury

The answer is A: **Bladder injury.** This patient most likely has an injury to his bladder. Injury to the urinary tract should be suspected with pelvic fractures. Signs and symptoms of bladder injury include gross hematuria, suprapubic pain/tenderness, and difficulty voiding. Gross hematuria is present in 98% of bladder injuries and is often found on insertion of a Foley catheter. Cystogram is obtained and, as shown in the image, reveals an intraperitoneal bladder injury with contrast outlining loops of bowel. Diagnosis of bladder injury can be made with CT imaging and/or a retrograde cystogram, with intraperitoneal extravasation visualized. The most common site of bladder rupture is the dome. If urethral injury is suspected, a retrograde urethrogram should be obtained prior to inserting a Foley catheter. Intraperitoneal bladder injuries require surgical repair. In some cases, extraperitoneal ruptures can be managed medically with simple catheter drainage.

(A) Hematuria is generally not a result of bowel injury. Furthermore, this patient's rectal examination shows no blood which makes a bowel injury less likely. (C) Femur fractures do not generally result in hematuria. (D) Although renal injury can cause gross hematuria, this patient does not have lower rib fractures, flank pain, or abdominal contusions. Furthermore, his difficulty voiding, lower mid abdominal tenderness, and pelvic fracture indicate a bladder injury as the more likely cause. In general, blunt traumatic renal injuries do not require surgery. (E) Urethral injury should be ruled out when urinary tract trauma is suspected. Signs of urethral trauma include blood at the meatus, which is an absolute contraindication to passing a Foley catheter until a retrograde urethrogram is performed and shows no urethra injury. A rectal examination may show a high riding prostate. This patient's presentation makes a bladder injury much more likely.

---

10 A 20-year-old male gang member is shot multiple times in the chest and abdomen. Prior to and during an emergent laparotomy, the patient receives 13 units of packed red blood cells and several liters of lactate Ringer solution. Halfway into the surgery, blood starts oozing from all dissected surfaces, exposed vessels, and IV insertion sites. Which of the following is the next best step in management?

(A) Abort the operation
(B) Administer platelets and fresh frozen plasma
(C) Continue blood transfusions as needed and complete surgery
(D) Send a D-dimer assay and administer antibiotics
(E) Send STAT coagulation labs

The answer is B: **Administer platelets and fresh frozen plasma.** This patient has received multiple units of packed red blood cells and crystalloid intravenous hydration. With this much volume replacement that does not contain platelets or clotting factors, coagulopathy is a common development. The next best step to control bleeding is to administer platelets and coagulation factors to help correct the patient's deficit. Surgery should continue, as this patient is in critical condition and will not survive unless bleeding is controlled.

(A) Aborting the operation would most likely result in the patient's death as his platelets and clotting factors have not been replaced and bleeding from the gunshot wounds has not been controlled. (C) Continuing blood transfusions would not correct the patient's coagulopathy and would most likely result in the patient's death. Platelets and coagulation factors should be replaced right away. (D) Although antibiotics should be administered, this patient's presentation is not consistent septic shock. Sending a D-dimer assay would not assist in this patient's acute management. (E) Sending for labs would delay proper treatment. The cause of this patient's coagulopathy is apparent without coagulation studies.

---

11   A 23-year-old primigravida female professional ice skater at 12 weeks' gestation is brought into the emergency department after falling during a triple axel maneuver. She arrives clutching her right upper leg and complains of severe pain. She says that she has a history of pain in this area and was recently diagnosed with a stress fracture on the shaft of her right femur. Despite warnings by her team physician to rest, especially during pregnancy, she admits that she has continued to ice skate. She denies loss of fluid, vaginal bleeding, or contractions. Her blood pressure is 130/80 mmHg, pulse 110/min, and respirations 18/min. Intravenous hydration is initiated and an x-ray ordered. During the physical examination, she starts to complain of difficulty breathing. Her vitals are taken again and reveal a blood pressure of 135/80 mmHg, pulse 150/min, and respirations 30/min. She appears acutely confused. Chest x-ray is obtained and is shown in *Figure 2-3*.

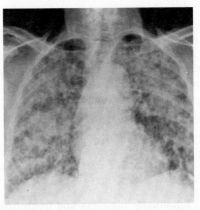

Figure 2-3

Which of the following is the most common cause of her new symptoms?

- **(A)** Amniotic fluid embolism
- **(B)** Fat embolism
- **(C)** Intravascular volume depletion
- **(D)** Fluid overload
- **(E)** Venous thromboembolism

The answer is B: Fat embolism. This patient is most likely suffering from a fat embolism. Acute signs in this patient include worsening tachycardia, tachypnea, dyspnea, and neurologic symptoms in the setting of long bone fracture. The diagnosis is often difficult, and can be made with clinical suspicion along with imaging (CT or ventilation/perfusion scan, the latter often used for pregnant patients). Chest x-ray shows bilateral air space consolidation. 24 to 48 hours after the injury, a petechial rash may form. Treatment is often supportive with maintenance of oxygenation, ventilation, and circulation. Early stabilization of bone fractures is recommended to minimize the amount of marrow embolization. Corticosteroids are sometimes used.

(A) Although this patient is pregnant, an amniotic fluid embolism is unlikely as the patient is not complaining of vaginal bleeding, loss of fluid, or contractions. Amniotic fluid embolization is rare and usually occurs during labor. (C) Intravascular volume depletion is unlikely in this patient since her blood pressure is increased. (D) Fluid overload can cause dyspnea, tachycardia, and tachypnea, but would not typically cause such acute neurologic complaints. Furthermore, this patient's blood pressure is normal and her symptoms better explained by a fat embolism. (E) Venous thromboembolism occurs in the setting of hypercoagulablilty, venous stasis, and endothelial damage (Virchow's triad). The source is usually the lower extremities. Pregnancy can increase the likelihood of venous thrombosis. However, this patient is young and has remained active. She has no complaints other than her femur fracture; thus, venous thromboembolism is an unlikely cause of her symptoms.

12 A 22-year-old man is stabbed in the back with a knife while at a party. He stumbles and collapses to the floor. A friend subsequently removes the knife and brings him to the hospital. He arrives in the emergency department fully conscious but complaining of difficulty moving his left leg. On examination, there appears to be a penetrating knife injury just left and lateral to his thoracic vertebrae, but angled slightly inward toward the spine. The patient has complete paralysis on the left side and loss of pain sensation on his right side distal to the injury. He is unable to feel a vibrating tuning fork on the left side of his body below the injury. Which of the following is the most likely cause of his neurologic complaints?

- **(A)** Anterior cord syndrome
- **(B)** Brown-Séquard syndrome
- **(C)** Syringomyelia

(D) Transection of the dorsal root ganglion

(E) Transection of the posterior spinal artery

The answer is B: Brown-Séquard syndrome. Based on this patient's neurologic symptoms, he has most likely suffered a hemitransection of the left side of the spinal cord (Brown-Séquard syndrome). Hemitransection would cut motor and vibration/proprioceptive fibers on the ipsilateral side and damage pain and temperature tracts from the contralateral side. The key to this question is to recall that pain and temperature sensory pathways cross over at the anterior white commissure and travel up on the opposite side via the spinothalamic tract.

(A) Anterior cord syndrome most often occurs in the setting of ischemia from aortic pathologic processes. The anterior spinal arteries obtain blood from the aorta and supply the anterior spinal cord. Symptoms include complete motor paralysis and loss of pain and temperature sensation on both sides below the level of the lesion. Proprioception and vibratory sensation remain intact since the dorsal columns obtain blood supply from the posterior spinal arteries. (C) Syringomyelia can occur from spinal cord injury and may result in dilation of the central canal. The classic presentation is bilateral loss of pain and temperature sensation at the level of the lesion ("cape-like" distribution). It most commonly occurs at C8 to T1. (D) Transection of a dorsal root ganglion would result in damage to sensor fibers in the distribution of the specific sensory nerve. (E) Posterior spinal artery ischemia is rare due to collateral blood supply. If it does occur, it would be characterized by loss of tendon reflexes and vibratory/proprioception below the lesion.

---

 13 A 42-year-old construction worker is helping build a commercial building when part of a concrete wall collapses onto him. He is rushed to the emergency department. His blood pressure on arrival is 95/60 mmHg. Examination shows multiple contusions and crush injuries. An airway is secured and intravenous lines are placed. Blood is drawn and sent to the lab. Which of the following laboratory abnormalities is most likely present in this patient?

(A) Hypercalcemia

(B) Hyperkalemia

(C) Hypokalemia

(D) Hypophosphatemia

(E) Metabolic alkalosis

The answer is B: Hyperkalemia. This patient has multiple crush injuries. The trauma results in cellular damage and release of intracellular contents. Laboratory analysis may show hyperkalemia, hyperphosphatemia, hypocalcemia, metabolic acidosis, myoglobinemia, and other abnormalities. Renal failure from rhabdomyolisis commonly occurs and can sometimes be prevented with aggressive hydration. Compartment syndrome is also a common occurrence and should be watched for. An electrocardiogram should be obtained to look for signs of hyperkalemia, as this can be quickly fatal. The patient's urine output and electrolytes should also be frequently monitored. In addition to intravenous hydration with normal saline, treatment for hyperkalemia in crush syndrome may include sodium bicarbonate, albuterol, kayexalate, and emergent dialysis.

(A) Hypocalcemia most commonly occurs in crush injuries due to calcium deposition in the damaged muscle, absorption of calcium by hypoxic tissues during reperfusion, and binding of calcium to the increased levels of phosphate. (C) Hyperkalemia, not hypokalemia, occurs in crush injuries. (D) As a result of crush injuries, phosphorus is released from damaged cells and may result in hyperphosphatemia. (E) Metabolic acidosis occurs in crush injuries due to tissue hypoxia, lactic acid, and release of amino acids from damaged cells. Metabolic alkalosis is generally not seen.

 14 A 35-year-old man jumps off a bridge to commit suicide. On arrival to the emergency department, he is spontaneously breathing, but multiple traumatic injuries are apparent including a deep gash with echymosis over his right scalp. His blood pressure is 90/65 mmHg, pulse 120/min, and respirations 25/min. The patient opens his eyes with sternal rubbing. He is making noise, but cannot be understood. He pulls his arm away when his wrist is flexed. What is this patient's Glasgow coma score?

(A) 3
(B) 8
(C) 10
(D) 13
(E) 15

The answer is B: **8.** The Glasgow coma score is useful for estimating the extent of neurologic damage in a trauma patient. It has three elements: eye, verbal, and motor response. The highest score is 15 (a fully awake individual) and the lowest score is 3 (fully comatose). A patient can be scored as follows:

Eye opening (four possible total points):

Opens spontaneously: 4
Opens in response to voice: 3
Opens in response to painful stimuli: 2
Does not open eyes: 1

Verbal response (five possible total points):

Oriented, normal: 5
Confused or disoriented: 4
Utters inappropriate words: 3
Makes incomprehensible sounds: 2
Makes no sounds: 1

Motor response (six possible total points):

Obeys commands: 6
Localizes pain: 5
Withdraws from painful stimuli: 4
Decorticate response (flexion posturing): 3
Decerebrate response (extension posturing): 2
Makes no movements: 1

This patient has eye opening with painful stimuli (2), incomprehensible sounds (2), and withdraws from painful stimuli (4) making his Glasgow coma score 8.

(A) A Glasgow coma score of 3 is too low for this patient. This would be a patient that does not open eyes at all, makes no sounds, and makes no movements. (C) A Glasgow coma score of 10 is too high for this patient. This score could represent a patient that opens the eyes in response to a voice, utters inappropriate words, and withdraws from painful stimuli. (D) A Glasgow coma score of 13 is too high for this patient. This score could represent a patient that opens the eyes spontaneously, is confused or disoriented, and can localize pain. (E) A Glasgow coma score of 15 would characterize a fully awake individual without any dramatic neurologic impairment.

 15 A 25-year-old woman is playing volleyball at a family reunion when she injures her shoulder. She says that she heard a "pop" while she was spiking the ball. She is now complaining of severe right shoulder pain. On examination, she is holding her right arm slightly abducted and externally rotated. She is unable to touch her left shoulder. There is a loss of contour over her right deltoid muscle. Her right radial pulse is palpated and she feels normal. An x-ray shows a subcoracoid position of the right humeral head. Which of the following structures is most commonly damaged in this type of injury?

(A) Axillary nerve
(B) Brachial artery
(C) Long thoracic nerve
(D) Radial nerve
(E) Subclavian artery

The answer is A: Axillary nerve. This patient has an anterior should dislocation. Anterior shoulder dislocations most commonly occur from blows to the upper extremity during abduction, extension, and external rotation (e.g, spiking a volleyball). It results in the humeral head being pushed forward out of the glenoid fossa. These patients will often find it painful to abduct and internally rotate the affected arm. The most commonly injured vascular or neurologic structures in an anterior dislocation include the axillary nerve and the axillary artery. Axillary nerve injuries will result in paralysis of the teres minor and deltoid muscles, resulting in loss of abduction, along with weak flexion, extension, or rotation of the shoulder. There may also be loss of sensation over the lateral upper arm.

(B) Brachial artery injury can occur following a supracondylar fracture of the humerus. (C) Long thoracic nerve injuries typically occur from blows to the ribs with an outstretched arm. Symptoms classically include the "winged" scapula. (D) Radial nerve injuries may occur after mid-shaft humerus fractures or after "Saturday night palsy" (falling asleep with one's arms hanging over the armrest of a chair compressing the radial nerve). (E) Subclavian artery injuries can occur from blunt or penetrating trauma to the shoulder region, but rarely occur from anterior shoulder dislocations.

16 A 29-year-old woman is shot with a .22 caliber rifle during a drive-by shooting. The bullet hits her in the posterior leg as she is running away. She arrives in the emergency department complaining of leg pain. Her blood pressure is 130/85 mmHg, pulse 110/min, and respirations 19/min. Examination shows a bullet hole in the posterior lateral upper leg with minimal bleeding and no exit wound. Her pulses are intact distal to the injury and her sensation below the wound is normal. An x-ray shows the bullet embedded in her biceps femoris muscle lateral to her femur. There are no apparent bone injuries. The patient says that her last tetanus shot was 7 years ago. Which of the following is the best treatment for this patient?

(A) Irrigation and cleaning of the wound
(B) Tetanus prophylaxis along with irrigation and cleaning of the wound
(C) Arteriogram of her leg vessels
(D) Surgical exploration of the wound
(E) Antibiotics, pain management, reassurance, and follow-up

The answer is B: Tetanus prophylaxis along with irrigation and cleaning of the wound. This patient has a low caliber gunshot wound to the lower extremity, but is stable and appears to be without major vascular or neurologic damage. The patient's wound should be irrigated and cleaned. In addition, tetanus prophylaxis should be given. Since the bullet is not near any major vascular structures, it may be left in place. Surgical exploration is not necessary. Antibiotics may also be prescribed depending on the injury.

(A) Although irrigation and cleaning of the wound are important, tetanus prophylaxis should be given to any serious or dirty wound if the last booster is greater than 5 years prior to the injury. (C) This patient's wound has not damaged any major vascular structures. Furthermore, her pulses are intact distal to the injury. Arteriogram of the leg vessels is not needed. (D) Surgical exploration is not needed since the bullet is low caliber and not in close proximity to major vascular or neurologic structures. (E) Although antibiotics, pain management, and follow-up may be important, cleaning of the wound and tetanus prophylaxis are also required.

---

 17 An 11-year-old boy with a history of asthma is playing outside by his grandmother's house when he is stung by several bees. He is seen in the emergency department 20 minutes later complaining of difficulty breathing. His blood pressure is 70/50 mmHg, pulse 120/min, and respirations 25/min. He is actively wheezing and his face seems swollen. There are multiple bee sting sites over his body. What is the next best step in management?

(A) Diphenahydramine
(B) β-Agonist inhaler
(C) Intramuscular epinephrine
(D) Intravenous calcium gluconate
(E) Subcutaneous epinephrine

The answer is C: Intramuscular epinephrine. This patient is having an anaphylactic reaction to a bee sting. Bee stings cause more deaths in the United States than any other form of envenomation. With previous exposure, patients may potentially have a type 1 hypersensitivity reaction (IgE mediated) with subsequent vasodilation, bronchospasm, laryngospasms, angioedema, and possible respiratory arrest. Serious reactions such as this one should be managed with injection of epinephrine. Intramuscular injection (best performed in the thigh) results in rapid absorption and higher plasma levels than subcutaneous injection.

(A) Diphenahydramine is helpful for more local reactions or to decrease the size and discomfort of the stings, but does adequately help anaphylactic shock. (B) β-Agonist inhaler may help if this patient was having an acute asthma attack. This patient's symptoms are not consistent with an asthma attack. (D) Intravenous calcium gluconate is used in the management of black widow spider bites. (E) Although subcutaneous epinephrine does have some efficacy in treating anaphylactic shock, it takes longer to be absorbed and results in lower levels of plasma epinephrine than intramuscular injections.

---

 18 A 30-year-old woman is involved in a multivehicle car accident. She is brought to the emergency department via ambulance. On arrival, her Glasgow coma score is 7. Her blood pressure is 70/30 mmHg, pulse 140/min, and respirations are 24/min. She has several large bruises over her face and neck with a large forehead laceration that is mildly bleeding. Her neck veins are flat. Her extremities are cold and clammy, but have no apparent injuries. A chest x-ray shows clear lungs, a normal cardiac silhouette, and a fractured right fifth rib. Which of the following is the most likely cause of her hypotension?

(A) Acute subdural hematoma
(B) Femur fracture and bleeding
(C) Intraabdominal bleeding
(D) Myocardial injury
(E) Spinal cord shock

The answer is C: Intraabdominal bleeding. This patient is suffering from hypovolemic shock from hemorrhage. Of the options listed, only intraab-dominal bleeding could account for this patient's presentation. Hypovolemic shock can occur with 25% or more of blood volume loss. An average adult has 5 L of blood. Since no significant external hemorrhaging can be found in this patient, attention should be focused on finding an internal source. There are several places in the body that can accommodate enough blood to account for hypovolemic shock. These include the chest, abdomen, pelvic cavity, and more rarely hematomas within the thighs. Without other cues to look elsewhere, inside the abdomen is the best place to look for the bleeding in this patient.

(A) Although it is possible that this patient has an acute subdural hema-toma (her Glasgow coma score is only 7 and multiple head injuries are appar-ent), the brain cavity cannot accommodate enough blood to account for this patient's hypovolemic shock. (B) Although this option could potentially result in hypovolemic shock, a femur fracture and subsequent hematoma would be apparent on an external examination. (D) Myocardial injury can result in car-diogenic shock. This patient's presentation, especially the cold and clammy extremities and flat neck veins, is not consistent with cardiogenic shock. (E) Spinal cord injury may be present in this patient, but spinal cord shock often results in bradycardia, and warm skin due to dilatation of the blood vessels.

19 A 53-year-old man is involved in an all-terrain vehicle (ATV) accident in a remote area. Witnesses say that he was thrown from the ATV at high speed. He is airlifted to the closest hospital and is hypotensive on arrival. On examination, the patient has multiple bruises over the tho-rax and point tenderness over multiple ribs. The abdomen is tender and distended. A chest x-ray shows several rib fractures on both sides and an abdominal ultrasound shows blood in the abdominal cavity. On fur-ther workup, the spleen is found to have a grade 2 laceration, which is subsequently repaired. The patient is stabilized and appears to be doing well until postoperative day 2, when he starts to complain of chest pain and dyspnea. A chest x-ray shows a "white-out" appearance in both lung fields. What is the most likely diagnosis?

(A) Atelectasis
(B) Hemothorax
(C) Pneumonia
(D) Pneumothorax
(E) Pulmonary contusions

The answer is E: Pulmonary contusions. Findings of respiratory distress and a "white-out" appearance of the lungs on x-ray 24 to 48 hours after blunt chest trauma is most likely caused by pulmonary contusions. Pulmonary contusions are defined by injury to the lung parenchyma leading to edema and blood collection in the alveoli. This in turn causes increased pulmonary vascular resistance, decreased lung compliance, and inflammation. Management is primarily supportive with fluid restriction, diuretics, and respiratory support. Intubation and mechanical ventilation may be required.

(A) Atelectasis is extremely common after surgery. It is often a result of general anesthesia and surgical manipulation, which leads to temporary diaphragmatic disruption. It is also a very common cause of early postoperative fever. Chest x-ray findings in more severe atelectasis will show signs of lobar collapse including displacement of natural fissures and other structures. However, atelectasis does not appear as a "white out" on chest x-ray. (B) Although hemothorax could cause respiratory distress and increased density on x-ray, it would typically be unilateral and accompanied by hypotension. Other chest x-ray findings indicating hemothorax would include blunting or obliteration of the costophrenic angle and air-fluid interfaces. (C) Pneumonia can occur postoperatively, but would most likely present with fever. It usually does not occur this early. (D) Pneumothorax would not have x-ray findings of a bilateral "white-out" appearance.

20 A 43-year-old morbidly obese man is stabbed with a pocketknife during an argument with his teenage son. He is brought to the emergency department distressed and yelling "I'm gonna kill that boy!". His blood pressure is 150/85 mmHg, pulse 105/min, and respirations 19/min. On examination, there is a small penetrating wound to the right of the umbilicus with minimal bleeding. There is superficial tenderness over the stab wound site and the rest of his abdomen is nontender. A rectal examination shows no blood. Which of the following is the next best step in management of this patient?

(A) CT scan of the abdomen
(B) Focused abdominal sonography for trauma
(C) Immediate laparotomy
(D) Referral for family counseling
(E) Sterile wound exploration

The answer is E: Sterile wound exploration. This patient has a penetrating stab wound to the abdomen that may or may not have penetrated into the peritoneal cavity. There are several clues here that would indicate that the knife did not penetrate into the peritoneal cavity. First, pocket knives generally have short blades. Additionally this man is morbidly obese (increased abdominal thickness) and is hemodynamically stable. He has no signs of peritoneal irritation or bowel evisceration. Due to these factors, the next best step in management is sterile wound exploration to visualize the depth of the knife tract. If the posterior rectus fascia in this case is found to be adequately visualized and intact, then the patient can be safely discharged home after proper wound care.

(A) Although CT imaging may show peritoneal penetration in some cases, it is generally not sensitive enough in the evaluation of small anterior penetrating abdominal wounds to be helpful, especially in obese individuals. (B) This patient has no signs of peritoneal irritation and is hemodynamically stable. These findings along with other clues that indicate a superficial wound make abdominal ultrasound unnecessary. (C) Immediate laparotomy would most likely be performed if this patient was hemodynamically unstable and had signs of peritoneal irritation. (D) Referral for family counseling might be appropriate after other more acute issues (such as the stab wound) are addressed.

 21 A 25-year-old man is shot in the chest by an assailant. He is brought by rescue squad to the emergency department. He is awake, alert, and combative. He arrives complaining of moderate shortness of breath. His blood pressure is 115/70 mmHg, pulse 103/min, and respirations are 20/min. Physical examination reveals a single bullet hole in the outer left chest with a exit wound just lateral to the scapula. There are no breath sounds on the left lung base and the left chest base is dull to percussion. A chest x-ray shows obliteration of the costophrenic angle on the left side. A chest tube is placed which immediately drains 200 mL of blood. Although the patient's vitals remain stable, another 50 mL of blood is recovered over the next hour. Which of the following is the next best step in management?

(A) Close observation and continued monitoring of chest tube drainage
(B) CT scan of the chest
(C) Emergent thoracotomy at bedside
(D) Exploratory thoracotomy in the operating room
(E) Ventilation perfusion scan

The answer is A: **Close observation and continued monitoring of chest tube drainage.** This patient has a penetrating wound to the upper left chest and symptoms of a hemothorax. However, the patient remains stable and the amount of blood draining from the chest tube is decreasing and below the value requiring surgical exploration. In general, surgical exploration should be considered if there is evacuation of more than 1,000 mL of blood immediately after tube thoracotomy, continued bleeding from the chest tube at a rate of greater than 150 to 200 mL over 2 to 4 hours, and/or repeated blood transfusion requirements to maintain hemodynamic stability of the patient.

(B) Although CT scanning can be helpful for quantification of blood amount or diagnosis when an x-ray is unequivocal, it is generally not needed when the diagnosis has already been made, the patient is stable, and the amount of blood draining from the chest tube is minimal and decreasing. (C) Emergent bedside thoracotomy is generally indicated in thoracic injuries when survival rate without immediate intervention is low. It is not needed in this patient who is hemodynamically stable with mild blood loss. (D) Exploratory thoracotomy would be indicated if this patient was hemodynamically unstable, had greater than 1,000 mL of blood loss immediately after chest tube placement, or had increasing and/or significant continued bleeding from the chest tube. (E) Ventilation perfusion scans are sometimes helpful in the diagnosis of pulmonary embolism. It would not be indicated in this case.

---

22)   A 32-year-old man is involved in a single vehicle accident where his vehicle hit a tree. He is unconscious immediately after the accident, but briefly regains consciousness during the ambulance ride to a large trauma center. On arrival to the emergency department, he is now comatose. He is intubated and started on intravenous hydration. Examination shows a fixed and dilated right pupil. Which of the following is the next best step in management?

(A) Administer intravenous mannitol
(B) CT scan of the head
(C) Induce hypoventilation
(D) MRI imaging of the head, neck, and lumbar spine
(E) Neurosurgical consultation and emergent craniotomy

The answer is B: CT scan of the head.   This patient is most likely suffering from an acute subdural hematoma. After securing and airway and stabilizing circulation, the most important next step in head trauma is emergent non-contrast CT scanning of the head. This will establish the diagnosis of an acute subdural hematoma and will often show a hyperdense crescent-shaped mass between the skull and the surface of the cerebral hemisphere. The hematoma may push on the brain and cause herniation or other mass effects, as evidenced by this patient's fixed and dilated pupil. Treatment will involve a neurosurgical consultation with surgical decompression.

(A) Prior to emergent decompression, medical therapy may be initiated to reduce intracranial pressure. One approach is using osmotic diuretics such as mannitol. It is not indicated for long-term use. (C) Hyperventilation, not hypoventilation, may be used to decrease intracranial pressure. It works by decreasing cerebral blood flow. (D) MRI is less useful than CT imaging in acute subdural hematoma due to the time it takes to obtain the study and lack of equipment in the suites for emergent resuscitation. (E) Although a neurosurgical consult followed by emergent craniotomy is the correct treatment of an acute subdural hematoma, the diagnosis should be first established with CT imaging.

23 A 23-year-old college student is stabbed in the neck during an argument with a roommate. He arrives in the emergency department complaining of difficulty speaking and coughing up blood. He appears confused. His blood pressure is 130/75 mmHg, pulse 107/min, and respirations 19/min. Examination of his neck shows a penetrating wound just superior and left of the cricoid cartilage with the knife still in place. Over the course of the trauma examination in the triage bed, a lump forms next to the wound that seems to be pulsating and expanding. An airway is immediately secured and large bore intravenous lines established. Blood has already been sent to the laboratory for type and cross. Which of the following is the next best step in management?

(A) Admission with observation in critical care unit
(B) Angiography
(C) Direct laryngoscopy
(D) Immediate removal of the knife with applied pressure
(E) Immediate surgical exploration of the neck

The answer is E: Immediate surgical exploration of the neck. This patient has a penetrating injury to zone 2 of his neck, which contains many vital structures. Patients who are exsanguinating from a zone 2 neck wound, have a stroke, or have evidence of an expanding hematoma should have immediate exploration of the neck to control the bleeding. Neck wounds with an expanding hematoma in either zone 1 or 3 of the neck can sometimes be initially imaged with emergent angiography or CT angiography, although may also require immediate surgical exploration.

(A) Admission and observation in critical care area may be needed after surgery, but is not the next best step in management of this patient. (B) Angiography is the gold standard for evaluating stable patients with penetrating wounds to zones 1 and 3 of the neck. (C) Direct laryngoscopy might be indicated in this case as the patient may have an airway injury. However, this patient's airway has now been secured with intubation and the possible major vessel injury in the neck should be addressed now. (D) Removal of objects protruding from the neck should not be done in the emergency department. It is possible that the knife is currently preventing significant blood exsanguination. The knife may be carefully removed in the operating room during surgical exploration.

24 A 35-year-old transient man with a history of alcohol abuse is trying to jump from a moving train when his backpack is caught on the door. He falls out of the train and has an uncontrolled landing where he says that he hit his head. The patient arrives in the emergency department fully immobilized on a long board with a semirigid collar in place. He is complaining of leg pain, but denies pain in his back or neck. His breathing is clear and his oxygen saturation is 99% 1 L of oxygen. His blood pressure is 115/75 mmHg, pulse 80/min, and respirations 15/min. His pupils are round and reactive to light and accommodation and there is mild bruising over his left temple. His right leg is mildly tender at the knee joint. Which of the following is a contraindication to clearing the cervical spine and removing the collar without additional imaging?

(A) Bruising over the temple
(B) History of alcohol abuse
(C) Impaired motor function of his right knee
(D) Normal sensation and reflexes
(E) Presence of posterior midline tenderness

The answer is E: **Presence of posterior midline tenderness.** Most trauma patients are suspected of having cervical spinal injury until proven otherwise. Cervical trauma often occurs from hyperflexion, hyperextension, vertical compression, or lateral rotation of the neck during an injury. It is possible that this patient injured his neck and he should be checked for signs of spinal injury. Examination involves assessing midline tenderness, sensation, motor function reflexes, and performing a rectal examination. Examination findings that suggest spinal injury include pain with movement, tenderness, gaps or steps in the spine, edema or bruising over the spine, or spasm of associated muscles. Patients without these symptoms can be cleared assuming other risk factors (such as increased age, mechanism of injury, falls greater than 1 m, axial loads on the spine, high-speed or dramatic injuries) are not present.

(A) Mild bruising over the left temple does not necessarily indicate neck or back trauma. (B) Patients that are intoxicated should have imaging to assess the cervical spine. A history of alcohol abuse does not necessarily mean the patient is intoxicated. (C) This patient sustained a knee injury; thus, impaired function of his right knee might be expected. This is not a contraindication to clearing the cervical spine without additional imaging. (D) Normal sensation and reflexes would imply an intact spinal cord.

 25 A 32-year-old woman is brought to the emergency department after being stabbed by her husband in the left abdomen. She complains of abdominal pain localized to the knife injury. On examination, there is a defect in the left abdominal wall with several protruding loops of small bowel. Her airway is clear and she is not complaining of difficulty breathing. Her blood pressure is 135/85 mmHg, pulse 95/min, and respirations 14/min. Which of the following interventions is the next best step in management?

(A) Abdominal ultrasound
(B) CT scan of the abdomen
(C) Diagnostic peritoneal lavage
(D) Immediate laparotomy
(E) Reduce the bowel back into the abdomen and close the defect

The answer is D: Immediate laparotomy. This patient has an obvious penetrating injury to the abdomen with evisceration. She is stable, but the abdomen needs to be surgically explored and any injuries if found, repaired. Other imaging modalities will most likely not be helpful in this case and may only serve to delay care.

(A) Abdominal ultrasound imaging is not necessary in this case as the injury is apparent and it would only serve to further delay care. (B) CT imaging of the abdomen is not necessary for the same reason as above. (C) Diagnostic peritoneal lavage is most useful in the case of questionable abdominal bleeding in an unstable patient. It would not be helpful in this case. (E) Some trauma centers have advocated immediate reduction with closure of the defect with evisceration since many laparotomies are found to be negative for additional injury. However, recent studies have shown prompt operative intervention to be the best management. An exception might be applied to a select few patients with only omentum evisceration and benign abdominal findings.

Acute Abdomen

1 A 57-year-old woman presents to the emergency department with abdominal pain. She reports a 1-day history of dull, aching abdominal pain that has gradually worsened over the last 24 hours. Her pain does radiate to her back. She has had nausea, vomited numerous times, and has had no appetite. She has a past medical history of hypertension, gastroesophageal reflux disease (GERD), and long-standing alcohol abuse. She is noted to be febrile, but hemodynamically stable. Physical examination reveals a supine motionless female. Abdominal examination reveals a distended abdomen, and tenderness with guarding. CT scan is obtained and is shown in *Figure 3-1*.

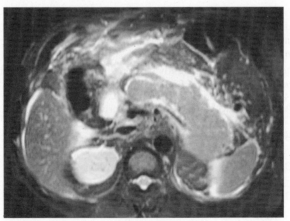

Figure 3-1

Which of the following choices represents the ideal management for this patient?

(A) Appendectomy
(B) Exploratory laparotomy

(C) NPO management with IV hydration and IV pain control

(D) Renal ultrasound

The answer is C: NPO management with IV hydration and IV pain control. A diagnosis of acute pancreatitis should always be considered in a patient with abdominal pain and a history of alcoholism. The presentation of acute pancreatitis varies, but the pain is typically in the epigastrium, described as a dull worsening ache, and radiating to the back 50% of the time (as a retroperitoneal organ). Physical examination reveals an acute abdominal picture with distention, guarding, tenderness. Rarely, jaundice or icterus may be noted on the patient. Some physical findings tested in necrotizing pancreatitis include the Cullen sign and Grey-Turner sign. The CT scan shows enlargement of the pancreas and pancreatic edema. Management in pancreatitis includes pain control, NPO management, and intravenous fluids.

(A) An appendectomy would be performed for a patient presenting with acute appendicitis. This is clearly not appendicitis based on the patient's clinical history, and the physical examination findings. (B) An "ex lap" would be a valid option in an acute abdominal situation in which the patient was not hemodynamically stable (i.e., with acute abdominal hemorrhage). Other than her fever (common in pancreatitis), her vital signs are normal. (D) A renal ultrasound would be indicated if renal stones or an obstructing ureteral stone was suspected. These pathologies typically produce flank or flank and groin pain, respectively, which is not described by this patient.

2 After writing admission orders for the patient from the previous question, you present the patient to your attending physician. Your attending demands to know if this patient's status is "severe." Which of the following data currently best predict the prognosis for the patient from the previous question?

(A) Age, white blood cell count, serum glucose, serum LDH, and aspartate aminotransferase (AST)

(B) Age, white blood cell count, hematocrit (Hct) change, serum calcium, and alanine aminotransferase (ALT)

(C) Hct change, serum calcium, base deficit, white blood cell count, and LDH

(D) Hct change, BUN, serum calcium, PaO$_2$, base deficit, and fluid sequestration

The answer is A. Age, white blood cell count, serum glucose, serum LDH, and AST. There are many sets of criteria that stage acute pancreatitis (e.g., Ranson, APACHE). While there is no standard, the Ranson criteria are frequently tested. These criteria collect two sets of data, one at admission, and another 48 hours later to determine severe disease states. Each criterion is assigned a single point value. Scores of 5 or greater have a 50% mortality, 15% for scores 2 to 3, and minimal for scores less than that. Admission criteria include age over 55 years, WBC greater than 16,000/µL, blood glucose greater than 200 mg/dL, serum LDH greater than 350 IU/L, and AST greater than 250 IU/L. The 48-hour criteria include hematocrit decrease by 10%, BUN increase of 8 mg/dL, serum calcium lower than 8 mg/dL, PaO_2 less than 60 mmHg, base deficit greater than 4 mEq/L, and estimated fluid sequestration greater than 600 mL.

(B) These criteria are a mix of both sets of Ranson criteria, but note that AST (not ALT) is regarded in the Ranson criteria. (C) Similarly, these criteria are a mix of both Ranson criteria sets, but all variables are individually correct. (D) Note that these are the correct criteria for those recorded at 48 hours, but this question is in regard to the patient's admission and current prognosis.

3 You are called to see a 48-year-old woman who was admitted for abdominal pain. She noted the onset of diffuse abdominal pain 2 days prior with nausea, diarrhea, vomiting, and chills. She has past medical history of GERD, hypertension, and hepatitis C acquired from intravenous drug abuse. She is febrile but hemodynamically stable and appears jaundiced. Abdominal examination reveals spider angioma, distention, tympany, and a fluid wave. She exhibits tenderness with guarding throughout. Which of the following is the most likely diagnosis?

(A) Acute cholecystitis
(B) Acute appendicitis
(C) Pancreatitis
(D) Perforated viscus
(E) Spontaneous bacterial peritonitis (SBP)

The answer is E: Spontaneous bacterial peritonitis (SBP). This question is strongly hinting that this patient has an acute abdominal picture in the presence of ascites (distended tympanic abdomen with fluid wave) due to her hepatitis (history of IV drug abuse, spider angioma). Given the combination of this history and these findings, a diagnosis of SBP must be entertained. This involves bacterial seeding of the ascitic fluid, and can present in this manner.

(A) This is an atypical presentation for acute cholecystitis, but perhaps tempting given the jaundice as a possible sign of obstructive biliary disease. The history and the angiomatous signs noted make the jaundice more likely due to cirrhosis. (B) This is an atypical presentation for acute appendicitis. While included in the differential, this is not the most likely diagnosis. (C) This is the most tempting incorrect answer with the presence of jaundice in this patient; however, jaundice is an infrequent finding in acute pancreatitis (despite it being commonly tested). Pancreatitis typically presents with epigastric pain and is associated with gallstone disease or alcoholism. (D) This is a possible diagnosis that should also be considered, but less likely than SBP given the history and the findings described in this patient. Causes include peptic ulcer disease, appendicitis, and diverticulitis.

4 A 23-year-old male medical student presents to the emergency department concerned that he has appendicitis. He noted the sudden onset of right lower quadrant pain while playing tennis 3 hours prior. He immediately stopped playing with some relief, but his pain gradually worsened and he vomited several times. He reports being tender. He is otherwise healthy and takes no medications. Vitals include a temperature of 100.9°F, heart rate 97 beats/min, respiratory rate 17 breaths/min, blood pressure 124/79 mmHg, oxygen saturation 99%. Physical examination reveals absent bowel sounds, exquisite abdominal tenderness over the right lower quadrant with tenderness and rebound. There is a firm mass noted in that area. Which of the following is the most likely diagnosis?

(A) Acute appendicitis
(B) Acute herniated bowel
(C) Acute mesenteric ischemia (AMI)
(D) Rectus sheath hematoma
(E) Urinary obstruction

The answer is D: Rectus sheath hematoma. This question serves to both remind you of the diagnosis of muscle hematoma and portray its clinical similarity to acute appendicitis. Rectus muscle hematomas often involve nausea and vomiting, low-grade fever, and an acute abdominal picture. In this patient, the onset of abdominal pain during strenuous activity and the palpable mass on examination both point to a rectus sheath hematoma. Surgical consultation can be made to determine the extent of damage as well as if the injury is severe enough to indicate surgical repair.

(A) Acute appendicitis is a tempting distracter here for many reasons, including the location of the pain, the associated gastrointestinal symptoms, the low-grade fever, and the physical examination findings. This is less likely, however, given the associated activity with onset, and the palpable mass. (B) If a hernia was to present in this manner, it would do so secondary to incarceration with or without strangulation. Presumably, we would be provided the medical history including a preexisting hernia (or chronic abdominal pain) that preceded this incident. (C) AMI typically involves an embolus that blocks blood flow to the bowel. Given the fairly healthy state of this medical student, this is unlikely. (E) A urinary obstruction produces pain secondary to distention of the renal collecting system, the ureter, or the bladder. While the location of this pain may indicate a ureteral stone, the presence of a superficial palpable mass makes this less likely.

5 A 37-year-old woman presents to the emergency department with a 14-hour history of right lower quadrant pain. She reports that she first experienced central abdominal pain before some associated nausea and vomiting following dinner last evening. Upon awakening this morning, her pain had moved to her lower right abdomen and was worse with movement. She vomited twice this morning. She specifically noted that her pain was exacerbated by the bouncing of her car during her drive here. CT scan is obtained and is shown in *Figure 3-2*.

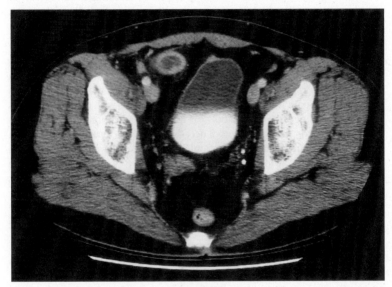

Figure 3-2

You proceed to do a physical examination. Which of the following statements best defines Rovsing sign?

(A) Right lower quadrant pain due to drainage of a gastric or duodenal ulcer

(B) Right lower quadrant pain following hip extension against resistance with the knee in full extension

(C) Right lower quadrant pain following internal rotation of the right leg with the hip and knee flexed

(D) Right lower quadrant rebound tenderness following left lower quadrant palpation

The answer is D: Right lower quadrant rebound tenderness following left lower quadrant palpation. The many physical examination findings in acute appendicitis are frequently tested and can be helpful in further eliciting the location of the inflamed appendix (as it varies from patient to patient). Rovsing sign describes palpation of the left lower quadrant that elicits rebound tenderness in the right lower quadrant. It does not specify the appendiceal location. The CT scan reveals a thickened appendix with edema and inflammatory changes.

(A) This statement defines a Valentino sign, and is unique in that the pathology differs from the remaining choices. This is a fairly outdated term, but still referenced casually and for testing purposes. (B) This statement describes a positive psoas sign, which is helpful in revealing a "retrocecal" or retroflexed appendix which happens to lie inflamed on the belly of the psoas muscle. (C) This statement describes a positive obturator sign. The obturator sign is helpful is diagnosing a patient with "pelvic" appendicitis.

6 A 51-year-old gentleman presents with abdominal pain. He describes an aching, cramping sensation in his lower abdomen that began 11 hours ago. His pain worsened and he became nauseous with multiple episodes of vomiting and watery stools. He takes no medications and has no surgical history. He complains of occasional anxiety. Examination reveals a febrile, tachycardic man, motionless and in obvious pain. Tenderness is maximal in the lower left quadrant. Voluntary guarding is present. The remainder of the examination is normal. The pathophysiology of this disease is best described by which of the following?

(A) Chronic atherosclerotic disease of the mesenteric vessels causing ischemia
(B) Inflammation and perforations at weak outpouchings of the colon
(C) Poorly understood mechanism involving modifiable risk factors such as low-fiber diet and chronic constipation
(D) Transmural inflammation and perforation causing abnormal adherence to an adjacent structure

The answer is B: Inflammation and perforations at weak outpouchings of the colon. This patient is presenting with a classic case of acute diverticulitis. Recall that the pathophysiology of diverticulitis occurs in the presence of diverticulosis. Though the mechanism is not completely elicited, inflammation and macro- or microperforations occur through these preexisting diverticula. Obstruction, fistulae formation, and necrosis can all be involved.

(A) This statement describes the pathophysiology of chronic mesenteric ischemia. We would expect to see pertinent risk factors including CAD and PVD. Pain from chronic mesenteric ischemia is typically chronic, associated with meals, and causes food aversion with subsequent weight loss. The abdominal examination is often normal. (C) This is a tempting answer as it describes the pathophysiology of diverticulosis, a condition necessarily preceding the development of diverticulitis. While it appears tricky, it is a helpful and educative distinction to make. (D) This statement describes the general pathophysiology of fistula formation. A fistula can develop secondary to diverticulitis but is not necessarily involved. A fistula describes the pathology of two abnormally joined viscous organs (e.g., enterovesical fistula). This is not the mechanism of diverticulitis.

7 A 19-year-old girl presents for sudden-onset abdominal pain that has worsened over the past 9 hours. It is worst over her right lower abdomen where it started. She has no associated nausea or vomiting, and she denies sexual activity. She has no past medical or surgical history. Examination reveals tachycardia, a young woman in acute distress, and a tender abdomen with guarding and rebound over the right lower quadrant. She is hemodynamically stable. Which of the following is the next best step in management?

(A) Exploratory laparotomy
(B) Serum β-hCG analysis
(C) Serum amylase and lipase levels
(D) CT of the abdomen
(E) MRI of the abdomen and pelvis

The answer is B: Serum β-hCG analysis. The best management step for this patient is to rule out pregnancy and the possibility for an ectopic pregnancy. This diagnosis must be entertained in the acute abdomen of a woman of child-bearing age. Verification should be obtained with a serum level of β-human chorionic gonadotropin. Though emphasis and trust are always placed in the patient history, this is one item that should always be verified.

(A) Exploratory laparotomy would be a suitable management option in a patient who is hemodynamically unstable with suspected intraperitoneal injury. This is not the case in this patient, as we are told that she is stable. (C) Serum amylase and lipase are highly sensitive and specific for suspected cases of acute pancreatitis. Pancreatitis classically involves a history of alcoholism or gallstone disease and typically presents with epigastric pain with or without radiation to the back. Jaundice is uncommonly associated but can be present. (D) CT of the abdomen is definitely within the scope of management of this patient, but only after verification of a nonpregnant state. Proceeding with this test would pose a radiation risk to the developing fetus. This unnecessary radiation should be delayed until ectopic pregnancy is ruled out. (E) MRI of the abdomen and pelvis is a viable option, given the lack of radiation in concerns of the fetus, but other safe imaging modalities (e.g., ultrasound) would be more appropriate initially (all after a negative hCG level).

8 A 16-year-old girl presents to the emergency department with abdominal pain and vomiting. She describes the onset yesterday while in school, occurring near her umbilicus. Her pain was made worse by walking home. She napped without relief and awoke with the pain in her lower abdomen. She has not eaten but vomited 2 hours ago. She is febrile and tachycardic. Abdominal examination reveals tenderness in the right lower quadrant with rebound and guarding.

Her white blood cell count is 16.2. A pregnancy test is negative. CT of the abdomen shows an inflamed retrocecal appendix. The pain currently being described by this patient can best be defined as what type of pain?

(A) Peritoneal pain
(B) Rebound pain
(C) Referred pain
(D) Somatic pain
(E) Visceral pain

The answer is D: Somatic pain. This case is describing another case of acute appendicitis in which this woman's pain has progressed from her umbilicus to her right lower quadrant. Based on this symptom and her peritoneal signs (rebound tenderness and guarding), we can confidently say that she is experiencing somatic pain caused by inflammation of the peritoneum (i.e., peritonitis). This is caused by inflammation of the appendix in contact with the peritoneum, allowing localization of the pain via somatic-type nociceptors (pain fibers).

(A) While she is experiencing peritonitis, this is not considered "peritoneal pain," which is not a typical pain-type classification. (B) Rebound pain, or rebound tenderness, describes a physical diagnostic sign indicating the presence of peritonitis. Rebound tenderness describes the subjective sensation of pain by the patient upon release of palpation pressure. This patient exhibits rebound tenderness but this is not a classic type of pain per se. (C) Referred pain describes pain that is sensed in an area that differs from its true origin. The classic examples of referred pain include left upper arm and jaw pain suffered in angina, and pain subjectively localized to an amputated limb (phantom pain). No referred pain is currently occurring in this patient. (E) Visceral pain in acute appendicitis is classically described by the vague periumbilical pain at the onset of the disease. Visceral pain is very poorly localized without direct peritoneal irritation and is instead based on the embryologic development of the mesenteric nervous system.

---

9 A 53-year-old man presents to the emergency department with a 4-hour history of immediate onset left lower quadrant pain. The patient admits to associated nausea and vomiting following the onset of his pain. He has a past medical history of hypertension, GERD, type II diabetes mellitus, and chronic constipation. He has never had surgery. Physical examination reveals a patient in acute distress and writhing in pain. Abdominal examination reveals voluntary guarding and rebound tenderness worst in the left lower quadrant. An upright abdominal film reveals subdiaphragmatic air. Which of the following signs or symptoms is atypical for the picture of acute abdomen?

(A) Nausea and vomiting following the onset of pain
(B) Pain located in the left lower quadrant
(C) Sudden-onset abdominal pain
(D) The patient writhing in pain
(E) Voluntary guarding

The answer is D: The patient writhing in pain. This vignette paints a clinical picture of clear-cut peritonitis, or acute abdomen. It is essentially asking you to recall the classically cited "motionless" patient who is suffering from acute abdomen. This patient, however, is described as "writhing in pain," a sign more associated with renal colicky conditions caused by pathology such as renal calculi. This finding, though possible, is atypical.

(A) Nausea and vomiting following the onset of pain is classic for peritonitis, and often cited as one of the classic symptomatology progressions in acute appendicitis. This is in contrast to the pain that follows nausea and vomiting, which could be suggestive of muscle injury following retching. (B) Diverticulitis and perforation of a diverticulum are both classically associated with left lower quadrant pain. Both are possible and likely diagnoses in this clinical scenario, and therefore this finding does not point away from a peritonitis diagnosis. (C) The sudden, acute onset of pain in "acute" abdomen is a very real possibility, and is very commonly noted in this condition. Noting this symptom should not steer you away from diagnosing an acute abdomen. (E) While voluntary guarding (as opposed to involuntary guarding) is thought to be more under patient control, both signs are indicative of an acute abdomen scenario. This, as the other findings, should not steer you away from this diagnosis.

 10 You are called to the emergency department to see a 31-year-old G_1P_0 woman at 27 weeks' gestation. She has been seen by the obstetric service who verified a normally progressing and uneventful pregnancy thus far. She is experiencing right upper quadrant abdominal pain of 9-hour duration associated with nausea and vomiting. Ultrasound of her gallbladder, liver, and bilious structures was unremarkable. Right renal ultrasound was read as normal. Abdominal examination reveals tenderness in the right upper quadrant with guarding and rebound. Which of the following is the most likely diagnosis?

(A) Acute acalculous cholecystitis
(B) Acute appendicitis
(C) HELLP syndrome
(D) Preeclampsia
(E) Right renal colic

The answer is B: Acute appendicitis. The correct answer is acute appendicitis. This question serves to remind you that the anatomical changes of the obstetric patient can skew the classic appearance of many conditions.

With the presence of a fetus, the appendix may elevate dramatically and can cause pain at the right midabdomen or even the right upper quadrant. Acute appendicitis is the most common reason for surgical exploration in a gravid woman, and appendectomy is safest during the second trimester. For these reasons, this atypical presentation of acute appendicitis is frequently tested.

(A) This is a drawing distraction because this patient's pain is situated at the right upper quadrant. Additionally, "acalculous" or stone-free pathology suggests that radiologic studies like ultrasound may be normal. In fact; ultrasonography in acalculous cholecystitis still reveals classical cholecystitis signs, but without the stones (sensitivity and specificity near 70%). (C) HELLP syndrome (hemolysis, liver enzymes, low platelet count) is a variant of pre-eclampsia. Right upper quadrant pain during HELLP syndrome can occur due to capsular distention of the liver. The incidence of liver distention is infrequent relative to appendicitis. (D) Preeclampsia is a complication of pregnancy involving hypertension and proteinuria. Most of the pathophysiology is involved with medium-sized vasculature pathology. Liver distention more commonly occurs in association HELLP syndrome, a severe variant of pre-eclampsia. (E) While right renal colic would definitely be included in the differential diagnosis, we are told that this patient underwent a right renal ultrasound which appeared normal. We would expect some abnormality (calculus, ureteral calculus, hydronephrosis, etc.) to be present with this condition.

---

 11 You are consulted to see a 29-year-old man who was admitted for shortness of breath secondary to a mediastinal lymphoma. His CD4 count was measured at 56 cells/mm^3 and subsequent workup confirmed HIV positivity. He is currently complaining of extreme abdominal pain that started yesterday. He describes it as vague and aching. Palpation reveals diffuse abdominal tenderness with rebound. Which of the following is the most common cause of nonsurgical abdominal pain in patients with AIDS?

(A) Infectious enteritis
(B) Kaposi sarcoma
(C) Non-Hodgkin lymphoma (NHL)
(D) Pancreatitis
(E) Sclerosing cholangitis

The answer is A: Infectious enteritis. This question is testing your knowledge on abdominal pain workup in a patient with AIDS, whose pathology is definitely altered with this disease state. The presentation can strongly vary as well, as patients with AIDS manifest pain differently, and peritoneal signs can be altered as well. The most common cause of nonsurgical abdominal pain is infectious enteritis, with cytomegalovirus (CMV), *Mycobacterium avium* complex (MAC), and *Cryptosporidium* comprising over 30% of the cases.

All causes of acute abdominal pain (appendicitis, cholecystitis, diverticulitis, peptic ulcer disease (PUD)) must still be considered. (B) Kaposi sarcoma would be included in the differential diagnosis, but comprises a much small number of cases relative to infectious enteritis. (C) NHL is the second most common cause of nonsurgical abdominal pain in patients with AIDS. While it appears more common than MAC and *Cryptosporidium* individually, infectious enteritis stills outweighs it as a whole, which this question is asking. (D) Pancreatitis is the third most common nonsurgical cause of abdominal pain in patients with AIDS (after infectious enteritis and NHL). Like NHL, it is more common than MAC and *Cryptosporidium* enteritis, but less common than infectious enteritis in general. (E) Sclerosing cholangitis is not necessarily at a higher frequency in patients with AIDS than the general population, but still represents a "nonsurgical" cause of abdominal pain. It is far from being more common than infectious enteritis in this patient population.

---

12 A 40-year-old G_2P_2 obese woman is 1 day postoperative following a laparoscopic cholecystectomy. She has been hemodynamically stable, a febrile, and without complaints. She is receiving Lovenox, ambulating with assistance, and performing incentive spirometry with nursing supervision. Her pain has been well controlled. This morning, she noticed constant nagging shoulder pain upon awakening. Her vitals are normal and stable. She denies shortness of breath and leg pain. Which statement best describes the pathophysiology involved?

(A) Normal pain following positioning for a laparoscopic procedure
(B) Pulmonary embolism
(C) Referred pain due to bilious leakage of the cystic duct
(D) Referred pain due to subdiaphragmatic air

The answer is D: Referred pain due to subdiaphragmatic air. The most likely answer here, given that this patient underwent a laparoscopic procedure, is referred shoulder pain secondary to subdiaphragmatic air. Any gas remaining postoperatively sits under the diaphragm and causes irritation. The Kehr sign is the phenomenon describing shoulder pain secondary to peritoneal fluid or air; it is based on the anatomical overlap between the nerve roots of the phrenic nerve and the cervical nerves innervating the dermatomes around the shoulder (specifically C3 and C4).

(A) Postoperative patients may experience "appropriate" abdominal tenderness and soreness, but there is no basis for shoulder pain. Furthermore, we are not given any reason to believe that the patient suffered a musculoskeletal complication while sedated. (B) While pulmonary embolus would be a concern in a patient postoperatively, there are many pieces of information that argue against it. She is receiving deep venous thrombosis (DVT) prophylaxis, she is not experiencing either shortness of breath or leg pain, and her vitals are stable (tachycardia is an extremely sensitive sign for pulmonary embolus). (C) Bilious leakage of the ductal remnant in this procedure could, in theory, produce Kehr sign as a peritoneal fluid collection; however, the incidence of referred shoulder pain due to residual gas is much more common, and therefore a better answer.

 13 A 60-year-old African American man comes to the emergency department for sudden-onset, diffuse abdominal pain. He describes the pain as diffuse, 10/10, and sharp in nature that maximized within a few seconds. He has a past medical history of CABG × 2, diabetes treated with Metformin, and atrial fibrillation treated with warfarin. Vitals reveal tachycardia at 106. Abdominal examination reveals a normal abdomen, absent bowel sounds, and no tenderness. His INR today is 1.3. Which of the following is the most likely diagnosis?

(A) Hemoperitoneum due to hemorrhagic bowel
(B) Mesenteric ischemia
(C) Myocardial infarction (MI)
(D) Pancreatitis
(E) SBP

The answer is B: Mesenteric ischemia. Acute mesenteric ischemia (AMI) results from acute cessation of blood flow to the bowel. Risk factors associated include coronary artery disease and peripheral vascular disease. In AMI, arterial embolism to the bowel is the most common cause, with atrial fibrillation being the most common concomitant disease. The classic description is "pain out of proportion to the exam," which is the case with this patient, as the examination appears normal. Peritoneal signs begin to surface only after necrosis of the bowel occurs.

(A) Hemorrhage of the bowel is a tempting choice given the patient's use of warfarin for his atrial fibrillation history. However, recall that a therapeutic INR is between 2 and 3; furthermore, because he is subtherapeutic (INR 1.3), we should more concerned with emboli or thrombi (causing AMI), not hemorrhage. (C) This patient has serious risk factors for MI including his coronary artery disease; therefore, MI must be included on your differential and should be ruled out with serial troponins. The presentation described, however, is fairly classic for mesenteric ischemia, making it more likely. (D) Pancreatitis is classically described as a dull, aching abdominal pain in the epigastric area. Risk factors include the presence of gallstones or current alcoholism. Serum amylase and lipase levels are a very effective means of diagnosis. (E) SBP is typically found in the setting of ascites, which does not seem to be present in this patient. SBP has a range of presentations, but does involve abdominal pain usually of an acute gradual onset.

 14 A 57-year-old man is brought to the hospital by an rescue squad team. He had been complaining of abdominal pain radiating to his back. The pain began following dinner. Some hours later, his abdominal pain became "tearing" and he became diaphoretic. He described immediate dizziness and collapsed. Vital signs in the emergency department reports a lowest in the emergency department reports a lowest blood pressure of 90/47 mmHg and a fastest heart rate of 106 beats/min. This patient takes hydrochlorothiazide–lisinopril and as needed sildenafil. Abdominal examination reveals a pulsatile mass. What is the next best step in management?

(A) Abdominal ultrasonography
(B) Chest x-ray (CXR)
(C) Computed tomography (CT) of the abdomen
(D) Exploratory laparotomy
(E) Transesophageal echocardiogram (TEE)

The answer is D: Exploratory laparotomy. This question provided the classic presentation and triad (hypotension, pulsatile mass, and abdominal pain) of abdominal aortic aneurysm (AAA). Additionally, this patient is the classic patient to present with AAA, as he is male, has hypertension (note the medication), and smokes. The question asks for the next step in management of this patient. Given his hypotension (blood pressure of 90/47 mmHg) and tachycardia, he is hemodynamically unstable and must proceed to exploratory laparotomy.

(A) Abdominal ultrasonography is the ideal screening test for those patients at risk of developing AAA. Given this patient's risk factors of smoking, hypertension, and his age, he would have been an ideal candidate for screening. Abdominal ultrasound is not ideal in a hemodynamically unstable patient. (B) CXR is a potential means of diagnosis in patients with thoracic aortic aneurysm, where it can reveal widening of the aortic knob. Thoracic aortic aneurysms present with stabbing chest pain that radiates to the back. (C) CT of the abdomen would be a reasonable option in a patient suffering from a suspected AAA who is hemodynamically stable. However, this patient is not, and requires immediate intervention. (E) Transesophageal echocardiography would confirm a suspected diagnosis or thoracic aortic aneurysm (likely following the CXR as an initial study). Thoracic aortic aneurysms present with stabbing chest pain that radiates to the back. Transesophageal examinations are preferred to transthoracic ones based on the proximity to the great vessels.

15. A 43-year-old G_4P_4 obese woman reports to her local emergency department following an intense session of tailgating that involved abundant grilling and celebrating. After her meal, she began having immediate right upper quadrant pain and vomited. She denied red or yellow-green vomitus. Vitals reveal a fever of 102°F. Abdominal examination reveals right upper quadrant tenderness and voluntary guarding. Ultrasound of the area reveals biliary sludging, and gallbladder thickening. There is microlithiasis present. Which of the following statements best describes Murphy sign?

(A) Cessation of inspiration with deep palpation of the right upper quadrant

(B) Painless palpable gallbladder

(C) Referred shoulder pain secondary to diaphragmatic irritation

(D) Right upper quadrant tenderness due to application of an ultrasound probe

(E) Tenderness in the right upper quadrant with deep palpation assisted by inspiration

The answer is A: Cessation of inspiration with deep palpation of the right upper quadrant. Murphy sign is a commonly tested physical examination phenomenon and frequently misinterpreted. A patient is first asked to fully expire as the examiner places his hand in a deep palpation position at the right upper quadrant. The patient is then asked to fully inspire. Traditionally, a positive Murphy sign refers to the cessation of patient inspiration due to pain. Inspiration causes downward movement of the diaphragm, which causes sudden pain when it contacts the inflamed gallbladder.

(B) Palpable gallbladder typically describes Courvoisier sign, a sign suggestive of carcinoma of the head of the pancreas. The head of the pancreas leads to obstruction of the common bile duct, leading to gallbladder dilatation. The process is typically painless, as it involves a chronic, slowly occurring process (desensitizing the nociceptors). (C) This statement describes Kehr sign, which can occur in a wide variety of cases of peritonitis. Kehr sign is unique in that it is referred pain which occurs in the abdominal cavity based on the overlapping nerve roots that innervate the diaphragm as well as sensory nerves of the shoulder. (D) This is a distracting statement, as it describes the sonographic Murphy sign, which is considered a variant of the Murphy sign. It does not necessarily involve cessation of patient inspiration. It is slightly different from the classically tested Murphy sign. (E) This statement describes the frequent misinterpretation by students (that the role of inspiration is only to elicit right upper quadrant tenderness). Correctly stated, however, a positive Murphy sign describes cessation of inspiration by the patient.

---

 16 A 15-year-old boy presents to the emergency department following 3 hours of abdominal pain. His pain is located around his umbilicus. Following the onset of pain, he became nauseous and vomited. Abdominal examination reveals diffuse abdominal tenderness. His white blood cell count is 16. CT of the abdomen reveals an inflamed appendix in the normal location in the right lower quadrant. What best explains the location for the visceral pain at this location in this particular patient?

(A) Greater splanchnic nerve innervations via T5–T9
(B) Lesser splanchnic nerve innervations via T9–T11
(C) Least splanchnic nerve innervations via T9–T11
(D) Least splanchnic nerve innervations via T11–L3

The answer is B: Lesser splanchnic nerve innervations via T9–11. Recall from the chapter that the basis for the location of visceral pain is embryologically based. Foregut, midgut, and hindgut structures are innervated by the greater, lesser, and least splanchnic nerves, respectively. These structures correlated with nerve roots in the T5–T9, T9–T11, and T11–L3, respectively. As a midgut (distal duodenum to transverse colon) structure, the most appropriate answer for appendicitis is the lesser splanchnic nerve, which accurately corresponds to the T9–T11 dermatome.

(A) The greater splanchnic nerve innervates the foregut (esophagus to proximal duodenum) structures. It is associated with the T5–T9 nerve roots. This is not the correct nerve associated with appendiceal visceral pain. (C) The least splanchnic nerve innervates the hindgut (descending colon to anus) structures. It is associated with the T11–L3 nerve roots, not the T9–T11 nerve roots. This answer is incorrect for multiple reasons. (D) The least splanchnic nerve innervates the hindgut (descending colon to anus) structures. It is associated with the T11–L3 nerve roots. This is not the correct nerve associated with appendiceal visceral pain.

17 You are called to see a 32-year-old woman who recently underwent a cesarean delivery. Her complaints include chills, dizziness, and extreme abdominal pain. Vitals include a temperature of 39°C, heart rate of 107 beats/min, respiratory rate of 17 breaths/min, blood pressure of 106/98 mmHg, and normal oxygen saturation. Examination reveals a nervous, diaphoretic woman. There are no bowel sounds during the abdominal examination, and a focal mass is palpated in the left lower quadrant. There is diffuse tenderness. White blood cell count is reported to be 18.2. Which of the following is the most likely diagnosis?

(A) Abdominal abscess
(B) Acute appendicitis
(C) Acute cholecystitis
(D) Postpartum eclampsia
(E) Uterine atony

The answer is A: Abdominal abscess. This postpartum woman is most likely suffering from a pelvic abscess following contamination from her recent cesarean section. Abdominal and pelvic abscesses present with abdominal pain, fever or chills, and a white blood cell count. A focal palpable mass may or may not be present. Abdominal abscesses, as infections, can proceed to a sepsis-like picture involving hypotension. A white blood cell count further speaks to the process.

(B) Acute appendicitis is the most common indication for surgical intervention in the gravid woman. While aspects of this picture could possibly suggest complication of appendicitis with abscess formation, her pain is left sided. Furthermore, this is a less likely diagnosis given her recent surgery. (C) Cholecystitis does have an association in the gravid and parous woman as well as the postoperative period. However, the presentation is strikingly different than the one provided here (pain location, mass location, etc.). Her recent procedure makes other diagnoses more concerning. (D) Eclampsia describes the condition of preeclampsia (hypertension and proteinuria) along with the presence of grand-mal seizures. It is treated with magnesium, but is ultimately expected to resolve with delivery of the child. This is different than the condition described. (E) Uterine atony describes a condition where the uterus fails to regain tone immediately following delivery of the child. A laxed, enlarged uterus on examination would reveal the diagnosis. This is quite different than what is presented.

---

 18 A 52-year-old woman travels to the emergency department complaining of unbearable reflux. She describes her discomfort as following her dinner this evening, but unaffected by the over-the-counter medications which usually alleviate her GERD-like symptoms. She also admits to nausea as well as weakness and tingling in her left arm. She denies chest pain and shortness of breath. Her medications include metformin and insulin, omeprazole, and escitalopram. Which of the following characteristics most strongly masks the presentation of myocardial infarction (MI) in this patient?

(A) Age
(B) Depression
(C) Diabetes mellitus
(D) GERD
(E) Taking over-the-counter antacids

The answer is C: Diabetes mellitus. Diabetes, female gender, and advanced age are known risk factors for "atypical angina (lacking the crushing, localized chest pain)," and therefore these are patient populations you should treat extra-cautiously. One theory for the occurrence of atypical angina in diabetics relates to the neurovascular effects this disease has systemically. In the setting of abdominal pain and/or discomfort, angina with or without MI must be considered, particularly in these patient populations.

(A) Advancing age is a risk factor for atypical angina. Typically, this effect manifests in the elderly. A patient who is 52 years old may certainly have age-related atypical angina, but diabetes would far outweigh this age-related risk. (B) Depression does not appear to be a risk factor for atypical angina, as diabetes is. On the other hand, the major psychiatric condition that clouds the condition of angina is panic disorders, whose symptoms can appear identical. (D) Symptoms of GERD (abdominal upset, nausea, retrosternal burning, etc.) are often the one described during atypical angina (if present). The presence of GERD, however, does not predispose a patient to atypical angina. There is danger, however, should a patient confuse atypical angina with his or her "typical reflux symptoms." (E) Over-the-counter antacids do not mask symptoms of angina. When taking a complete history, pain due to angina will not be relieved by antacids, but will instead be relieved with nitroglycerin prescribed to patients who have high cardiovascular risk.

19 A 45-year-old man is brought to the emergency department by paramedics. He was at an amusement park today when he collapsed and was found to be diaphoretic and experiencing extreme abdominal pain. He reports that he had been experiencing abdominal pain and constipation for the entire day and avoiding meals accordingly. He takes no medications. He had a cholecystectomy 3 years prior. Vitals are normal. Abdominal examination reveals diffuse tenderness with guarding and rebound. Chest x-ray reveals subdiaphragmatic air. Which of the following actions is the best next step in management?

(A) Conservative management
(B) Exploratory laparotomy
(C) Diagnostic and therapeutic endoscopy
(D) Laparoscopic appendectomy

The answer is B: Exploratory laparotomy. Always be able to recognize this CXR finding for both testing and practical purposes. This film exhibits "free air," or subdiaphragmatic air. This finding is pathognomonic for a perforated viscus (presumably bowel) until proven otherwise. This is an indication for immediate exploratory laparotomy.

(A) Conservative medical management is an option in postoperative ileus or the early stages of a suspected bowel obstruction in stable patients. Because the free air in this film indicates a perforation, likely secondary to obstruction based on the history, exploratory laparotomy is indicated. (C) Endoscopy can be diagnostic and therapeutic for intussucception (when the bowel "sleeves" on itself). This diagnosis is more common in the pediatric population. Free air would not be an expected finding in intussusception unless necrosis occurs. (D) Laparoscopic appendectomy would be indicated for cases of acute appendicitis. Based on this history and the description of this patient's symptoms, this is not acute appendicitis. Furthermore, a laparoscopic approach would be less than ideal given a suspected perforation.

20 An 80-year-old woman presents to the emergency department with abdominal pain. She describes the pain as crampy in nature and of a 48-hour duration. Her last meal exacerbated her pain, which preceded bilious vomiting that alleviated her pain. She has since avoided meals. Her medications include omeprazole, loratadine, albuterol, and Miralax. Surgical history includes cholecystectomy and appendectomy, both more than 10 years ago. Examination reveals a distended abdomen with increased bowel sounds, diffusely tender with voluntary guarding. Air–fluid levels are seen on the flat and upright abdominal x-ray. Which of the following is the most likely diagnosis?

(A) Iatrogenic cecal volvulus
(B) Iatrogenic small bowel obstruction
(C) Internal bowel herniation through the falciform ligament
(D) Postoperative ileus

The answer is B: **Iatrogenic small bowel obstruction.** Patients with bowel obstructions often present with colicky abdominal pain worse with eating, relieved by vomiting (which can be bilious), and acute constipation. Air–fluid levels are the classic radiologic finding. The most common cause of bowel obstruction in developed countries is iatrogenic due to postoperative adhesions in patients with previous surgeries. In complete bowel obstruction, small bowel obstructions far outnumber large bowel obstruction.

(A) Cecal volvulus would be a specific type of large bowel obstruction and therefore less common than small bowel obstructions in general. Furthermore, cecal volvuli involve other risk factors (high fiber diets, chronic recumbency), with postoperative adhesions being a less significant factor. (C) While patients with bowel herniation through the falciform ligament do indeed present with bowel obstruction symptoms, they extremely rarely account for obstruction (<0.2%). This is not, therefore, the most likely diagnosis. (D) Postoperative ileus describes the obstructive-like picture that occurs acutely after surgery. This patient's surgical history is distant, which makes this diagnosis impossible. Additionally, postoperative ileus tends to present more subtly and is associated with discomfort rather than acute pain onset.

---

 21 A 57-year-old woman presents to her physician for a routine health maintenance examination. She has a prior medical history of hypothyroidism, diabetes mellitus, and hypertension. Her surgical history includes open cholecystectomy 20 years prior, and laparoscopic appendectomy 7 years prior. Blood pressure is 130/84 mmHg and pulse is 76 beats/min. Physical examination is normal other than a right subcostal scar, and three small laparoscopic incisions which appear healed. Which statement listed below best defines McBurney point?

(A) Two-thirds the distance from the left anterior superior iliac spine (ASIS) to the umbilicus
(B) Two-thirds the distance from the right ASIS to the umbilicus
(C) Two-thirds the distance from the umbilicus to the left ASIS
(D) Two-thirds the distance from the umbilicus to the right ASIS

The answer is D: Two-thirds the distance from the umbilicus to the right ASIS. This question is testing basic abdominal anatomy, specifically that of McBurney point, the location commonly overlying the inflamed appendix in acute appendicitis. McBurney point lies between the umbilicus and the right ASIS, specifically two-thirds the distance toward the ASIS. A McBurney incision is located here (at the point of maximal tenderness) perpendicular to this line.

(A) This statement does not accurately describe McBurney point, as this point overlies the appendix, which is located on the right. (B) While closely describing McBurney point, the problem with this statement is that the point lies closer to the ASIS than the umbilicus. This statement is describing the point being closer to the umbilicus. (C) This statement does not accurately describe the McBurney point, as this point overlies the appendix, which is located on the right.

22 A 52-year-old woman presents to her physician with epigastric pain of sudden onset. She describes it being in a similar location to the gnawing sensation she experiences with meals but now is much worse. Her current medications include omeprazole, loratadine, and a multivitamin, and she reports a history of *H. pylori* infection. Physical examination reveals significant abdominal tenderness in the mid-epigastrium with involuntary guarding and mild rebound tenderness. What is the most appropriate next step in the management of this patient?

(A) Colonoscopy, limited to rectosigmoid region
(B) CT of the pelvis
(C) Esophagogastroduodenoscopy (EGD) to duodenum
(D) Upright abdominal plain film x-ray (AXR)

The answer is D: Upright abdominal plain film x-ray (AXR). This patient's history of *H. pylori* makes peptic ulcer disease very likely, which should raise concern for perforation of a preexisting ulcer. This is further supported with the sudden onset of abdominal pain in the epigastrium. An upright AXR in the setting of perforation can be very specific if it reveals subdiaphragmatic air. As an inexpensive diagnostic approach, it is the best first step.

(A) Colonoscopy is incorrect. The patient's history, symptoms, and examination indicate that the pathology involved is the upper gastrointestinal tract. A colonscopy, therefore, would contribute little to this diagnosis. (B) Computer tomography would be the next best step if the abdominal film appears normal. A CT study would provide more specifics about the perforation including size, severity, and location. In a stable patient, it could be useful in addition to an abdominal film for preoperative intraabdominal details. (C) In the setting of a perforation (as in peptic ulcer perforation), and diverticulitis (when microperforations exist or can occur easily), endoscopy is contraindicated. This would therefore be not an ideal management step, though it is addressing the relevant organ.

23 A 53-year-old man presents to the emergency department because of abdominal pain. He describes worsening cramping pain in his left lower abdomen of 8-hour duration. He had been nauseous with diarrhea for 24 hours. He has a past medical history of hypertension, peptic ulcer disease status post *H. pylori* eradication, and history of renal lithiasis. His medications include hydrocholorothiazide, rabeprazole, and over-the-counter Miralax. He has never had a colonoscopy. His last renal calculus episode was 19 years prior. Physical examination reveals a temperature of 38.2°C, blood pressure of 140/70 mmHg, and pulse of 110 beats/min. He has abdominal tenderness and guarding over his left lower quadrant. What is the most appropriate next step in the evaluation of this patient?

(A) Colonoscopy limited to rectum and sigmoid colon
(B) CT of the abdomen and pelvis
(C) Esophagogastroduodenoscopy (EGD)
(D) No further diagnostic testing is necessary given this clinical diagnosis
(E) Magnetic resonance imaging (MRI) of the abdomen and pelvis

The answer is B: CT of the abdomen and pelvis. Given the symptoms and physical examination findings, this patient is most likely suffering from acute diverticulitis. While he is lacking a previous diagnosis of diverticulosis, we are also told he has never had a colonoscopy. His Miralax use suggests constipation, a condition that may predispose to diverticulosis (or may been a symptom of the disease itself). CT is the diagnostic gold standard for acute diverticulitis based on sensitivity and specificity. CT studies reveals colonic stranding, thickening of bowel, and other involved processes (e.g., abscess, phlegmon, fistulae, etc.).

(A) Colonoscopy is relatively contraindicated in diverticulitis. There is a significant risk of bowel perforation through an affected diverticula. This patient is already showing signs of perforation based on peritoneal signs. (C) Despite having a history of peptic ulcer disease, perforation of a peptic ulcer is a less likely diagnosis given the location of this patient's pain. Furthermore, patients with peritoneal signs due to an ulcer perforation would proceed to exploratory laparotomy, not EGD, which is contraindicated. (D) The diagnosis is not certain. While this would deviate from the classic, typical presentation of renal calculus disease (involving renal or ureteral colic on the patient's left side), it is still a possibility given this patient's history. Further workup is required. (E) MRI would contribute little to this clinical picture. The patient has a fairly classic presentation and physical examination findings for diverticulitis. Given renal calculus disease is included in the differential based on his history, CT would first be more appropriate to determine which is the cause.

A 16-year-old boy presents to the ambulatory care center of the emergency department with right lower quadrant pain. He first noted the onset of pain 10 days prior while doing homework, which worsened over 1 day. He experienced a warm sensation with relief of his pain 2 days after onset. His pain subsided for some time, but began to recur 2 days prior to presenting. He noted fever and chills, nausea, and vomiting. Examination reveals a tachycardic, febrile young man in no acute distress. Abdominal examination reveals right lower quadrant tenderness with guarding. CT scan reveals appendiceal rupture with a walled-off abscess. Which of the following is the ideal treatment given the findings in this patient?

(A) Conservative management
(B) Interval appendectomy
(C) Laparoscopic appendectomy
(D) Open appendectomy

The answer is B: Interval appendectomy. Select cases of acute appendicitis are prone to rupture; rupture predisposes to abscess formation and possible sepsis. In cases where the abscess is effectively walled off, it is established that interval appendectomy (appendectomy 8 to 12 weeks after allowing the abscess to "cool off") is the gold standard in the pediatric population. Variations on this standard treatment include whether or not to administer antibiotics, and whether or not to begin with percutaneous drainage.

(A) Conservative management is partially correct, in that interval appendectomy involves 8 to 12 weeks of conservative management prior to removal of the appendix. This answer is incorrect because it does not mention the appendectomy that occurs later; therefore **B** is a better answer. (C) Laparosopic appendectomy would be ideal in an uncomplicated case of acute appendicitis. A walled off abscess is more so an indication for interval appendectomy. (D) Open appendectomy would be an option for acute appendicitis. In the pediatric population, however, laparoscopic would be the preferred approach. A walled off abscess, however, is more so an indication for interval appendectomy.

 A 16-year-old male is brought to the emergency department by his parents for right-sided abdominal pain. He reports that the pain started 2 hours prior while doing sit-up drills during gym class at school. He became nauseous and vomited after being picked up by his parents. He reported alleviation of pain sitting upright in the car. He has no prior medical or surgical history. Blood pressure is 118/78 mmHg and pulse is 68 beats/min. Physical examination reveals a young man in acute distress. The right lower quadrant of his abdomen is diffusely tender without guarding or rebound tenderness. The WBC count is 7800/mm^3. Which of the following is the best first step in attaining a diagnosis?

(A) Complete physical examination
(B) CT of the abdomen
(C) MRI
(D) Scrotal ultrasound
(E) Upright KUB film

The answer is A: **Complete physical examination.** This question is modeled after a published case report of a case of testicular torsion that presented with abdominal pain only. While this clinical picture is atypical for this scenario, it is irrelevant, since further workup for this patient (and any patient) should start with a complete, head-to-toe physical examination. Remember to include testicular torsion as a differential for abdominal pain, and to always complete the history and physical prior to other diagnostics.

(B) CT is a reasonable choice given the symptom of abdominal pain. While this would not provide the diagnosis of testicular torsion, it would rule out other diagnoses for right-sided abdominal pain such as appendicitis. (C) MRI is incorrect. This would take place well after a complete history and physical examination. Additionally, CT would take precedence. (D) A scrotal ultrasound would be recommended for this patient, as this is describing a case of testicular torsion. However, scrotal ultrasound would take place after a complete physical examination, including a urogenital examination. (E) An abdominal plain film showing the kidneys, ureters and bladder (KUB) film, or "kidneys, ureters, bladder" x-ray is similar to an abdominal plain film and is useful in beginning a workup for a patient with suspected renal or ureteral stones. While it is urologic it nature, it has no bearing in testicular torsion, and would not occur before a complete physical examination.

Hernias

1 A 25-year-old woman presents with pain in her thigh that started yesterday. She also reports an area of swelling in her thigh that has increased in size over the last few days. Her body temperature is 38°C, blood pressure 126/75 mmHg, pulse 76 beats/min, and respirations 15 breaths/min. On physical examination, there is a palpable bulge felt below the inguinal ligament. CT scan is obtained, and a representative image is shown in *Figure 4-1*:

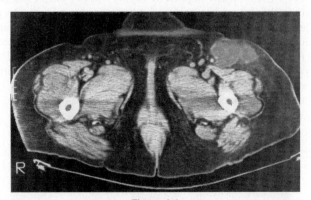

Figure 4-1

Which of the following is not a risk factor associated with this patient's problem?

(A) Chronic constipation
(B) Chronic cough
(C) Female sex
(D) Obesity
(E) Previous cesarean delivery

The answer is E: Previous cesarean delivery. This patient is presenting with signs and symptoms consistent with a femoral hernia. Femoral hernias are characterized by protrusion of abdominal contents (usually small bowel) below the inguinal ligament through the femoral canal. They are most common in elderly female patients (although they are relatively uncommon as a whole making up approximately 3% of hernias). In addition to female sex, risks for femoral hernias include obesity and any condition that increases intraabdominal pressure such as constipation or coughing. While a previous cesarean delivery or other abdominal surgeries may increase the risk for incisional hernias, they do not increase the risk of femoral hernias. CT scan shows fluid-filled loops of bowel along the course of the saphenous vein.

(A) Chronic constipation results in frequent elevations in intraabdominal pressure and has been associated with an increased risk of femoral herniation. (B) Similar to above, chronic cough (often a result of smoking) can also increase the risk for femoral hernias. (C) Women are more likely to suffer from femoral hernias than men. One reason for this disparity may be related to weakened abdominal musculature from pregnancy. (D) Obesity places extra strain on the abdomen, which in turn can lead to herniation.

2   A 51-year-old man presents with nausea, vomiting, and a fever of 101.8°F. On further inquiry, he admits that he has not had flatulence in 24 hours and has no bowel movements for a week. On physical examination, he appears acutely ill. Bowel sounds are absent and there is an erythematous and painful mass protruding from a defect in his right groin. His laboratory studies show a WBC count of 19,500/mm³, a lactate dehydrogenase level of 350 IU/L, and a BUN/Cr ratio of 35. After three attempts, the physician fails to reduce the mass. CT scan of the abdomen is obtained and is shown in *Figure 4-2*.
Which of the following is the next best step in management?

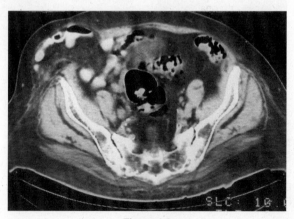

Figure 4-2

(A) Continue attempts at manual reduction
(B) Nasogastric suction and close observation
(C) Start intravenous cefoxitin
(D) Start intravenous vancomycin
(E) Urgent abdominal MRI scan

The answer is C: Start intravenous cefoxitin. This patient is most likely suffering from a strangulated inguinal hernia and will need initiation of broad-spectrum antibiotics and urgent surgery. In this patient, the CT scan was obtained which shows that the hernia is just lateral to the inferior epigastric vessels. Cefoxitin is a good choice of antibiotic for strangulated hernias since it covers both gram-negative and anaerobic organisms.

(A) Emergent initial management of suspected incarcerated hernia is attempts at manual reduction. When the patient appears toxic and two to three attempts at reduction are unsuccessful, strangulation should be suspected and further reduction should not be attempted. Continued attempts at manual reduction are not indicated in this patient since three attempts have already been made without success and strangulation is likely. (B) Nasogastric suction and close observation have been used in cases of patients with absent to very mild symptoms. Observation would not be appropriate in a toxic-appearing patient. (D) While vancomycin covers gram-positive organisms well, the most common infectious complications of strangulated hernias involve gram-negative and/or anaerobic organisms. (E) An abdominal CT scan sometimes helps with diagnosing questionable hernias, especially Spigelian or obturator hernias. However, a CT scan is not necessary in this case since the diagnosis is clear. In this patient, the CT scan was obtained which shows that the hernia is just lateral to the inferior epigastric vessels. MRI is inferior to CT in terms of visualization of abdominal pathology other than cancer. Thus, CT would be the preferred imaging modality for this patient.

---

3 A 52-year-old woman with a long history of smoking and chronic obstructive pulmonary disorder (COPD) complains of a "lump" in her upper thigh that increases in size when standing. Her body temperature is 37.3°C, blood pressure 130/75 mmHg, pulse 65 beats/min, and respirations 15 breaths/min. On physical examination, there is a mass on the lateral aspect of the pubic tubercle that appears to be protruding through the femoral canal. It is neither painful to palpation nor erythematous and can be easily reduced. An elective repair is scheduled. When performing surgery, which of the following structures are important landmarks that make up the boundaries of the femoral canal?

(A) Cystic duct, common hepatic duct, cystic artery
(B) Inguinal ligament, external oblique aponeurosis, transversalis fascia, conjoint tendon
(C) Inguinal ligament, inferior epigastric vessels, rectus muscle
(D) Inguinal ligament, pectineal ligament, lacunar ligament, femoral vein
(E) Pubic symphysis, ischiopubic ramus, ischial tuberosities

The answer is D: Inguinal ligament, pectineal ligament, lacunar ligament, femoral vein. This patient most likely has a femoral hernia which protrudes through the femoral canal. The femoral canal is bordered by four major structures: anterosuperiorly by the inguinal ligament, posteriorly by the pectineal ligament, medially by the lucunar ligament, and laterally by the femoral vein. The entrance to the canal is via the femoral ring.

(A) These structures make up the borders of Calot triangle, which are important landmarks for gallbladder surgery. (B) These structures are the borders of the inguinal canal, the pathway in which an indirect inguinal hernia may occur. (C) These structures make up the borders of Hasselbach triangle, through which direct hernias may occur. (E) These structures make up the borders of the urogenital triangle.

4   A 45-year-old man presents with a palpable inguinal mass that has slowly increased in size over the last several months. After a thorough workup, the patient is diagnosed with an indirect inguinal hernia and scheduled for elective repair. When counseling this patient about the risks of surgery, which of the following is the most common complication of hernia repair?

(A) Excessive bleeding
(B) Hernia reoccurrence
(C) Intestinal injury
(D) Pulmonary embolism
(E) Wound infection

The answer is B: Hernia reoccurrence. In addition to ecchymosis, hernia reoccurrence is one of the most common complications of hernia repair. For inguinal hernia repair with primary herniorrhaphy or hernioplasty, reoccurrence rates may range from less than 1% to 15%. If one or more reoccurrences have already occurred, the reoccurrence rate approaches 20%. Other factors that increase the rate of reoccurrence include smoking, obesity, older age, diabetes mellitus, arteriosclerosis, steroids, and any other conditions that increase intraabdominal pressure (chronic cough, chronic obstructive pulmonary disorder (COPD), postnasal drip, etc.).

(A) Although excessive bleeding is a potential complication of hernia repair, it is relatively uncommon. (C) Intestinal injury is a potential complication of hernia repair, especially if the surgery is open. However, it is far from the most common complication. (D) Pulmonary embolism is a potential complication of any major surgery and is most common in those with prolonged bed rest. It is not as common as hernia reoccurrence postoperatively after hernia repair. (E) Wound infection is a potential complication of any surgery, but relatively uncommon with hernia repair. It more often occurs in repairs of reoccurring hernias and patients undergoing mesh repairs.

5 A 3-day-old male infant is brought by his mother to the physician after she notices a scrotal "bulge" that appears during the day and disappears at night. She has also noticed his scrotum swell when he cries. Other than the bulge, she reports her baby has been acting normally. On physical examination, the baby's right scrotum appears enlarged. It is nonpainful to palpation and there is no erythema. Transillumination reveals a solid mass within scrotum that can easily be pushed back into the abdomen. Which of the following is the best management of this infant's condition?

(A) Elective surgical repair
(B) Emergent surgical repair
(C) Medical management
(D) Observation for 12 months
(E) Reassurance

The answer is A: **Elective surgical repair.** This infant most likely has a congenital inguinal hernia. The definitive management of inguinal hernias is surgical repair. The timing of the surgery depends on whether the hernia is reducible or not. A history of a reducible mass, such as in this patient, should be repaired promptly but is not emergent. Manual reduction should be attempted and elective surgical repair scheduled. While awaiting surgical evaluation, the caretakers should be informed of signs and symptoms of incarceration, as this has been reported in up to 13% of children awaiting surgical repair. Incarcerated hernias require reduction as quickly as possible to avoid strangulation.

(B) Emergent surgical repair is required in strangulated or nonreducible incarcerated inguinal hernias. (C) Medical management is not appropriate for inguinal hernias. There are no medications that have shown to be beneficial. (D) Observation may be appropriate for umbilical hernias in infants, but is not appropriate for inguinal hernias as they almost never resolve on their own. (E) Reassurance is not appropriate, as congenital inguinal hernias usually do not resolve without intervention. Additionally, inguinal hernias have an increased risk of incarceration or strangulation; thus repair is necessary.

6 A 65-year-old man with a history of multiple abdominal surgeries complains of a bulging abdominal mass that has been becoming progressively worse over the last several months. He reports that his bowel movements are normal. His body temperature is 36.9°C, blood pressure is 135/80 mmHg, pulse 80 beats/min, and respirations 13 breaths/min. On physical examination, there is a bulging, erythematous, and painful mass in the upper right quadrant over a previous surgical incision. Open surgical repair using mesh is planned with access through the anterolateral wall. What is the order of abdominal layers that the surgeon must transverse before gaining access to the abdominal cavity?

(A) Skin, external oblique, internal oblique, superficial fascia, transversus, transversalis fascia, peritoneum

(B) Skin, superficial fascia, external oblique, internal oblique, transversus, transversalis fascia, peritoneum

(C) Skin, superficial fascia, internal oblique, external oblique, transversus, peritoneum, transversalis fascia

(D) Skin, superficial fascia, transversus, external oblique, internal oblique, transversalis fascia, peritoneum

(E) Skin, transversalis fascia, superficial fascia, external oblique, internal oblique, transversus, peritoneum

The answer is B: Skin, superficial fascia, external oblique, internal oblique, transversus, transversalis fascia, peritoneum The layers of the anterolateral abdominal wall from superficial to deep are:

1. Skin
2. Superficial fascia (Camper then Scarpa)
3. External oblique muscle
4. Internal oblique muscle
5. Transverse abdominal muscle
6. Transversalis fascia
7. Peritoneum

(A) This order is incorrect. (C) This order is incorrect. (D) This order is incorrect. (E) This order is incorrect.

---

 7 A 2-year-old boy is brought to the pediatrician by his mother for a routine well-child checkup. During the physical examination, the pediatrician notices that there is no palpable testicle on the right side. After a thorough workup, he is diagnosed with right cryptorchidism. Which of the following is an ectopic site where a testicle may be potentially found outside the normal path of dissension?

(A) Femoral canal
(B) Infrarenal
(C) Inguinal canal
(D) Intraabdominal
(E) Suprascrotal

The answer is A: Femoral canal. During fetal development, the testicles migrate from inside the abdomen (starting below the kidney) through the inguinal canal and into the scrotum. Transinguinal migration usually occurs by 28 to 40 weeks' gestation. Overall, approximately 3% of full-term male newborns have cryptorchidism. The rate is much higher in that of premature male newborns, approaching 30%. The most common ectopic sites where the testicle may deviate from the normal pathway of descent include the perineum, femoral canal, superficial inguinal pouch, contralateral scrotal pouch, and the suprapubic area.

(B) Infrarenal testicles are part of the normal path of descent. (C) The inguinal canal is part of the normal path of descent. (D) Intraabdominal cryptochordism is not an ectopic location as the testicles travel through the abdomen and through the inguinal canal. (E) Suprascrotal location is not outside of the normal pathway of descent.

8 A 24-year-old man presents for a preemployment physical. During the genital examination, the physician readily palpates a soft mass that protrudes through the superficial inguinal ring and into the scrotum while the patient coughs. Which of the following is the most likely diagnosis?

(A) Indirect inguinal hernia
(B) Direct inguinal hernia
(C) Femoral hernia
(D) Paraumbilical hernia
(E) Littré hernia

The answer is A: Indirect inguinal hernia. This patient most likely has an indirect inguinal hernia, which is the most common type of hernia in both men and women worldwide. Indirect hernias are a result of failure of embryologic closure of the deep inguinal ring (a persistent process vaginalis) after the testicle has completely descended. The hernia sac consists of peritoneum extending through the inguinal ring (lateral to the inferior epigastric vessels) to the spermatic cord in men or round ligament in women, which creates a path in which bowel or omentum may transverse. Patients usually present with a bulge in the groin that is palpable at the top or within the scrotum that is exacerbated by increasing intraabdominal pressure.

(B) In contrast to indirect hernias, direct inguinal hernias are most often acquired and result from weakness in the lower abdominal wall. Direct hernias transverse medially to the inferior epigastric vessels. They have a lower incidence of strangulation and incarceration when compared to indirect since a peritoneal sac is usually not involved. (C) Unlike indirect hernias but similarly to direct hernias, femoral hernias are often acquired. They are more common in older women as a result of age and stress (childbirth) on the abdominal musculature. Femoral hernias are usually a result in weakness within the femoral triangle. The hernia emerges below the inguinal ligament and often presents as a mass in the lower groin or thigh. Femoral hernias have a high rate of strangulation and require early repair. (D) Paraumbilical hernias are most often acquired and occur next to the umbilicus. They occur more often in women. Risk factors, among others, include obesity and pregnancy. (E) Littré hernia involves herniation of a Meckel diverticulum through an abdominal defect. They are most common in men and usually occur on the right side. Repair of Littré hernias involves resection of the diverticulum and herniorrhaphy.

9 A 6-month-old infant is brought by his grandmother to the physician after she notices a "bump sticking out near his belly button." She admits that it has been there since birth, but is worried since it doesn't seem to be going away. His previous well-child visits have been unremarkable. His vitals are within normal limits. On physical examination, there is a 2×2 cm^2 soft swelling over the umbilicus that bulges when the baby cries and is flat at rest. Which of the following is the next best step in management?

(A) Elective surgery
(B) Emergent surgery
(C) Observation and reassurance
(D) Reduce and maintain reduction with adhesive tape
(E) Ultrasound of the abdomen

The answer is C: Observation and reassurance. This infant has an umbilical hernia, a common malformation present in newborns. It is caused by delayed closure or failure to close the umbilical ring. It has a higher incidence among black children and may also occur more frequently in congenital hypothyroidism, fetal hydantoin syndrome, Beckwith-Wiedmann syndrome, and polysaccharide metabolic disorders. Although umbilical hernias in infants can be quite large, they are most often benign and usually resolve by age 2 to 3. If the hernia does not resolve, then the defect may be surgically repaired. The method of repair depends on the defect size where larger defects may require prosthesis.

(A) Elective surgery would be appropriate if this patient's umbilical hernia failed to close after conservative management. (B) Emergent surgery might be appropriate if there was evidence of incarceration or strangulation. This patient is symptom free and conservative management is the treatment of choice. (D) Placing objects or tape over the hernia does not assist in closure. Furthermore, objects may erode the skin and cause additional harm. (E) Ultrasound does not typically have a role in the diagnosis of umbilical hernias. The diagnosis here is not in doubt and ultrasound is not indicated.

10 A 73-year-old woman with a history of stress incontinence complains of hip pain, nausea, vomiting, and failure to pass stool for the last 7 days. She says that these same symptoms have happened several times before, but usually resolved after 1 to 2 days. Her body temperature is 37.6°C, blood pressure is 145/75 mmHg, pulse 100 beats/min, and respirations 19 breaths/min. On physical examination, there is pain in the anteromedial thigh when the hip is actively or passively extended and externally rotated. The pain is decreased with thigh flexion. There is no swelling appreciated in the inguinal region or leg. CT imaging will most likely reveal what type of hernia in this patient?

(A) Direct inguinal hernia
(B) Femoral hernia
(C) Incisional hernia
(D) Indirect inguinal hernia
(E) Obturator hernia

The answer is E: Obturator hernia. This patient most likely has an obturator hernia, a rare variety of abdominal hernia that usually occurs in elderly women (due to a wider pelvis) and has a high rate of morbidity and mortality. They occur in increasing frequency with pelvic floor weakness. Several examination findings are associated with obturator hernias, including the Howship-Romberg and Hannington-Kiff signs. The Howship-Romberg sign is positive when there is pain in the medial thigh that is worse with extension, adduction, or medial rotation and decreased with thigh flexion. The Hannington-Kiff sign is more specific (but less known) and is characterized by an absent adductor reflex in the thigh. Regardless of clinical signs, the diagnosis is best achieved with CT imaging which will show herniation of abdominal viscera into or through the obturator canal. Laparoscopic or open repair should be performed early to minimize morbidity and mortality.

(A) A direct inguinal hernia occurs through weak points in the abdominal fascia medial to the inferior epigastric vessels. Direct hernias do not contain a sac. Men and older individuals that are overweight are more likely to have direct inguinal hernias. Imaging studies are usually not required in the workup as the defect can be visualized on examination. (B) Femoral hernias are almost always acquired and, like direct inguinal hernias, do not contain a hernia sac. The defect occurs in the femoral canal. They usually occur in older thin women. Patients may experience pain aggravated by bending or lifting. Femoral hernias may be visualized and palpated in the anterior thigh and have a high rate of incarceration and strangulation. (C) Incisional hernias develop at the site of previous operations and are usually asymptomatic. They present as a bulge at the site of a previous incision that is worsened by standing or increasing intraabdominal pressure. Even after repair, recurrence rates are greater than 20%. (D) Indirect inguinal hernias are the most common type of hernia and are characterized by abdominal viscera protruding through the inguinal canal. They occur lateral to the inferior epigastric vessels. Many indirect hernias are asymptomatic and often present as a bulge in the groin. If strangulation or incarceration is present, pain is usually present in the groin area rather than the thigh. Imaging studies are not required in the workup as they can often be appreciated on examination.

11　A 55-year-old woman presents with left thigh swelling that is becoming progressively worse over the last several days. Her past medical history is remarkable for obesity and diabetes mellitus. She has a 40-pack-year history of smoking. Her body temperature is 37.2°C, blood pressure 140/85 mmHg, pulse 65 beats/min, and respirations 14 breaths/min.

On physical examination, she appears well. An abdominal examination reveals a 2×3 cm^2 mass in the medial thigh that protrudes below the inguinal ligament. There is no erythema or pain with palpation and the mass can be easily reduced. She is subsequently diagnosed with a femoral hernia. Which of the following characteristic of femoral hernias is the primary reason for early repair?

(A) Compression of the femoral artery
(B) Compression of the femoral vein
(C) High rate of strangulation
(D) Increased risk of forming an enterovascular fistula
(E) Increased risk of malignancy

The answer is C: **High rate of strangulation.** Femoral hernias have a high rate of incarceration and strangulation. This is most likely a result of the small-defined space in which protrusion may occur and its proximity to rigid structures such as the inguinal ligament, Cooper ligament, and its lacunar attachments. Thus, prompt repair of femoral hernias is recommended after diagnosis. For nonemergent surgery, an infrainguinal approach is often utilized for repair. For emergent surgery, a high approach to allow better access and visualization of the bowel is used.

(A) Compression of the femoral artery may rarely occur in a femoral hernia, but is not the primary reason for early repair. (B) Compression of the femoral vein may rarely occur in a femoral hernia, but is not the primary reason for early repair. (D) Enterovascular fistula is a potential but extremely rare complication of a femoral hernia. (E) Femoral hernias are not known to be associated with an increased risk of malignancy.

---

 12) Which of the following structures separate the boundaries of a direct and indirect inguinal hernia?

(A) Cooper ligament
(B) Inferior epigastric vessels
(C) Inguinal ligament
(D) Rectus abdominis muscle
(E) Superficial epigastric artery

The answer is B: **Inferior epigastric vessels.** Direct and indirect inguinal hernias are often defined anatomically by their relation to the inferior epigastric vessels. Direct inguinal hernias occur medially to the vessels (from a weak spot in the fascia of the abdominal wall) and indirect occur laterally (via a patent processus vaginalis).

(A) Cooper ligament (also called the pectineal ligament) is an extension of the lacunar ligament and rungs along the pectineal line of the pubic bone. It is often utilized in hernia repair since it is strong and holds sutures well. (C) The inguinal ligament does not separate indirect and direct inguinal hernias as both defects occur at or above the inguinal ligament. (D) The rectus abdominis muscle is a large paired muscle that runs vertically on each side of the anterior abdominal wall. It does not separate indirect and direct inguinal hernias. (E) The superficial epigastric artery distributes blood to the superficial fascia and skin of the lower abdominal wall. It originates below the inguinal ligament and passes through the femoral sheath. It is found between Camper and Scarpa fascia. The inferior, not superficial epigastric artery is a major separating landmark between direct and indirect inguinal hernias.

13 A 16-year-old boy is brought to the emergency department with fever, chills, and failure to pass stool for the last 8 days after a weight lifting competition at school. He is currently complaining of right scrotum pain that has gradually increased over the last week. His body temperature is 38.5°C, blood pressure 130/80 mmHg, pulse 100 beats/min, and respirations 20 breaths/min. He appears toxic and dehydrated. On examination, there is a tender and erythematous mass protruding into the right testicle. Normal saline and broad-spectrum antibiotics are initiated and emergent surgery prepared. Which of the following segments of bowel is most likely involved in this patient's herniation?

(A) Ascending colon
(B) Descending colon
(C) Duodenum
(D) Ileum
(E) Sigmoid colon

The answer is D: Ileum. Mobile segments of small bowel are the most common portion of bowel to be involved in indirect hernias. In addition, from the choices above, the ileum is the only mobile portion of bowel that could herniate on the left side.

(A) Ascending colon is fixed to the abdominal wall and is less commonly involved in hernias. (B) Like the ascending colon, the descending colon is also fixed to the abdominal wall and unlikely to be involved in herniation, especially on the right side. (C) The duodenum is fixed to the posterior and superior abdominal wall and would unlikely be involved in an inguinal hernia. (E) Although the sigmoid colon is mobile, it is more commonly involved in left inguinal hernias than right.

14 A 51-year-old man complains of colicky abdominal pain and distention for the last several days. He reports he has also been vomiting and has not had a bowel movement for 5 days or passed flatulence for the past 24 hours. His body temperature is 37.5°C, blood pressure 140/90 mmHg, pulse 105 beats/min, and respirations 23 breaths/min. On physical examination there are high-pitched bowel sounds heard

over a nonreducible bulge in the right lower quadrant. Which of the following is the next best step in management?

(A) Abdominal ultrasound
(B) Barium contrast study
(C) Intravenous cefazolin
(D) Intravenous hydration and emergent surgery
(E) Nothing by mouth, intravenous hydration, and observation

The answer is D: Intravenous hydration and emergent surgery. This patient is presenting with signs and symptoms of small bowel obstruction and possible strangulation. Thus he should receive intravenous hydration and emergent repair of the inguinal hernia.

(A) Abdominal imaging is not required when clinical suspicion is high. ultrasound (US) is best used to narrow the differential in scrotal masses or masses below the inguinal ligament. (B) Clinical suspicion is high in this case and imaging studies are not necessary to make the diagnosis. Additionally, barium studies should be avoided in patients with suspected complete small bowel obstruction. (C) Intravenous antibiotics may be given in suspected cases of strangulated hernias and in some cases of incarcerated hernias. However, cefazolin is a poor choice as first-generation cephalosporins do not have broad enough coverage. (E) Although nothing by mouth and intravenous hydration would be initial steps in the management of this patient, observation would be a poor choice of action and may result in death.

15   A 43-year-old man undergoes an open laparotomy after a single gunshot wound to the abdomen. The patient is found to be bleeding from a vessel injury in the transverse colon mesentery. The vessel is successfully repaired. Several days after surgery it is noted by the medical student that abundant salmon-pink colored fluid is leaking from the incisional site. Over the next couple of days, the amount of fluid draining from the site increases and an intestinal bulge under in the incision site is visualized. Which of the following is the best step in management?

(A) Broad-spectrum antibiotics and wound culture
(B) Continued observation
(C) Early ambulation
(D) Operative wound exploration
(E) Placement of a wound vacuum

The answer is D: Operative wound exploration. This patient most likely has wound dehiscence with an early incisional hernia. Wound dehiscence continues to be a major cause of morbidity and mortality after abdominal surgery. The incidence of fascial disruption following abdominal surgery ranges from 0.4% to 3.5% (depending on the type). In almost all cases, wound dehiscence is accompanied by an abundant salmon-pink serous discharge. Failure to correct the defect may result in evisceration, which is a surgical emergency. Preoperative factors that predispose patients to wound dehiscence include (among others) male sex, increased age, emergency operations, and obesity. Prevention of wound dehiscence is key and can be avoided with simple running techniques for closure, absorbable sutures, including all layers of the abdominal wall in the closure, taking adequate wound "bites" with sutures and placing the proper amount of tension. When fascia disruption is suspected, the patient's wound should be explored in the operating room and repaired as necessary.

(A) Although broad-spectrum antibiotics and wound culture may be necessary if wound infection is present, it will not fix wound dehiscence. (B) Continued observation is not appropriate as this patient's dehiscence is worsening. (C) Early ambulation may in fact worsen this patient's dehiscence, as it will result in increased intraabdominal pressure. (E) Placement of a wound vacuum may worsen this patient's condition since negative pressure outside the abdomen will provide additional incentive for the bowel to herniate.

16 A 53-year-old obese woman with a history of diabetes mellitus presents with an intermittent pain and a progressively enlarging mass in the left lower quadrant. Her body temperature is 37.5°C, blood pressure 130/85 mmHg, pulse 65 beats/min, and respirations 16 breaths/min. On physical examination, there is a 5 × 3 cm² reducible mass located adjacent to the iliac crest, which is best seen when the patient stands up. In addition, there is persistent point tenderness over the mass. An abdominal CT scan shows a ventral herniation of abdominal viscera through the linea semilunaris. Which of the following is the most likely diagnosis?

(A) Direct inguinal hernia
(B) Hiatal hernia
(C) Indirect inguinal hernia
(D) Obturator hernia
(E) Spigelian hernia

The answer is E: **Spigelian hernia.** This patient is most likely suffering from a spigelian hernia. Spigelian hernias are an uncommon form of ventral hernias that protrude between the attachment of the internal oblique and transversus abdominis muscle to the rectus sheath (semilunar line or "linea semilunaris"). Patients often present with swelling or pain in the mid to lower abdomen. Since they occur submuscularly, they may not be palpable and are thus difficult to clinically diagnose. Imaging with abdominal ultrasound (preferred) or CT may be helpful. Peak incidence is at age 50. Repair is performed using an open tension-free approach similar to incisional hernias. When present, they will often lead to incarceration and require urgent surgical repair.

(A) Direct inguinal hernias are most often acquired and result from weakness in the lower abdominal wall. Direct hernias transverse medially to the inferior epigastric vessels. They have a lower incidence of strangulation and incarceration when compared to indirect since a peritoneal sac is usually not involved. Imaging is usually not required in the diagnosis. (B) A hiatal hernia is the protrusion of the top of the stomach into the thorax through a tear or weakness in the diaphragm. (C) Indirect inguinal hernias are the most common type of hernia. Abdominal contents protrude through the inguinal canal and they originate lateral to the inferior epigastric vessels. Many indirect hernias are asymptomatic and often present as a bulge in the groin. If strangulation or incarceration is present, pain is usually present in the groin area rather than the thigh. Imaging studies are not required for diagnosis. (D) Obturator hernias are a rare variety of abdominal hernias that most often occur in elderly women. They occur when abdominal viscera protrude through the obturator canal. The diagnosis is best achieved with CT imaging. Laparoscopic or open repair should be performed as soon as possible since they are associated with high morbidity and mortality.

 A 29-year-old man presents with a new bulging mass in the groin. Workup reveals an inguinal hernia. Which of the following types of traditional repairs is associated with the lowest rate of recurrence?

(A) Bassini repair
(B) Lichtenstein repair
(C) McVay repair
(D) Modified Bassini repair
(E) Shouldice repair

The answer is B: Lichtenstein repair. Tension-free repairs and those using meshes have a significantly decreased rate of hernia reoccurrence. One popular tension-free method is the Lichtenstein repair, which involves placing a flat anterior overlying mesh. Patients receiving this type of repair usually go home within a few hours of surgery and can often resume normal activity within 1 to 2 weeks of the operation. Reoccurrence rates with the Lichtenstein repair range from less than 1% to 5%.

(A) The original Bassini repair is a "tension" repair in which the edges of the defect are sewn together without a mesh. The original Bassini (unmodified) repair involved opening the oblique aponeurisis through the external inguinal ring and resecting the cremasteric muscle from around the spermatic cord. For inguinal ligament repair, the conjoint tendon is approximated to the inguinal ligament. This type of repair is no longer used in developed nations since recurrence rates are high (5% to 15%). (C) McVay method of hernia repair is a method that was historically used for femoral and inguinal hernias. It involved incising the transversalis fascia and exposing the pectineal ligament. The conjoined tendon was then sutured to the pectineal ligament.

Additionally, a portion of the inguinal floor was repaired by approximating the inguinal ligament to the conjoined tendon. This repair is not commonly used since it is a higher tension repair and associated with higher rates of hernia recurrence. Recurrence rates are similar to Bassini repair and range from 5% to 15%. (D) A modified Bassini repair is similar to the original Bassini with suturing the conjoined tendon to the inguinal ligament. However, in contrast to the original, it does not involve opening the transversalis fascia or removing the cremasteric muscle. In addition, the divided transversalis fascia is not part of the suture repair. (E) The Shouldice repair is also a modification of Bassini repair. It utilizes four continuous layers of sutures with fine wire and removal of the cremasteric muscle. Recurrence rates are reported from less than 1% up to 7%. However, these statistics may be favorably skewed by the strict selection criteria, which exclude many patients with comorbidities.

---

18 A 3-month-old infant presents at the pediatrician's office for a well-child checkup. He was born at 32 weeks' gestation due to placental abruption, but did well in the hospital. His development since has been unremarkable. On today's visit, the mother is concerned about her son's "growing boy part." She admits that her son's left testicle will grow in size during the day and decrease in size at night. Physical examination reveals a swollen left testicle that is nontender to palpation. Which of the following is the next best step in diagnosis?

  (A) Measurement of serum beta-HCG and alpha-fetoprotein
  (B) Pelvic CT imaging
  (C) Reassurance
  (D) Scrotal ultrasonography
  (E) Transillumination of the scrotum

The answer is E: Transillumination of the scrotum. The first step in evaluating any scrotal mass is with physical examination (palpation) and transillumination. This patient will most likely have a hydrocele, but an inguinal hernia should be ruled out. A hydrocele is a collection of fluid within the process vaginalis that produces swelling within the scrotum and/or inguinal canal. Transillumination of a hydrocele will show fluid in the tunica vaginalis. In general, neonates with a hydrocele can be observed until age 2 if there is no discomfort, continued enlargement, or secondary infection. If a hernia is present, the risk of incarceration or strangulation is significant (especially with a history of prematurity) and it should be repaired as soon as possible.

(A) Measurements of serum tumor markers may be appropriate if a solid nonmobile mass was found attached to the testicle. This is not common in children at this age. (B) Pelvic CT imaging would not be the initial step as it is expensive. Less invasive and basic tests, like transillumination, should be performed initially. (C) Although this may be a hydrocele and require observation and reassurance, more serious conditions like inguinal herniation should be ruled out first. (D) Although scrotal ultrasonography may eventually be helpful in some conditions, more basic clinical tests like transillumination should be initially performed.

---

19 A 56-year-old man presents with acute abdominal pain, nausea, and vomiting. He has a history of a partial colectomy 10 years prior for localized adenocarcinoma of the colon. Before the current episode, he reports not having a bowel movement for the last 7 days. On physical examination, his previous surgical incision site appears well healed and intact. There is a small swollen bulge at the incision site that is tender on palpation. A CT scan of the abdomen shows only a small portion of the circumference of small bowel entrapped in a small defect under the previous incision site. Which of the following is the most likely diagnosis?

(A) Indirect inguinal hernia
(B) Littré hernia
(C) Morgagni hernia
(D) Richter hernia
(E) Spigellian hernia

The answer is D: Richter hernia. Richter hernias occur when only a part of the intestinal wall (antimesenteric border) protrudes through a defect in the abdominal wall. In addition to bowel obstruction, these hernias may still result in necrosis or perforation of the intestinal wall and peritonitis. Unfortunately signs of intestinal obstruction are often absent. CT imaging may show a bowel loop positioned in the middle of a defect, although diagnosis is often not made until surgery.

(A) Although an indirect inguinal hernia may present similarly, the CT findings are not characteristic of this type of hernia. (B) Littré hernia is a hernia involving a Meckel diverticulum. (C) Morgagni hernia occurs when abdominal contents pass through the thorax through a weakness in the diaphragm. (E) Spigellian hernias occur through the semilunar line and under the aponeurisis of the external oblique just medially to the rectus muscle.

---

20 Which of the following nerves provides sensation to the scrotum and penis, is found alongside the spermatic cord, and should be preserved during hernia surgery?

(A) Genitofemoral nerve
(B) Hypogastric nerve
(C) Ilioinguinal nerve
(D) Obturator nerve
(E) Pudendal nerve

The answer is C: Ilioinguinal nerve. The ilioinguinal nerve (branch of L1) runs along and outside the spermatic cord. It provides sensory fibers to the skin of the superior scrotum and root of the penis. Damage to this nerve should be avoided during hernia surgery.

(A) The genitofemoral nerve lies on the anterior surface of the psoas major and passes through the deep inguinal ring and inguinal canal. It supplies motor fibers to the cremaster muscle and elicits elevation of the testis via the cremaster reflex. (B) The hypogastric nerve lies inferior to the common iliac vessels and is involved in pain from pelvic viscera. (D) The obturator nerve passes through the obturator canal to innervate the muscles and provide sensation of the medial thigh. (E) The pudendal nerve is part of the sacral plexus. It passes through the pudendal canal and provides motor innervation to several pelvic muscles and sensation to the skin of the scrotum, labium, clitoris/penis, and anus.

 A 65-year-old woman presents to the ambulatory care clinic with progressive swelling in her thigh. Her pulse is 90 beats/min and blood pressure is 130/86 mmHg. She has no other complaints. After a thorough physical examination and workup, a femoral hernia is diagnosed. An elective repair of the femoral hernia is scheduled. During surgery, which of the following is the most likely space in which a femoral hernia will be identified?

(A) Between the femoral artery and vein
(B) Between the femoral nerve and artery
(C) Between the femoral vein and lymphatics
(D) Rectovesical pouch
(E) Retropubic space

The answer is C: **Between the femoral vein and lymphatics.** Femoral hernias occur within the femoral canal, below the inguinal ligament. From laterally to medially, the femoral triangle contains the femoral nerve, artery, vein, a space, and the lymphatics. Femoral hernias occur in the space between the vein and lymphatics.

(A) The femoral artery and vein lie next to each other and do not provide enough space for the hernia to occur here. (B) The femoral nerve is outside the femoral canal and is not involved in a femoral hernia. The femoral artery is found lateral to the femoral vein and is not a border of the femoral hernia. (D) The rectovesical pouch is the space between the rectum and bladder. It is not involved in a femoral hernia. (E) The retropubic space is an extraperitoneal space between the pubic symphysis and bladder. It is not involved in a femoral hernia.

 A 75-year-old man with a history of muscle invasive bladder cancer undergoes a cystoprostatectomy and ileal conduit urinary diversion. Following the surgery, the patient develops a parastomal hernia. Which of the following surgical methods greatly reduces parastomal hernia occurrence?

(A) Generous size of the stomal incision
(B) Placing stoma lateral to the rectus sheath
(C) Tension suturing
(D) Utilizing large bowel
(E) Utilizing small bowel

The answer is E: **Utilizing small bowel.** Parastomal hernias may occur after stomal construction since an artificial point of weakness is made in the abdominal wall. If the weakness is great enough, the abdominal contents may protrude through the defect and often into the subcutaneous tissue. Some studies show that the rate of parastomal hernia may be as high as 30% following stomal construction. Factors that increase the risk of parastomal herniation include (1) placement of the stoma lateral to the rectus sheath, (2) poor abdominal muscle tone (pregnancy, aging, etc.), (3) creation of an oversized stomal incision, (4) factors that increase intraabdominal pressure such as chronic cough or ascites, (5) location of the stoma in a midline incision, and (6) wound infection. Small bowel has the lowest rate of parastomal herniation. Multiple methods are described for parastomal hernia repair including meshes, localized fascia repair, and moving the stoma to a different site in the abdomen.

(A) Larger stomal incisions are associated with an increased risk of parastomal herniation. (B) Placement of the stoma lateral to the rectal sheath is associated with an increased risk of parastomal herniation. (C) Tension suturing is associated with an increased risk of parastomal herniation. Tension-free techniques are most often used when constructing stomas. (D) Use of large bowel for stoma formation is associated with an increased risk of parastomal herniation.

 23 A 47-year-old man with cirrhosis secondary to chronic and ongoing alcoholism presents to the emergency department with worsening abdominal distention and a new umbilical hernia. His body temperature is 36.9°C, blood pressure 146/85 mmHg, pulse 70 beats/min, and respirations 18 breaths/min. On physical examination, there is an enlarged firm and nodular liver. A shifting fluid wave can be percussed within the abdomen. A large umbilical hernia is apparent with skin ulceration and necrosis over the hernia and around the umbilicus. Which of the following is the next best step in management?

(A) Intravenous fluid hydration and broad-spectrum antibiotics and observation
(B) Emergent liver transplantation
(C) Primary umbilical hernia repair
(D) Umbilical hernia repair with peritovenous shunt
(E) Watchful waiting

The answer is D: **Umbilical hernia repair with peritovenous shunt.** This patient most likely has an umbilical hernia that is exacerbated by his ascites. Since there is skin breakdown and necrosis of the hernia, repair is a necessary and urgent part of this patient's management. However, repair of the hernia should be accompanied by treatment of his ascites since failure to do so would most likely make the repair unsuccessful. Of the choices above, only using a peritovenous shunt along with hernia repair would address both problems. In stable patients, treatment of ascites should precede hernia repair.

(A) Although intravenous hydration and broad-spectrum antibiotics may be part of this patient's management, avoiding correction and observing the patient could be disastrous. (B) This patient would not be a candidate for liver transplant due to his current alcoholism. (C) Primary umbilical hernia repair without addressing the ascites would result in a very high rate of repair failure. (E) Reassurance is not appropriate as this patient's condition is quite serious.

 24 A 52-year-old woman presents to the emergency department with colicky abdominal pain and a left lower quadrant bulge that is difficult to reduce. She reports not having a bowel movement for the last several days. After a thorough workup involving CT imaging of her abdomen, she is diagnosed with a Spigelian hernia. Which of the following describes the path of a Spigelian hernia?

(A) Between the internal oblique and transversus abdominis muscle, anterior to the external oblique aponeurisis

(B) Between the internal oblique and transversus abdominis muscle, posterior to the external oblique aponeurisis

(C) Medial to the inferior epigastric vessels

(D) Lateral to the inferior epigastric vessels

(E) Through the obturator canal

The answer is B: **Between the internal oblique and transversus abdominis muscle, posterior to the external oblique aponeurisis.** Spigelian hernias are an uncommon form of ventral hernia that protrudes between the attachment of the internal oblique and transversus abdominis muscle to the rectus sheath (semilunar line). Patients often present with swelling and/or pain in the mid to lower abdomen. Since they occur submuscularly, they may not be palpable on examination and are thus difficult to clinically diagnose. Imaging with abdominal ultrasound (preferred) or CT may be helpful. Peak incidence is at age 50. Repair is performed using an open tension-free approach similar to repair of incisional hernias.

(A) Although Spigelian hernias do occur between the internal oblique and transversus abdominis muscle, they are posterior (not anterior) to the external oblique aponeurisis. (C) Indirect inguinal hernias originate lateral to the inferior epigastric vessels and protrude through the inguinal ring. (D) Direct inguinal hernias originate medial to the inferior epigastric vessels (in Hesselbach triangle) though a weak point in the fascia of the abdominal wall. (E) Obturator hernias occur through the obturator canal.

25) A 41-year-old male carpenter presents to his primary care physician because he fears that he has suffered an inguinal hernia. He complains of right inguinal pain with deep coughing. Risk factors for inguinal hernias in this patient may include:

(A) Anorexia nervosa
(B) Chronic obstructive pulmonary disease
(C) Hypertension
(D) Irritable bowel syndrome
(E) Sedentary lifestyle

The answer is B: Chronic obstructive pulmonary disease. Heavy straining and increased pressure are contributory factors to the development of inguinal hernias. Chronic obstructive pulmonary disease leads to chronic forceful coughing, which can lead to increased pressure.

(A) Anorexia nervosa is not known to be a predisposing factor for hernias. (C) Hypertension is not known to be a predisposing factor for hernias. (D) Irritable bowel syndrome is not known to be a predisposing factor for hernias. (E) Sedentary lifestyle is not known to be a predisposing factor for hernias.

5

Esophagus and Stomach

1 A septuagenarian man receiving palliative care in an extended care
facility begins to develop recurrent pneumonias. A barium swallow
study is completed and reveals an obvious outpouching within the left
neck between the levels of the pharynx and the esophagus. An imaging
study is obtained and is shown in *Figure 5-1*.

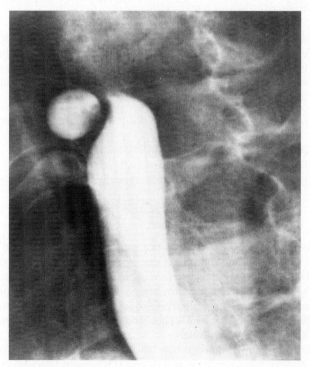

Figure 5-1

Which of the following is the most likely diagnosis?

(A) Meckel diverticulum
(B) Traction mid-esophageal diverticulum
(C) True diverticulum
(D) Zenker diverticulum

The answer is D: Zenker diverticulum. A Zenker diverticulum is an out-pouching that occurs at the junction of the pharynx and esophagus, usually seen in the elderly, and typically first noticed secondary to dysphagia. The imaging study shows that the diverticulum is in the proximal esophagus. Though aspiration resulting in pneumonia is infrequent, it can occur. It is easily diagnosed with a barium study. Given the weakness of the diverticulum, endoscopic approaches are avoided.

(A) A Meckel diverticulum (also a true diverticulum) typically presents in childhood or presents as a bowel obstruction in adults. (B) Mid-esophageal traction diverticulum is a true diverticulum that can be asymptomatic or present with dysphagia that has a different location than that described. (C) A Zenker diverticulum is a pulsion (or false) diverticulum and therefore not a true diverticulum (as is mid-esophageal diverticulum).

2 A 42-year-old man with longstanding alcoholism is brought to the emergency department by his family after vomiting large volumes of bright red blood. Bedside esophagoscopy reveals tearing of the mucosa near the gastroesophageal junction (GEJ). Which of the following statements regarding this condition is true?

(A) Diagnosis cannot be established without the use of computed tomography (CT) scanning
(B) Endoscopy is not only diagnostic but also therapeutic
(C) The disease is usually fatal
(D) The morbidity of this disease typically necessitates surgical intervention
(E) The presentation of this disease is an indication to screen for *Helicobacter pylori*

The answer is B: Endoscopy is not only diagnostic but also therapeutic. Mallory-Weiss syndrome is due to mucosal bleeding near the GEJ, typically due to retching and often seen in patients with alcoholism (or severe vomiting). The disease course is fairly benign. This condition can be both diagnosed and treated endoscopically. Endoscopic treatment is typically successful with balloon tamponade, sclerotherapy, banding, hemoclipping, electrocoagulation, or heater probe application.

(A) A CT scan would contribute little to this clinical picture. (C) Fatality due to Mallory-Weiss syndrome is very rare. (D) Surgical intervention, which involved ligation, is required only for rare cases that fail endoscopic management.

(E) *H. pylori* is not involved in the pathogenesis of this condition, as it is caused by an increased pressure gradient across the GEJ due to increased intraabdominal pressure.

3 A 50-year-old man presents to the emergency department following the sudden onset of constant back and abdominal pain following prolonged vomiting over the past few days. He denies hematemesis. Physical examination of the oral cavity is unremarkable, but palpation of the chest reveals crepitus, and auscultation reveals crunching sounds with individual respirations. Which of the following is the best first step in diagnosis?

(A) CT scan
(B) CT scan with intravenous contrast
(C) Esophagoscopy
(D) Oral contrast study with barium
(E) Oral contrast study with Gastrografin

The answer is E: Oral contrast study with Gastrografin. The physical examination findings described in this clinical vignette, specifically subcutaneous emphysema and palpable air in the mediastinum (so-called Hamman crunch), are classic for Boerhaave syndrome. Note the similar history to the Mallory-Weiss syndrome described above. In contrast to Mallory-Weiss syndrome, Boerhaave syndrome typically involved full-thickness tears of the esophagus whose bleeding resolves spontaneously. While the most common cause of Boerhaave syndrome is iatrogenic secondary to upper endoscopy, it can occur due to similar causes of Mallory-Weiss syndrome (trauma, heaving, retching, etc.). The gold standard for diagnosis of Boerhaave syndrome is an oral contrast study with water-soluble contrast (e.g., Gastrografin).

(A) While CT can be effective in diagnosing esophageal rupture, the low cost and high sensitivity of a water-soluble contrast study make CT a less ideal choice of study. (B) Not only would CT be less ideal for reasons stated above, but also the use of contrast would contribute little to this scenario. (C) Upper endoscopy can be effective in determining the extent of damage, but air introduced into the esophagus can worsen the patient's condition. (D) Barium should be avoided due to complications involving extravasation into the mediastinum.

4 A 22-year-old woman is brought by rescue squad to the emergency department following a failed suicide attempt. You are told on arrival that she consumed a copious amount of an unidentified household cleaner and was found covered with vomitus. She is febrile with otherwise normal vitals, writhing in pain on her stretcher, and unable to provide any information. Oral examination reveals erythema and hypersalivation. Which of the following is the most crucial step in treatment of this patient?

(A) Administration of an emetic
(B) Encouragement of oral hydration
(C) Esophagoscopy
(D) Surgical intervention with resection of involved esophageal portions

The answer is C: Esophagoscopy. Esophagoscopy should be performed first to examine the entire lining of the esophagus and assess the damage done by the offending agent. Assessment of damage can help to determine the treatment plan as well.

(A) Antiemetics should also be avoided as vomiting can "twice-expose" the esophageal lining and increase the likelihood for perforation of a weakened mucosal lining. (B) Oral hydration can be dangerous in this situation, where the substance is not identified, and water could cause further damage if proper neutralizing agents (for acidic or alkaline agents) are not given. (D) Surgical resection of damaged esophagus may be indicated for stenosis or fistulae, but only after thorough examination and diagnosis via esophagoscopy.

5 An 86-year-old woman post mastectomy returns to your clinic for scheduled follow-up. On review of systems, you learn that she has had an unintentional weight loss of 15 pounds and has developed acute onset of dysphagia with occasional regurgitation. Further questioning reveals that her dysphagia occurs with both solids and liquids, and that her dysphagic pain is relieved with nitroglycerin that was given to her by her cardiologist. Her pain is not related to physical exertion. Physical findings, including a thorough cardiovascular examination, are normal. An upper GI series is obtained and a representative image is shown in *Figure 5-2*:
Which of the following is the most likely diagnosis?

(A) Achalasia
(B) Gastroesophageal reflux disorder (GERD)
(C) Stable angina
(D) Type I hiatal hernia
(E) Zenker diverticulum

The answer is A: Achalasia. The symptoms described in this vignette are classic for those of achalasia, where an aperistaltic esophagus and unrelaxed lower esophageal sphincter lead to patient complaints. Dysphagia to solids and liquids, regurgitation, and weight loss secondary to bothersome meals are classic findings. The relief of pain by nitroglycerin is due to the drug's effect on sphincter tone (and can also be a finding in diffuse esophageal spasm). Physical examination is typically normal. The esophagogram shown reveals the infamous "bird's beak deformity."

(B) Though symptoms of GERD could be similar to those described here (dysphagia, regurgitation), this discomfort would not be relieved by

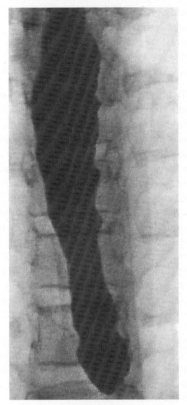

Figure 5-2

nitroglycerin and not be so acute. (C) While a cardiovascular workup is definitely indicated, this chest pain would not be diagnosed as "stable" angina given it lacks relation to physical exertion. (D) Most type I hiatal hernias are asymptomatic unless they lead to GERD symptomatology. (E) Finally, Zenker diverticula are typically asymptomatic unless progressive where they are associated with dysphagia that is localized cervically.

A 27-year-old man presents to your clinic with postprandial retrosternal burning and nausea. His symptoms occur nightly, are worse after large meals, and commonly occur when he lies recumbent following dinner. He has never sought treatment for this apparently new problem. He has a benign past medical and surgical history. His family history is noncontributory. He consumes two to three cups of coffee per day and drinks an occasional beer (one to two per week) with dinner. Which of the following is the best means to establish this patient's diagnosis?

(A) Electrocardiogram
(B) Esophagogastroduodenoscopy (EGD)
(C) Oral contrast study with barium
(D) Trial of therapy with sublingual nitroglycerin
(E) Twenty-four-hour pH monitoring of the esophagus

The answer is E: Twenty-four-hour pH monitoring of the esophagus.
The young gentleman in this question is presenting with the classic symptoms of GERD, and the diagnosis is fairly straightforward. The question redirects, however, to ask means of diagnosis (a redirect commonly used on USMLE examinations). The gold standard for diagnosing GERD is a 24-hour esophageal pH monitor, where a pH less than 4.0 for 1.3% of the day (proximal esophagus) or 4.2% of the day (distal esophagus) is sufficient for a diagnosis.

(A) An electrocardiogram (EKG) would be useful to diagnose angina when it is present (or at least induced with an exercise or pharmacologic stress test). (B) An EGD would be useful for GERD refractory to treatment, or as a means to assess longstanding GERD complications (i.e., Barrett esophagus). (C) A barium swallow study would be useful in cases of GERD attributable to another cause (e.g., hiatal hernia). (D) Finally, while a therapeutic trial is useful for GERD in the primary care setting (and typically the USMLE answer of choice given the cost-effectiveness), an inappropriate medication is listed in this answer.

  The patient in the previous question stem returns to your clinic following the outpatient diagnostics you arranged. Which of the following is the ideal management of this patient assuming that your suspected diagnosis is confirmed?

(A) Endoscopic dilatation and/or stenting
(B) Nissen total fundoplication
(C) Pharmacologic therapy with ranitidine
(D) Pharmacologic therapy with omeprazole
(E) Watchful waiting

The answer is D: Pharmacologic therapy with omeprazole. We are told that the patient from the previous question returns with a positive diagnosis for presumptive GERD, and we are asked the ideal treatment for this disease. In addition to conservative measures (avoidance of caffeine, alcohol and smoking, elevating the head of the bed, etc.), medications are the mainstay of treatment. While H_2-receptor blockers (e.g., ranitidine) are effective for occasional GERD symptoms, we are told that this patient experiences nightly symptoms.

(A) Endoscopic dilatation would be appropriate if other pathology was reported (achalasia, advanced cancer with compromised function, Schatzki ring, etc.) but there is no indication for this invasive procedure. (B) A Nissen fundoplication is very effective in correcting and reversing pathology involved with symptomatic hiatal hernias, but again, nothing indicates the presence of such pathology. (C) Proton pump inhibitors (PPIs, e.g., omeprazole) are recommended for daily symptoms and have become the first-line drug for patients with GERD. (E) Finally, watchful waiting is not appropriate given a confirmed diagnosis of GERD, as complications include Barrett esophagus, a disease state that predisposes to esophageal cancer (specifically esophageal adenocarcinoma).

---

 8 A 61-year-old Caucasian man has decided to transfer the care of his esophageal cancer to your facility. Records indicate that this patient was diagnosed with esophageal adenocarcinoma based on numerous biopsies collected during EGD 3 weeks prior. He indicates to you that he has an extensive GERD history that he self-treated with occasional, over-the-counter antacids for years. An extensive physical examination reveals lymphadenopathy in his right supraclavicular region. Three nodes measure greater than 2 cm. They are fixed, matted, and hard upon palpation. Which is the most accurate stage of this man's disease based on the tumor, nodes and metastasis (TNM) (AJCC) classification system?

(A) Stage I
(B) Stage II
(C) Stage III
(D) Stage IV
(E) Stage V

The answer is D: Stage IV. This is the classic patient for an esophageal cancer (a Caucasian man in his sixth to seventh decade). He also indicates the classic history for esophageal adenocarcinoma, that is, longstanding, poorly treated GERD. Based on AJCC's TNM staging system, metastatic esophageal cancer in general (adenocarcinoma or squamous cell carcinoma) is noted by the presence of distant organ or nodal involvement (M1b) or nodal involvement of the celiac of supraclavicular lymph nodes (M1a). Typically, metastatic disease (M1 or greater) is classified at stage IV disease, which this gentleman unfortunately has. Note that right-sided supraclavicular lymphadenopathy is more associated with esophageal cancers. This patient will likely proceed to palliative chemotherapy, radiation, or combination therapy.

(A) Stage I esophageal cancer lacks nodal involvement and is reserved for T1 disease. (B) Stage II includes T3 disease without nodal disease, or T2 disease with nodes. (C) Stage III is diagnosed in the presence of T4 disease (cancer beyond the adventitia into adjacent structures) or for T3 disease (into the adventitia only) with nodal involvement. (E) There is no stage V based on the AJCC classification system.

9 A 47-year-old woman returns to your office following upper endoscopy secondary to longstanding, refractory GERD. A review of the operative report indicates that red, velvety patches of esophageal mucosa were noted at the level of the GEJ. Multiple biopsies were taken. Review of the corresponding pathology report indicates the presence of Barrett esophagus. You communicate to the patient her increased risk for esophageal malignancy and the need for continued medical, possible surgical, therapy. Which of the following statements most accurately describes the pathological findings in Barrett esophagus?

(A) Abnormal squamous maturation with numerous intraepithelial eosinophils

(B) Invasion of dysplastic glandular cells into the lamina propria

(C) Metaplasia from a columnar epithelium to a squamous epithelium

(D) Metaplasia from a squamous epithelium to a columnar epithelium

(E) Multinucleated giant endothelial cells with cystoplasmic inclusion bodies

The answer is D: Metaplasia from a squamous epithelium to a columnar epithelium. This patient undergoes appropriate endoscopic evaluation for her longstanding refractory GERD symptoms. Endoscopic evaluation reveals the classic gross description of Barrett esophagus (red, velvety changes near the GEJ) and pathology indicates as such. Barrett esophagus describes metaplasia (cell morphology change) from the native squamous epithelium of the distal esophagus to a columnar lining similar to that of gastric mucosa. Recall that Barrett esophagus predisposes to esophageal adenocarcinoma (not squamous cell carcinoma).

(A) The presence of eosinophilic infiltrates does not describe Barrett esophagus but indicates eosinophilic esophagitis, which can be present with GERD. (B) Note that an invasion of dysplastic cells into the lamina propria is by definition invasive disease (i.e., cancer) and not a predisposing lesion such as Barrett esophagus. (C) The change of Barrett esophagus occurs with squamous to columnar metaplasia, not columnar to squamous metaplasia. (E) Finally, multinucleated cells with cellular inclusions are classic for HSV or CMV infection; in this case, viral esophagitis in a likely immunocompromised patient.

10 A 39-year-old man is being followed up by you and your surgical colleagues for longstanding GERD and a suspected hiatal hernia. His symptoms include dysphagia and postprandial fullness. He has been taking omeprazole for 6 months without alleviation of symptoms. No endoscopic diagnostics have been attempted. Results from his video barium esophagram reveal a stable GEJ with herniation of the stomach beyond the diaphragm. Which of the following is the most likely current working diagnosis?

(A) Type I (sliding) hiatal hernia
(B) Type II (paraesophageal) hiatal hernia
(C) Type III (mixed) hiatal hernia
(D) Type IV (mixed with other organ involvement) hiatal hernia

The answer is B: **Type II (paraesophageal) hiatal hernia.** This patient undergoes a barium esophagram study for a suspected hiatal hernia causing his GERD symptoms. The description of a nonmobile GEJ with herniation of the stomach into the thorax is the classic description of a paraesophageal hernia (or a type II hiatal hernia). Though paraesophageal hernias are rare, surgical correction is needed to avoid herniation and strangulation.

(A) Note that type I hiatal hernias are typically asymptomatic. (C) By definition, the GEJ is mobile in type III hiatal hernias. (D) In type IV (mixed) hiatal hernia, the GEJ is also mobile.

 11 A 56-year-old woman with longstanding history of alcohol-induced end-stage liver disease (ESLD) presents to the emergency department with diffuse hematemesis. On admission, her systolic blood pressure is 85 with an undetected diastolic. On examination, she has altered mental status, an extensive amount of blood covering her clothing, and dried blood over her oral mucosa. She appears jaundiced and cachectic. A report from the emergency department physicians indicates that she has vomited 750 cc of bright red blood since her arrival 30 minutes prior. Which of the following is the most appropriate next step in management?

(A) A trial of medical management with continuous intravenous octreotide
(B) Emergent surgery with creation of a portocaval shunt
(C) Endoscopic balloon tamponade
(D) Endoscopic band ligation of varices
(E) Transjugular intrahepatic portosystemic shunting (TIPS)

The answer is D: **Endoscopic band ligation of varices.** Here we have a classic history for an esophageal variceal bleed: a patient with alcohol-induced cirrhosis who presents with hematemesis. Because mortality can be as high as 50% in initial variceal bleeds, and this woman is already exhibiting hypotension secondary to acute blood loss, this is an emergent situation. First-line therapy in actively bleeding esophageal varices is endoscopic hemorrhage control with band ligation or sclerotherapy given that effectiveness approaches 80%.

(A) While octreotide and other somatostatin analogues are effective pharmacologic agents, their efficacy is most evident when used in conjunction with endoscopic management; therefore, medical treatment alone is inappropriate. (B) Surgical creation of shunts that decrease portal venous hypertension (e.g., portocaval) has mostly been replaced by the less invasive TIPS procedure. (C) Endoscopic balloon tamponade is far from first-line therapy, and is recommended when endoscopic, pharmacologic, and transjugular therapies are not available. (E) Finally, while TIPS is effective, it is best suited for patients that continue to hemorrhage following attempted endoscopic ligation with octreotide.

12 A 39-year-old woman presents to her primary care physician for heart burn. She has a medical history of rheumatoid arthritis and systemic lupus erythematosus (SLE), both of which are currently being treated by her rheumatologist. She reports to you that she is ANA positive. Prior to conducting your physical examination, which of the following findings would you expect to find in this patient?

(A) Absence of ganglion cells on rectal biopsy
(B) Bird's beak narrowing on esophagram
(C) Positive antimitochondrial antibodies
(D) Sclerodactyly

The answer is D: Sclerodactyly. Patients with a history of autoimmune disease (e.g., rheumatoid arthritis, lupus) verified with positive serology (antinuclear antibody (ANA) titers) with esophageal symptoms suggestive of a dysmotility disorder should be evaluated for CREST syndrome (calcinosis cutis, Raynaud phenomenon, esophageal dysmotility, sclerodactyly, telangiectasia). CREST syndrome, or scleroderma in general, causes fibrotic changes of the esophageal sphincter and leads to aperistalsis with resultant esophageal symptoms. Sclerodactyly is classically found in both disease states.

(A) Absence of ganglionic cells in the rectum is pathognomonic for Hirschsprung disease, a GI malformation commonly diagnosed in children. (B) A bird's beak narrowing on barium esophagram is the classic finding for achalasia, which is possible but less likely given the medical history. (C) Finally, positive testing of antimitochondrial antibodies describes the serology associated with primary biliary cirrhosis which produces no esophageal symptoms.

13 Your surgery service is consulted to 51-year-old woman in the emergency department who is a long-term patient at a psychiatric institution. She recently began complaining of the inability to tolerate oral intake, and projectile vomiting associated with meals. CT of the abdomen obtained in the emergency departments reveals immense distention of the stomach, which is full of contents including hair. Which of the following is the most appropriate intervention to be executed by the surgical team?

(A) Gastrectomy
(B) Splenectomy
(C) Endoscopic therapy
(D) Vagotomy and pyloroplasty
(E) Proton pump inhibitors and two antibiotic therapies for 3 weeks

The answer is C: Endoscopic therapy. A bezoar is an accumulation of undigested gastric material; those that contain hair are referred to as "tricho-bezoars." Patients subject to trichobezoars include the pediatric population and residents of psychiatric institutions. Large bezoars can present with signs and symptoms of gastric outlet obstruction (as seen in this clinical vignette). Most bezoars can be roughly debrided with the use of an endoscope; however, some must be decompacted surgically.

(A) Gastrectomy is a drastic management option regardless of the cause, and is the least likely correct answer here. (B) Splenectomy is completed unrelated to the pathophysiology, and we have no reason to believe that the spleen is pathologic (i.e., trauma, hypotension, meningeal sepsis) (D) Vagotomy and pyloroplasty are reserved for intractable cases of peptic ulcer disease (PUD). (E) The use of a PPI and antibiotics would be the therapy of choice for PUD associated with *H. pylori* infection, which is not described in this patient.

 14 A 63-year-old woman presents with dull, aching epigastric discomfort associated with nausea that occurs following meals for the past 11 months. She has noted alleviation with over-the-counter calcium carbonate. Her past medical history is significant for endometriosis and two cesarean sections, most recently 28 years prior. Vitals and physical examination are normal other than vague epigastric tenderness. Her stool guaiac test is positive. Her colonoscopies, up to date, have all been normal. Which of the following is the most appropriate next step in management?

(A) Acquisition of serum gastrin levels
(B) Drawing of serology for anti-*H. pylori* antibodies
(C) Diagnostic laparoscopy
(D) Medical management with omeprazole
(E) Esophagogastroduodenoscopy

The answer is E: Esophagogastroduodenoscopy. The gold standard in diagnosis of peptic ulcer disease (PUD), which is fairly straightforward given this patient's history and physical examination, is upper endoscopy. Upper endoscopy helps to differentiate stomach cancer and PUD, which prevent with similar symptoms along with gastrointestinal bleeding. Endoscopy allows biopsying of active ulcers to rule out malignancy and determine the involvement of *H. pylori* (commonly causative of PUD) with the Campylobacter-like organism CLO test. The hallmark of PUD management, therefore, is upper endoscopy.

(A) Assessing serum gastrin levels can be diagnostic of Zollinger-Ellison (ZE) syndrome, which typically presents as refractory PUD with severe, non-healing ulcers. (B) Assessing serology for *H. pylori* infection is an effective means to determine need for triple therapy, but since endoscopy should be performed, these data will be collected elsewhere. (C) Diagnostic laparoscopy would determine the extent of this patient's endometriosis, which is a distracter here given that her disease is clearly gastrointestinal-related. (D) While medical management with omeprazole is likely to follow formal diagnosis, upper endoscopy should first rule out a more serious disease (e.g., gastric adenocarcinoma) before treating presumptive PUD.

---

15) The patient in the previous question follows the management plan you selected. Results following this management plan confirm your suspected diagnosis, along with infection of *H. pylori*, the suspected causative agent. Which of the following is the most appropriate current treatment for this patient?

(A) Amoxicillin, clarithromycin, and omeprazole for 10 to 14 days
(B) Amoxicillin, clarithromycin, and omeprazole for 30 days
(C) Metronidazole, clarithromycin, and omeprazole for 30 days
(D) Metronidazole, tetracycline, and omeprazole with bismuth for 10 to 14 days
(E) Metronidazole, tetracycline, and omeprazole with bismuth for 30 days

The answer is A: Amoxicillin, clarithromycin, and omeprazole for 10 to 14 days. This question asks for the recommended therapy for eradication of *H. pylori*. This patient with diagnosed peptic ulcer disease (PUD) is confirmed to have *H. pylori* infection, a very common occurrence, and should therefore proceed to triple therapy of a PPI and two antibiotics (commonly amoxicillin and clarithromycin). Note that all of the answer choices are viable treatment options, but are not first line.

(B) The typical recommended duration of the medication is 10 to 14 days, but not as long as 30 days, which would be excessive. (C) Replacing amoxicillin with metronidazole is done for patients with a penicillin allergy, but we are not told this allergy exists. (D) Quadruple therapy with bismuth, a PPI, metronidazole, and tetracycline is reserved for *H. pylori* strains resistant to the first-line triple therapy. (E) Quadruple therapy is also effective if given for 10 to 14 days, and 30 days of treatment is unnecessary.

---

16) A 45-year-old gentleman with past medical history of GERD, PUD, hypertension, and obesity presents to your clinic for outpatient follow-up. He recently underwent therapy for eradication of documented *H. pylori* infection and has continued to take omeprazole daily as discussed with his physician previously. His home stool guaiac tests over

the past year have been negative. Which of the following patient symptoms helps to differentiate between gastric and duodenal ulcers in PUD?

(A) Alleviation of symptoms with dietary modifications
(B) Elimination of ulcerative lesions following *H. pylori* eradication
(C) Relationship between the severity of pain and the consumption of food
(D) Results from radiologic tests

The answer is C: Relationship between the severity of pain and the consumption of food. The classic subjective information that distinguishes duodenal and gastric ulcers (for board examinations, at least) is whether the patient's epigastric pain is alleviated with food (duodenal ulcers) or exacerbated by food (gastric ulcers). Note that none of the information provided about this patient is necessary to answer the question.

(A) Dietary modifications are not considered to be effective in PUD as they are in GERD. (B) While elimination of *H. pylori* can be more successful in treating duodenal ulcers (where *H. pylori* is more commonly attributable), eradication can effectively treat both, making this a less ideal answer. (D) Radiologic testing would contribute very little to the diagnosis of PUD, although radionuclide scans may eventually help to determine the source of a gastrointestinal bleed.

---

 17 An 87-year-old Japanese woman with a history of gastric adenocarcinoma status post partial gastrectomy presents with increasing fatigue. On examination, vitals are stable and notable for a heart rate of 117 beats/min. She has notable pallor compared to previous visits and her mucosa is strikingly pale throughout. Which of the following statements would accurately describe the results of the Schilling test in this patient?

(A) Administration of oral radiolabeled B_{12} with intramuscular B_{12} results in urine excretion of 30%
(B) Administration of radiolabeled vitamin B_{12} with intrinsic factor (IF) results in urine excretion of 30%
(C) Administration of radiolabeled vitamin B_{12} following 10 days of antibiotic therapy results in urine excretion of 30%
(D) Administration of radiolabeled vitamin B_{12} with 5 days of oral pancreatic enzymes results in urine excretion of 30%

The answer is B: Administration of radiolabeled vitamin B_{12} with intrinsic factor (IF) results in urine excretion of 30%. Undiagnosed anemia in a patient status postgastrectomy is classic for pernicious anemia, a megaloblastic anemia caused by deficiency of IF. IF is a cofactor necessary for B_{12} absorption that is normally produced by the parietal cells of the stomach.

The Schilling test is the classically tested diagnostic measure in pernicious anemia management. Administration of radiolabeled vitamin B_{12} along with an intramuscular administration normally results in urinary excretion between 10% and 40% (indicating sufficient oral absorption, as in choice A). However, in patients with pernicious anemia, urinary excretion is usually less than 10%, indicating poor absorption of the oral dose (presumably due to IF absence). Administration of B_{12} with IF corrects excretion to a normal range in patients with pernicious anemia, making choice B the correct answer.

(A) Again, this would be a normal result, since urine excretion between 10% and 40% indicates sufficient absorption from the intestine. (C) Those patients who restore normal B_{12} excretion following antibiotic treatment are diagnosed with bacterial overgrowth syndromes. (D) Patients who respond to pancreatic enzyme administration suffer from chronic pancreatitis and/or pancreatic insufficiency.

---

18 A 59-year-old Japanese American man is referred to your cancer care facility from a community hospital where he was suspected to have undiagnosed stomach cancer per subjective patient information. While he claims that his records were sent, the staff is apparently unable to locate the records in the office today. Which of the following is the best initial means to assess for advanced disease?

(A) Integrated PET/CT imaging
(B) MRI
(C) Staging laparoscopy
(D) Thorough history and physical examination

The answer is D: Thorough history and physical examination. Always attempt to answer USMLE-style questions with answers that are cost-effective as well as standard of care (versus expensive diagnostic measures and imaging). A thorough history and physical examination should be completed on all patients prior to formal diagnostics. This question should remind you that uncommon physical examination findings of patients with gastric adenocarcinoma are frequently tested, specifically lymphatic invasion (Sister Mary Joseph node, Virchow nodes, Krukenberg tumors, and the Blumer shelf).

(A) The integration of PET/CT is useful in determining the presence of metastatic disease as well as monitoring patients for recurrence or progression. (B) The use of MRI would have similar roles to the PET/CT integrated imaging, and would definitely not take place prior to a history and physical examination. (C) Similarly, staging laparoscopy is more useful in assessing more advanced stages of gastric adenocarcinoma (assessing local lymph nodes, the liver margin, etc.), but only after a thorough history and physical examination.

19 The patient in question 18 undergoes your initial assessment, and your findings suggest advanced-stage gastric adenocarcinoma. Which of the following is the best means of formally confirming the diagnosis?

(A) Abdominopelvic CT scan
(B) Oral barium study
(C) Serum tumor marker studies
(D) Upper endoscopy

The answer is D: Upper endoscopy. Following a thorough history and physical examination, gastric adenocarcinoma is best diagnosed by upper endoscopy with biopsy, considered the gold standard for diagnosis. CT scans for gastric adenocarcinoma are typically used for preoperative evaluation following diagnosis.

(A) The poor assessment of primary tumor invasion by CT makes it a poor initial diagnostic measure. (B) While barium studies can indicate filling defects along with infiltrating lesions of the gastric mucosa, it appears that endoscopy offers greater rates of sensitivity and specificity, and is therefore preferred. (C) Serum tumor markers for gastric adenocarcinoma include CEA and CA-125. Based on a lack of evidence, neither carcinogenic embryonic antigen (CEA) nor CA-125 has been shown to have sufficient diagnostic value (nor staging value for that matter) to affect clinical decision making.

20 A 25-year-old man who has recently undergone upper endoscopy for chronic dyspepsia and diarrhea was diagnosed with duodenal ulcer disease. Biopsies revealed no malignant involvement, and his Campylobacter-like organism (CLO) test was negative. One year following avoidance of nonsteroidal antiinflammatory agent (NSAID) and treatment with a PPI, his symptoms are unchanged. Which of the following results would confirm a suspected diagnosis of ZE syndrome?

(A) A marked increased in serum gastrin following administration of secretin
(B) Fasting serum gastrin levels greater than 1,000 pg/mL
(C) Gastric acid secretion measurements corresponding to the disease
(D) Nonfasting serum gastrin levels greater than 1,000 pg/mL

The answer is B: Fasting serum gastrin levels greater than 1,000 pg/mL. ZE (Zollinger-Ellison) syndrome is a condition whereby an underlying gastrinoma in the pancreas or small intestine contributes to gastric acid hypersecretion with complications including refractory PUD. Workup for multiple endocrine neoplastic (MEN) syndromes, specially MEN I, is required. Diagnosis of ZE syndrome occurs when fasting serum gastrin levels are found to be greater than 1,000 pg/mL.

(A) The secretin stimulation test is useful for patients with indeterminate results of serum gastrin levels (where an increase in serum gastrin following secretin is diagnostic of ZE syndrome). (C) The use of gastric acid secretion measurements is largely outdated in the diagnosis of ZE syndrome. (D) Finally, fasting (not nonfasting) gastrin levels are preferred for collection on three separate occasions, given the high variability of gastrin concentrations throughout the day.

---

 21 A 61-year-old African American woman has a history of refractory GERD. Her symptoms include dysphagia, heartburn, and nausea and have been consistent for 4 years. She has tried a numerous over-the-counter and prescription medications without relief. She reports a pertinent family history of gastric adenocarcinoma. Upper GI endoscopy reveals several polypoid lesions throughout the gastric mucosa. Pathology reveals hyperplastic polyps. Which of the following statements is true regarding this condition?

(A) Rates of concurrent adenocarcinoma are as high as 20%
(B) They are commonly associated with familial polyposis syndromes
(C) They are associated with a large artery that erodes the mucosa and causes massive hematemesis and hypovolemia
(D) Nitrate consumption is a risk factor for their development
(E) Resolution occurs with successful eradication of *H. pylori*

The answer is E: Resolution occurs with successful eradication of *H. pylori*. Hyperplastic polyps are a benign tumor of the stomach that commonly arise secondary to chronic atrophic gastritis. They are small (<2 cm), rarely undergo malignant transformation (1% to 3%), and respond with eradication of *H. pylori*. The incorrect answers in this question refer to other pathologies involving the stomach.

(A) Rates of adenocarcinoma as high as 20% are found in adenomatous polyps. (B) Stomach polyps commonly found in familial polyposis syndromes describe fundic gland polyps, a pathology that lacks malignant potential altogether. (C) An artery eroding through the gastric mucosa and contributing to a potentially dangerous bleed describes a Dieulafoy lesion. (D) And, finally, nitrate consumption (a substance found in smoked meats common to the Japanese diet) is a risk factor for the development of malignant adenocarcinoma.

---

 22 A 59-year-old man with a history of hypertension, obstructive sleep apnea, and type II diabetes mellitus presents with chronic complaints of reflux, belching, and excessive salivation with meals. His current medications include metformin, hydrochlorothiazide, and a multivitamin. He underwent laparoscopic cholecystectomy at age 48 years. He has no smoking history and drinks four to five beers on weekends. Which pharmacologic action is the mechanism of action for the most appropriate therapy for this patient?

(A) Decreased production of prostaglandins via inhibition of COX-1 and COX-2 enzymes

(B) Formation of a viscous gel along the gastric lining for protection against ulceration

(C) Histaminergic antagonist that decreases volume and concentration of gastric acid

(D) Irreversible blocking of the H^+/K^+-ATPase exchange pump at the gastric parietal cell

(E) Synthetic prostaglandin analogue that decreases acid secretion and increases bicarbonate secretion

The answer is D: Irreversible blocking of the H^+/K^+-ATPase exchange pump at the gastric parietal cell. This patient appears to have a fairly straightforward case of GERD, and we are told in the question that he is proceeding to medical management. While many drugs are useful for GERD, PPIs have become the first-line drug for patients with GERD based on efficacy. This question asks, therefore, for the mechanism of action of PPIs, with distracters being his medication list and past medical history. PPIs work by binding irreversibly to the H^+-K^+-ATPase exchange and reduce gastric acid secretion. Their efficacy is largely based on the fact that they act on the terminal source of acid secretion in the stomach (as opposed to H_2 antagonists, for example, which exert their mechanism upstream of hydrogen ion pumps).

(A) Decreased production of prostaglandins via inhibition of COX-1 and COX-2 enzymes describes nonsteroidal antiinflammatory agents (NSAIDs) causal link to gastritis, which is an adverse effect, and not a therapeutic mechanism. (B) Formation of a viscous gel along the gastric lining for protection against ulceration is the mechanism of action of sucralfate (a cytoprotective GERD drug). (C) A histaminergic antagonist that decreases gastric acid secretion would describe any H_2-receptor blockers.(E) Finally, a synthetic prostaglandin analogue that decreases acid secretion and increases bicarbonate secretion would be misoprostol (a prostaglandin E_1 (PGE_1) analogue).

---

23 A 48-year-old man presents to his primary care physician for his annual follow-up. He has a past medical history of gastroesophageal reflux, hypertension, and hypercholesterolemia. He underwent a right inguinal hernia repair 14 years prior. Review of systems reveals the onset of dark tarry stools 6 months prior. His most recent laboratory results reveal a hemoglobin level of 9.7 g/dL. His stool guaiac test is positive. What is the most likely explanation for these findings?

(A) Gastric adenocarcinoma
(B) GERD
(C) Epistaxis
(D) Low-dose daily aspirin
(E) Peptic ulcer disease

The answer is E: Peptic ulcer disease. The most common cause of an upper GI bleed regardless of age is PUD, which is causative as often as 40% of cases. This patient's previous diagnosis of GERD could simply be a misdiagnosis, which would explain the progression of his PUD to melena as well as anemia. His situation deserves a workup with upper endoscopy with biopsy, and likely, triple therapy.

(A) Gastric adenocarcinoma is undoubtedly included on this patient's differential, albeit at much lower rates compared to PUD. (B) While GERD is not a typical cause of an upper GI bleed, progression of GERD to Barrett esophagus may cause subtle blood loss via the GI tract. (C) Epistaxis is not a common cause of GI bleeds as this adult patient presents; however, it can be a source of massive, acute, intractable hemorrhages in patients with severe cirrhosis. (D) While low-dose daily aspirin as secondary prevention for cardiovascular disease is not a common cause of GI bleeding, it does have noteworthy risk in terms of GI bleeds, particularly in repeat GI bleeds and its risk, therefore, should be assessed per patient circumstances.

---

 24 A 65-year-old woman undergoes upper endoscopy secondary to chronic dyspepsia, epigastric pain, weight loss, and melena. Endoscopic exploration reveals multiple small ulcerative erosions, one larger than the remainder. Biopsies are undertaken and reveal chronic gastritis and the presence of *H. pylori*. The largest lesion appears as a "dense infiltrate of lymphocytes in the lamina propria with reactive B-cell follicles," and immunohistochemical staining is positive for CD19 and CD20. What is the most appropriate management for this patient?

(A) PET scan to determine extent of disease
(B) Radiation therapy
(C) Repeat endoscopic biopsy based on improper collection site
(D) Surgical resection of underlying malignancy
(E) Treatment of underlying infectious process

The answer is E: Treatment of underlying infectious process. The pathology describes a gastric MALToma (mucosa-associated lymphoid tissue), the most common extranodal lymphoma. Gastric MALTomas may transform into widespread malignant disease, but their pathophysiology is strongly related to chronic gastritis as well as *H. pylori* infection. Surprisingly, eradication of *H. pylori* successfully treats most patients and exhibits low rates of recurrence. Eradication of this infectious process, therefore, is the first-line form of treatment given that the disease only involves the lamina propria.

(A) A PET scan would be effective if metastatic disease was present (i.e., examination or biopsy suggested lymphomatous spread outside of the stomach). (B) Radiation therapy is effective for MALTomas and is an option for early-stage disease, but it is typically reserved for *H. pylori*-negative gastric

MALTomas. (C) While MALTomas can resemble the Peyer patches of the small intestine, we can be fairly certain given this patient's history and symptoms that this biopsy was obtained from the correct area. (D) Finally, surgical resection is rarely advised for gastric MALToma given the success of *H. pylori* treatment and radiation; furthermore, advanced disease proceeds to immuno- or chemotherapy, not surgery.

---

 25 A 35-year-old male bariatric patient who underwent Roux-en-Y gastric bypass 9-weeks prior presents for follow-up. Now he complains of sweating, lightheadedness, and chills after each meal. He seems disturbed when he informs you that during the last occurrence, he fainted while rushing to the bathroom to vomit. What is the most likely explanation for these findings?

(A) Anastomotic ulceration with subsequent leakage
(B) Conversion disorder
(C) Dumping syndrome
(D) Partial small bowel obstruction

The answer is C: **Dumping syndrome.** Dumping syndrome describes a common condition secondary to gastric bypass surgery, particularly the Roux-en-Y bypass. Symptoms are similar to those described here. Dumping syndrome is thought to be caused by rapid dumping of food into the Roux-en-Y limb with rapid distention of the small intestine with hyperosmolar food content that rapidly bypasses the stomach. It commonly occurs during this postoperative time period (10 weeks). Foods that provoke symptoms (sugar-laden foods) can be avoided for initial conservative measures, or antimotility drugs that slow the passage of food through the stomach can be used.

(A) Anastomotic ulceration is a rare complication of Roux-en-Y gastric bypass, but patients develop the complication quickly (within days) with signs of peritonitis and/or sepsis. (B) Conversion disorder as an answer choice entertains the idea that undergoing gastric bypass surgery is a major physiologic and psychiatric adjustment for the patient. Depression, not conversion disorder, can be a serious nonsurgical patient issue. (D) A bowel obstruction due to iatrogenic causes (postoperative adhesions) would be expected to occur much later than dumping syndrome; additionally, the presentation would be similar to any bowel obstruction (and thus different from this patient's symptoms).

Small Bowel

1. A 45-year-old man with a recent history of bowel surgery presents with abdominal pain, nausea, vomiting, and failure to have a bowel movement for the last several days. He describes the pain as intermittent. He had diarrhea at first but is now complaining of constipation. He is afebrile. His pulse is 95 beats/min and respirations 17 breaths/min. His laboratory studies show a mild elevation in leukocytes with a left shift and an elevated blood urea nitrogen. The remainder of his laboratory results are unremarkable. Plain radiography is shown in *Figure 6-1*.

   Which of the following is the next best step in management?

   (A) Abdominal CT scan
   (B) Intravenous hydration, nasogastric suction, and antibiotics
   (C) Immediate laparoscopy
   (D) Morphine sulfate
   (E) Promethazine

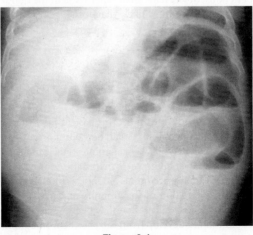

Figure 6-1

The answer is B: Intravenous hydration, nasogastric suction, and antibiotics. This patient is most likely suffering from a small bowel obstruction. Initial management should always include aggressive fluid resuscitation, bowel decompression, antibiotics (with coverage of gram-negative and anaerobic organisms), analegesics, and antiemetics. KUB reveals multiple dilated loops of small bowel with air–fluid levels. A nonoperative trial is indicated in all cases of suspected partial or simple small bowel obstruction. If complete small bowel obstruction is present or evidence of strangulation, surgical care with laparoscopy is indicated.

(A) Although abdominal CT scans are useful with the diagnosis of strangulated obstructions and working out the etiology of small bowel obstruction, this patient already has sufficient evidence for diagnosis and a clear etiology (recent surgery). An abdominal CT scan would be costly and unnecessary at this point. (C) Immediate laparoscopy would be required if there was evidence of strangulation or complete obstruction. (D) Morphine sulfate would be indicated to assist with pain. However, intravenous hydration is always the first step. (E) Promethazine is useful as an antiemetic for small bowel obstruction and may be indicated. However, intravenous hydration should always be the initial step.

 A 67-year-old man presents with vague abdominal discomfort, weight loss, and intermittent nausea that has been increasing over the last 6 months. He has a history of smoking but does not drink alcohol. His temperature is 36.7°C, blood pressure 130/80 mmHg, pulse 80 beats/min, and respirations 14 breaths/min. His physical examination is unremarkable. His stool is heme positive. Laboratory studies show a hemoglobin level of 10.5 g/dL. Although colonoscopy is unremarkable, an upper endoscopy reveals an annular mass in the duodenum. Which of the following is the most likely diagnosis?

(A) Adenocarcinoma
(B) Carcinoid tumor
(C) Lymphoma
(D) Sarcoma
(E) Squamous cell carcinoma

The answer is A: Adenocarcinoma. This patient has symptoms and diagnostic tests suggestive of a neoplasm. Small bowel tumors are exceedingly rare accounting for approximately 1% of gastrointestinal carcinomas. The most common neoplasm of the small bowel is metastatic. However, the most common primary tumor is adenocarcinoma. Adenocarcinomas are most common in the duodenum in the region of the ampulla of Vater. Tumors are usually annular or polypoid. Mucosal ulceration may be present.

(B) Carcinoid tumors develop from the enterochromografin cells and are most common in the appendix. The small bowel is the second most common location and usually occurs in the distal ileum. They begin as polypoid masses and may invade through the wall of the small bowel. Symptoms may initially occur from small bowel obstruction. Some tumors may secrete serotonin and other vasoactive substances which results in malignant carcinoid syndrome with irritable syndromes, diarrhea, bronchoconstriction, and flushing. (C) Lymphomas have a variety of morphologies and account for approximately 15% of small bowel cancers. (D) Sarcomas present most commonly with acute gastrointestinal bleeding. (E) Squamous cell carcinoma is extremely rare in the small bowel with only few case reports.

 3 A 1-year-old boy presents with chronic diarrhea, failure to thrive, poor growth, and difficulty feeding. Celiac disease along with several other conditions is suggested in the initial differential diagnosis. Which of the following antibodies are associated with a diagnosis of celiac disease?

(A) Anti-dsDNA
(B) Antiendomysial and antiglaiden
(C) Antimitochondrial and antiglaiden
(D) Anti-SRP and antitransglutaminase
(E) Antitopisomerase antibodies

The answer is B: Antiendomysial and antiglaiden. Celiac disease is a multifactorial autoimmune disease that primarily affects the small intestine. It is characterized by progressive atrophy and flattening of the small intestinal mucosa. In the pediatric population, symptoms often present before age 2. Gastrointestinal symptoms are very common and usually appear between 9 months and 24 months of age (when gluten is typically introduced into the diet). Chronic diarrhea, anorexia, abdominal distention and/or pain, poor growth, failure to thrive, and severe malnutrition may occur. Diagnosis may be made using several modalities including serum antibodies to the IgA endomysium and IgA tissue transglutaminase. These antibodies are highly sensitive and specific.

(A) Anti-dsDNA antibodies are found in patients with systemic lupus erythematosus. (C) While antiglaiden antibodies are found in patients with celiac disease, antimitochondrial antibodies are associated with primary biliary cirrhosis. (D) Although antitransglutaminase antibodies are associated with celiac disease, anti-SRP antibodies are associated with inflammatory myopathies. (E) Antitopisomerase antibodies are associated with scleroderma.

 4 A 42-year-old man is brought to the emergency department after a motor vehicle accident. He has multiple major injuries and is immediately brought into the operating room. During the surgery, it is found that a distal segment of small bowel is injured and it is subsequently removed. Which of the following arteries most likely supply this segment of bowel?

(A) Celiac artery and superior mesenteric arteries
(B) Inferior mesenteric artery and superior mesenteric arteries
(C) Middle and right colic arteries
(D) Pancreaticoduodenal and superior mesenteric arteries
(E) Superior mesenteric artery and left colic artery

The answer is B: Inferior mesenteric artery and superior mesenteric arteries. The blood supply to the majority of the small bowel is through the superior mesenteric artery. The proximal small bowel is supplied by branches of the celiac artery. The very distal part of the small bowel does receive some collateral flow from the iliocolic artery, which is a branch of the inferior mesenteric artery.

(A) Although branches of the superior mesenteric artery do supply the distal small bowel, the celiac artery does not. (C) Although the right colic artery does supply some blood to the distal small bowel, the middle colic primarily supplies the transverse colon and does not supply blood to the small bowel. (D) Although the superior mesenteric artery does supply the majority of the small bowel, the pancreaticoduodenal arteries (superior and inferior) supply blood to the duodenum and pancreas. (E) Although the superior mesenteric artery does supply blood to the small bowel, the left colic artery supplies the transverse and descending colon.

5 A 12-year-old boy presents with a small bowel obstruction several years after surgery for an appendectomy. During the exploratory laparotomy, several large lymph nodes are found in the paracaval and aortic area. Several of the nodes are removed and sent for pathologic diagnosis. Histology reveals sheets of small round and homogenous lymphocytes and a "starry sky" appearance. The tumor cells stain positive for CD19 and CD20 and strongly positive for Ki67. Which of the following is the most likely reason for the patient's small bowel obstruction?

(A) Acute myeloid leukemia
(B) Burkitt lymphoma
(C) Hodgkin lymphoma
(D) Lymphoid hyperplasia
(E) Previous surgery

The answer is B: Burkitt lymphoma. This patient's history and biopsy results are consistent with a small bowel obstruction secondary to Burkitt lymphoma. The histologic description of the Burkitt lymphoma is characterized by uniform and round cells with course chromatin, a thin rim of cytoplasm, very high mitotic rate (Ki67 is virtually 100% positive), diffuse growth pattern and B-cell lineage (CD19 and 20). It is often described as a "starry sky" appearance. The small intestine is a common site of Burkitt lymphoma in children and young adults. They may present with signs of small bowel obstruction due to the mass effect of the lymph nodes. Treatment for Burkitt lymphoma involves chemotherapy, which may include rituximab (a monoclonal antibody against CD20).

(A) While there are cases of small bowel obstruction in acute myeloid leukemia, the histologic appearance of the tumor above is not consistent with this diagnosis. (C) Hodgkin lymphoma may occur in the small bowel and cause symptoms of small bowel obstruction. The histologic description above is not that of Hodgkin lymphoma. (D) Lymphoid hyperplasia may cause small bowel obstruction and can occur in a variety of conditions including in reaction to gastrointestinal infection. Histology will show reactive lymphoid tissue rather than neoplastic changes. (E) While previous surgery is a common cause of small bowel obstruction in the general population, lymphatic obstruction from mass effect in the retroperitoneum is the likely cause in this patient.

 6 A 2-year-old boy presents with intermittent abdominal pain and crying. The mother reports the child has also been having sticky red stools with mucus and occasional vomiting. The child is afebrile. On examination, the pain is diffuse and there is a palpable "sausage"-shaped mass in the lower right quadrant. Which of the following is the next best step in management?

(A) Abdominal CT scan
(B) Abdominal radiograph
(C) Appendectomy
(D) Contrast enema
(E) Laparotomy

The answer is D: Contrast enema. This child is most likely suffering from intussusception. The peak age group for intussusception is 5 to 10 months, although it may occur later in life as well. The usual presentation is a child with intermittent abdominal pain, vomiting, and stools with blood and mucus often described as "current jelly stools." The condition is a medical emergency and should be treated as soon as possible. The initial management involves a contrast enema, which is both diagnostic and may be therapeutic in most cases. If reduction with contrast fails, surgery is indicated.

(A) Although an abdominal CT scan can easily diagnose a intussusception, they are costly and involve unnecessary doses of radiation. If imaging is needed, abdominal ultrasonography is the imaging modality of choice. (B) Although abdominal radiographs are inexpensive and fast, they have poor sensitivity for intussusception. However, abdominal radiography may be useful for ruling out other causes of abdominal pain including constipation and free-peritoneal air. (C) This patient's symptoms are not consistent with appendicitis; thus, an appendectomy is not indicated. (E) If a contrast enema fails to correct the problem, laparotomy may be indicated as the next step.

 7 A 68-year-old man with a history of diabetes mellitus and coronary artery disease presents with weight loss and worsening constipation over the last 6 months. He reports that on occasions he also suffers from nausea and abdominal cramping. He has a 30-pack-year history of smoking and drinks three beers daily. His current medications include metformin, aspirin, simvastatin, nitroglycerin, and metoprolol. On examination, his abdomen is distended and tympanic. A recent colonoscopy performed several months ago was unremarkable. Which of the following is the next best step in management?

(A) Capsule endoscopy
(B) Decrease dose of aspirin
(C) Decrease dose of metformin
(D) Discontinue nitroglycerin
(E) Upper gastrointestinal series with small bowel follow-through

The answer is E: **Upper gastrointestinal series with small bowel follow-through.** This patient's worrying symptoms of weight loss and constipation along with his history of smoking are concerning for cancer or another potentially serious disease involving the bowel. This patient will need a workup for malignancy including an upper gastrointestinal series. Upper gastrointestinal series with small bowel follow-through will show abnormalities in 53% to 83% of patients and is established as a useful imaging modality in patients with suspected small bowel malignancy.

(A) While capsule endoscopy may eventually be needed if other tests fail to identify the source of this patient's symptoms, it would not be the next best step. (B) Although aspirin and other nonsteroidal antiinflammatory drugs may cause bowel discomfort, it would not explain this patient's symptoms. (C) Although gastrointestinal complaints are commonly associated with metformin, they would not explain this patient's weight loss and other complaints. (D) Other than rare nausea, nitroglycerin is not associated with gastrointestinal symptoms.

---

8 A 33-year-old man with an unremarkable medical history complains of bloating, watery diarrhea, floating stools, poor appetite, and fatigue. On examination, he appears pale. The remainder of the examination is unremarkable. Laboratory studies reveal a macrocytic anemia with normal folate levels. The patient's stool has an elevated pH and D-lactic acid levels. A breath test reveals an early rise in hydrogen after ingestion of 14C glycocholic acid. Which of the following is the most likely diagnosis?

(A) Bacterial overgrowth
(B) Celiac disease
(C) Cystic fibrosis
(D) Irritable bowel syndrome
(E) Short bowel syndrome

The answer is A: Bacterial overgrowth. This patient is most likely suffering from bacterial overgrowth syndrome. Signs and symptoms include watery diarrhea, steatorrhea, bloating, abdominal pain, diarrhea, dyspepsia, and weight loss. Other symptoms may occur as a result of vitamin deficiencies including anemia from B12 deficiency. This patient's macrocytic anemia is most likely due to vitamin B12 deficiency. The typical workup for bacterial overgrowth syndrome includes eliminating causes of diarrhea, anemia, and malabsorption. In bacterial overgrowth, the stool is often acidic. D-lactic acidosis may occur and can be measured to help distinguish bacterial overgrowth from other causes of similar symptoms. Treatment includes antibiotics and nutritional support aimed at rebalancing the gut's natural flora. Tetracycline is the most common antibiotic used for this purpose.

(B) Celiac disease may present with similar symptoms as above and may also include steatorrhea and vitamin deficiencies. The diagnosis is usually made with biopsy and serum antibody studies. This patient's symptoms are not consistent with celiac disease. (C) Cystic fibrosis may appear with similar symptoms but would most likely present at a much earlier age. (D) Irritable bowel syndrome would not be associated with these findings. (E) Short bowel syndrome may present with similar symptoms. Patients usually have a history of Crohn disease, tumors, or previous bowel surgeries.

9 A 65-year-old man with a history of Crohn disease and multiple bowel surgeries presents with fatigue, nausea, diarrhea, and abdominal cramping. On examination he appears pale. There is stomatitis and glossitis apparent on a head and neck examination. Laboratory studies reveal iron deficiency anemia. His serum albumin is 2.1 g/dL. A C-reactive protein assay and erythrocyte sedimentation rate are normal. Which of the following is the most likely diagnosis?

(A) Active Crohn disease
(B) Anorexia nervosa
(C) Celiac disease
(D) Short bowel syndrome
(E) Small bowel malignancy

The answer is D: Short bowel syndrome. This patient is most likely suffering from short bowel syndrome. This may occur after multiple bowel surgeries and resections (such as in this patient). As the average small intestinal length is approximately 600 cm, studies have shown that any disease, which results in less than 200 cm of viable small bowel, may result in short bowel syndrome. This condition is common in patients with Crohn disease and a history of multiple bowel resections. Symptoms and clinical signs are often associated with malnutrition and may include vitamin deficiencies, fatty acid deficiencies, and mineral deficiencies.

(A) Although this patient may have active Crohn disease, it would usually be accompanied by an elevated CRP or ESR. Active Crohn disease is also often accompanied by rashes and joint pains. (B) Although anorexia nervosa may present with malnutrition, it is almost exclusively found in younger and usually female patients. Additionally these patients usually do not have a history of multiple bowel surgeries. (C) Celiac disease may present similarly to short bowel syndrome including malnutrition. However, dermatitis herpetiformes is the associated skin finding. Symptoms are usually associated with a gluten diet and occur in younger patients. Patients may have positive antitransglutaminase antibodies. (E) Small bowel malignancies may often present with similar symptoms. However, in this patient with a history of multiple small bowel surgeries, short bowel syndrome is much more likely.

10 A 31-year-old woman presents with abdominal pain that has occurred over the last year. She recalls that she often will have diarrhea and constipation within the same week. She has a history of depression. Her temperature is 37.1°C, blood pressure 120/82 mmHg, pulse 70 beats/min, and respirations 12 breaths/min. After a thorough workup, she is diagnosed with irritable bowel syndrome. Which of the following symptoms is least associated with irritable bowel syndrome?

(A) Back pain
(B) Bloating
(C) Headache
(D) Sensation of incomplete stool evacuation
(E) Weight loss

The answer is E: Weight loss. Irritable bowel syndrome is a clinical-based diagnosis of chronic bowel discomfort. Patients often complain of abdominal pain with frequent episodes of diarrhea, constipation, or both. Feeling of incomplete evacuation of stool is common as well as other chronic disorders such as fibromyalgia, depression, headaches, backaches, and other psychiatric disorders. The diagnosis that can be made based on the symptoms alone along with absence of certain worrying characteristics such as age greater than 50, gross blood in the stool, signs of infection, family history of bowel disease, and weight loss.

(A) Back pain is a common complaint in patients with irritable bowel syndrome. (B) Bloating and abdominal distention are a common complaint of patients with irritable bowel syndrome. (C) Headache and other chronic fatigue like symptoms are associated with irritable bowel syndrome. (D) One of the most common symptoms of irritable bowel syndrome is the sensation of incomplete stool evacuation.

11 A 62-year-old man presents with a history of coronary artery disease presents with weight loss, nausea, vomiting, and abdominal pain that starts after eating. He reports that these symptoms have been very stressful for him and more recently he has been fearful of eating due to the pain. On the abdominal examination, there is no rebound or guarding. Splanchnic angiography reveals narrowing of superior mesenteric artery. Which of the following is the best treatment for this man's condition?

(A) Bowel resection
(B) Limit eating to small meals low in fat content
(C) Long-term warfarin therapy
(D) Observation, regular exercise, and lifestyle changes
(E) Transaortic endarterectomy

The answer is E: Transaortic endarterectomy. Chronic mesenteric ischemia is a condition caused by atherosclerosis of the mesenteric arteries (most commonly the superior mesenteric artery) and is characterized by the triad of postprandial abdominal pain, food avoidance, and weight loss. The symptoms are caused by a gradual reduction in blood flow to the intestines. Since blood flow increases significantly during meals, symptoms may often present postprandial. It occurs most commonly in older patients with known atherosclerotic disease. Treatment includes surgical revascularization or stenting of the involved artery. Transaortic endarterectomy is one surgical approach that is often utilized in cases of superior mesenteric artery narrowing.

(A) Bowel resection may be needed in advanced cases of acute mesenteric ischemia, but is typically not performed unless the bowel becomes necrotic. (B) Although eating small meals and food low in fat content may be utilized in the treatment of chronic mesenteric ischemia, surgical management is the definitive treatment. (C) Medical management with long-term warfarin therapy is sometimes used in poor surgical candidates and patients who are not candidates for stenting. (D) Although regular exercise and lifestyle changes are important in the management of chronic mesenteric ischemia, observation in this patient would not be appropriate.

---

12 A 2-week-old neonate is brought into the emergency department with irritability and bilious vomiting. The infant was born at 39 weeks via vaginal birth without complications. He is afebrile and vital signs are within normal limits. On examination, the abdomen is distended and diffusely tender to palpation. There is hyperresonance with percussion. Upper gastrointestinal series is shown in *Figures 6-2A–C.*

Which of the following is the most likely diagnosis?

(A) Duodenal atresia
(B) Intussusception
(C) Necrotizing ileus
(D) Small bowel obstruction
(E) Volvulus

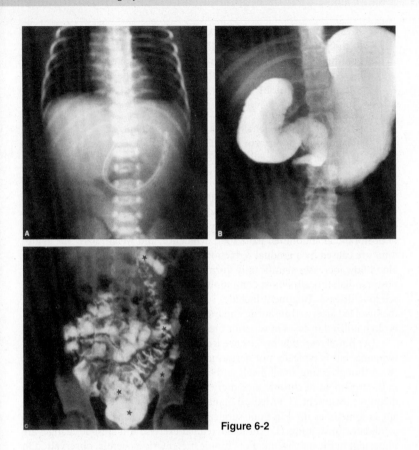

Figure 6-2

The answer is E: Volvulus. This neonate is most likely suffering from a midgut volvulus. A volvulus is characterized by rotation of the gut around its mesentery, which results in compromised blood flow. Volvulus is a surgical emergency and should be excluded in any infant presenting with bilious vomiting. In infants it is often due to congenital malrotation of the gut. The imaging study shows malrotation, midgut volvulus, and duodenal obstruction. Treatment includes insertion of a nasogastric tube, intravenous hydration, and antibiotics. Diagnosis may be established with an upper gastrointestinal series with barium contrast. Imaging will sometimes show a "spiral" or "cork-screw" tapering of contrast and an abnormal location of the superior mesenteric vessels.

(A) Duodenal atresia occurs in association with Down syndrome and often occurs a few hours after birth with bilious vomiting. Abdominal distention is absent. Imaging will often show the classic "double bubble" sign.

Treatment is surgical. (B) Intussusception is characterized by intermittent abdominal pain with vomiting and stools with blood and mucus. Stools are often described as "current jelly" in appearance. The condition is a medical emergency and should be treated as soon as possible. The initial treatment is a contrast enema, which is both diagnostic and may be therapeutic in most cases. If reduction with contrast fails, surgery is indicated. (C) Necrotizing ileus usually occurs 10 to 12 days after birth with distention, vomiting, and bloody stools. On examination, the abdomen will often be distended. Initial treatment involves nasogastric suction, intravenous support and nutrition, and antibiotics. If a trial of medical therapy fails, then surgical management is required. (D) Small bowel obstruction may also be characterized by abdominal distention. However, this patient's imaging is more characteristic of a volvulus.

---

13 A 4-year-old girl presents with bloody stools. She denies abdominal pain, fever, vomiting, or other symptoms. Her vitals are within normal limits. On examination, she appears happy and playful, but slightly pale. The remainder of the physical examination is unremarkable. Laboratory studies show a hemoglobin level of 8.5 g/dL. Which of the following tests will most likely reveal the diagnosis?

(A) Abdominal CT scan
(B) Arteriography
(C) Barium contrast study
(D) Plain radiography
(E) Technetium-99m pertechnetate scintiscan

The answer is E: Technetium-99m pertechnetate scintiscan. Meckel diverticulum is the most common congenital malformation of the small intestine. It is caused by incomplete obliteration of the vitelline duct. It most commonly presents as asymptomatic rectal bleeding in a child. However, other symptomatic presentations do occasionally occur including hemorrhagic shock, peritonitis, intestinal obstruction, and acute inflammation of the diverticulum. The imaging modality of choice is a Meckel scan using technetium-99m. The pertechnetate is taken up by the gastric mucosa in the Meckel diverticulum gastric mucosa and may be detected on imaging.

(A) Abdominal CT scanning is typically not helpful in the diagnosis of Meckel diverticulum because distinguishing the diverticulum from separate loops of bowel is extremely difficult. (B) Selective arteriography may sometimes be helpful when scintography and barium studies are negative, but are usually only helpful when bleeding is greater than 1 mL/min. (C) Barium contrast studies are usually unreliable in detecting a Meckel diverticulum, but may sometimes reveal a blind-ending pouch in the distal ileum. (D) Plain radiography is of limited value and is usually normal. Subtle signs evident on plain radiography may include signs of intestinal obstruction or perforation, which are uncommon complications of Meckel diverticulum.

14 A 33-year-old man with a history of psoriatic arthritis presents with abdominal pain, diarrhea, fever, and weight loss over the last 6 months. He reports that the abdominal pain is often relieved by defecation. He is currently afebrile and his other vital signs are within normal limits. On examination, there are several ulcers visible on his oral mucosa. Which of the following is not a typical characteristic of this patient's disease?

(A) Caseating granulomas on biopsy
(B) Cobblestone appearance
(C) Involvement of the ascending colon
(D) Involvement of the small bowel
(E) Transmural inflammation on biopsy

The answer is A: Caseating granulomas on biopsy. This patient is presenting with signs and symptoms of Crohn disease, a form of inflammatory bowel disease that can affect any part of the gastrointestinal tract from mouth to anus. There are numerous manifestations of Crohn disease that may include both gastrointestinal in nature and extraintestinal. Biopsy with histologic examination is important for confirming the diagnosis. Histology reveals transmural chronic inflammation and noncaseating granulomas. There may also be mucosal fragments and patchy ulcerations/erosions suggesting "skip lesions". Caseating granulomas are not a feature of Crohn disease and are more suggestive of tuberculosis.

(B) On endoscopy, the intestinal mucosa of Crohn disease patients is often described as appearing like a "cobblestone street" with areas of ulceration separated by areas of healthy tissue. (C) Crohn disease may involve the full length of the bowel including the ascending colon. (D) The terminal ileum is the most common segment of small bowel involved in Crohn disease. (E) Transmural inflammation is a characteristic of Crohn disease. In ulcerative colitis, the inflammation is limited to the mucosa.

15 An 82-year-old woman nursing home resident presents with worsening abdominal distention and crampy abdominal pain. Her medical history includes her current diagnosis of Alzheimer disease and arthritis. Her past surgical history is remarkable for a hysterectomy at age 45, cholecystectomy at age 39, and appendectomy at age 16. Workup reveals a small bowel obstruction. Which of the following is not a mechanical cause of small bowel obstruction?

(A) Abdominal adhesions
(B) Cancer
(C) Hernia
(D) Inflammatory bowel disease
(E) Narcotic medications

The answer is E: Narcotic medications. There are many potential causes of small bowel obstruction that are both mechanical and paralytic in nature. This patient has had multiple past abdominal surgeries suggesting abdominal adhesions as a potential mechanical cause of her symptoms. Other mechanical causes of small bowel obstruction include but are not limited to hernias, gallstones, inflammatory bowel disease, tumors, congenital malformations, volvulus, and foreign bodies. Paralytic causes include medications (opioids and other narcotics), mucosal infections, intestinal ischemia, surgery, kidney disease, and long-standing diabetes.

(A) Abdominal adhesions are the most common mechanical cause of small bowel obstruction. (B) Cancer may grow to occlude the small bowel lumen or push on the small bowel to cause obstruction. (C) Hernias may cause mechanical partial or complete bowel obstruction. (D) Small bowel obstruction is a common complication of Crohn disease.

 16 A 45-year-old man with a history of severe Crohn disease undergoes an operation with removal of a segment of diseased small bowel. During the surgery, the distal small bowel is found to be severely involved and is subsequently removed. Which of the following is not a potential problem associated with removal of the distal small bowel?

(A) Bile salt recycling
(B) Decreased water and electrolyte reabsorption
(C) Fat malabsorption
(D) Water-soluble vitamin deficiencies
(E) Vitamin B12 deficiency

The answer is D: Water-soluble vitamin deficiencies. The distal small bowel has a variety of functions and includes the functions specific to the terminal ileum. Resection of the distal small bowel may therefore result in impaired water and electrolyte absorption, bile salt enterohepatic recycling (resulting in fat malabsorption if stores are depleted enough), and vitamin B12 absorption. Water-soluble vitamins are primarily absorbed in the proximal small bowel and will thus not usually be affected by distal small bowel resection.

(A) Bile salt recycling is a primary function of terminal ileum. If the impairment is severe enough, bile acids may be depleted in the body resulting in fat malabsorption. (B) Resection of the distal ileum may severely impair water and electrolyte reabsorption. (C) Fat malabsorption may occur secondary to bile salt depletion with terminal ileum resection. (D) Vitamin B12 deficiency may occur when greater than 60 cm of distal small bowel is resected.

 17 A 35-year-old man with a history of Crohn disease undergoes bowel resection following an acute flare-up of his disease. The surgeon removes a 3-cm portion of the ileum and sends the specimen for pathologic evaluation. Which of the following describes the layers of the small bowel from inside to out that may be observed with histologic evaluation?

(A) Mucosa, circular muscle layer, submucosa, muscularis mucosa, longitudinal muscle layer, serosa
(B) Mucosa, muscularis mucosa, submucosa, circular muscle layer, longitudinal muscle layer, serosa
(C) Mucosa, muscularis mucosa, submucosa, longitudinal muscle layer, circular muscle layer, serosa
(D) Mucosa, submucosa, muscularis mucosa, circular muscle layer, longitudinal muscle layer, serosa
(E) Mucosa, submucosa, muscularis mucosa, longitudinal muscle layer, circular muscle layer, serosa

The answer is B: **Mucosa, muscularis mucosa, submucosa, circular muscle layer, longitudinal muscle layer, serosa.** The layers of the intestinal wall from inside to out are mucosa, muscularis mucosa, submucosa, circular muscle layer, longitudinal muscle layer, and serosa. The mucosa contains villi which are important for food absorption. Between the circular muscle layer and longitudinal muscle layer is the myenteric plexus.
(A) This is not the correct sequence of layers. (C) This is not the correct sequence of layers. (D) This is not the correct sequence of layers. (E) This is not the correct sequence of layers.

---

18 A 23-year-old man presents repeated episodes of abdominal pain that he has not been able to explain. On examination, there are multiple small, brown, and flat freckles around and inside the patient's mouth. After a thorough workup, the patient is found to have intussusception. Which of the following is not a characteristic of this patient's underlying disease?

(A) Autosomal dominant inheritance
(B) Increased risk of intestinal malignancy
(C) Lymphoid hyperplasia
(D) Multiple gastrointestinal hamartomas
(E) STK11/LKB1 mutation

The answer is C: **Lymphoid hyperplasia.** Peutz-Jeghers syndrome is a rare autosomal dominant condition characterized by the development of multiple hamartomatous polyps throughout the gastrointestinal tract and hyperpigmented macules on the lips and oral mucosa. Other problems associated with Peutz-Jeghers syndrome include bleeding and prolapse from the rectum, menstrual irregularities, gynecomastia in men, precocious puberty, hematemesis, and weakness due to anemia. Lymphoid hyperplasia is not a feature of Peutz-Jeghers syndrome. Due to increased incidence in a variety of cancers, patients with Peutz-Jeghers syndrome require close surveillance including esophogogastroduodenoscopy and colonoscopy every 2 years for gastrointestinal cancer, imaging of the pancreas yearly for pancreatic cancer, ultrasounds of the pelvis (women) or testicles (men) yearly for ovary and testicular cancer, mammography for breast cancer, and pap-smears for cervical cancer.

(A) Peutz-Jeghers syndrome is indeed inherited in an autosomal dominant fashion. (B) Patients with Peutz-Jeghers syndrome have a 15-fold increase in the incidence of malignancy and thus require increased surveillance as described above. (D Multiple gastrointestinal hamartomas is a core feature of Peutz-Jeghers syndrome. (E) Peutz-Jeghers syndrome is caused by a germline mutation in the STK11/LKB1 gene on chromosome 19 (a tumor suppressor gene).

---

19 A 13-year-old girl presents with nausea, vomiting diarrhea, and fever for the last day. She reports that she ate potato salad the previous day that had been sitting on the counter for several hours. On examination, she appears moderately ill and dehydrated, but is able to rehydrate orally. She is diagnosed with bacterial gastritis. Which of the following is not an important mechanism of defense found in the small bowel against invading bacteria?

(A) Gut-associated lymphoid tissue
(B) Mucin production
(C) Native bacteria
(D) Paneth cells
(E) Tight junctions

The answer is C: Native bacteria. Although there may be some bacteria present in the small intestine in normal individuals, it is generally sterile in the majority of the population. While native bacteria may be a protective mechanism against invading bacterial growth in the large intestine, it is not an important mechanism in the small intestine.

(A) Gut-associated lymphoid tissue is an important component of the small bowel for host defense. In fact, it is the largest mass of lymphoid tissue in the human body. (B) Mucin production is an important defense mechanism against invading bacteria. They compose the initial barrier that bacteria encounter in the intestinal tract. (D) Paneth cells are the principle epithelial cell of the small intestine. They secrete a variety of immune factors including defensins, lysozymes, phospholipase 2, and other important molecules involved in host defense. (E) Tight junctions between epithelial cells in the small intestine prevent bacteria from invading between cells and are an important component of intestinal defense against bacteria.

20 A 34-year-old man presents with arthralgias, abdominal pain, diarrhea, and weight loss over the last several months. He describes the joint pain as migrating from one joint to another. He also reports that his stools float and he occasionally suffers from fevers and chills. On examination, there is generalized lymphadenopathy and several areas of skin hyperpigmentation. A biopsy of the small intestine reveals villous atrophy and multiple macrophages containing periodic acid–Schiff-positive deposits in the lamina propria. Which of the following is the most likely diagnosis?

(A) Abdominal angina
(B) Celiac disease
(C) Crohn disease
(D) Hartnup disease
(E) Whipple disease

The answer is E: **Whipple disease.** This patient is most likely suffering from Whipple disease. This disease is a systemic disease caused by infection with the bacterium *Tropheryma whippelii*. Symptoms are often secondary to malabsorption along with joint, CNS, and cardiovascular manifestations. Small bowel biopsy is an essential part of the diagnosis and is characterized by an intestinal lamina propria packed full of periodic acid–Schiff-positive macrophages. Polymerase chain reaction (PCR) may also be used in the diagnosis. The mainstay of treatment is antibiotic therapy with trimethoprim–sulfamethoxazole, penicillin G, streptomycin, amoxicillin, or chloramphenicol. Surgery should be avoided in the treatment of these patients.

(A) This patient's systemic symptoms are not typical of abdominal angina. (B) Celiac disease may have gastrointestinal complaints similar to Whipple disease and may also have systemic symptoms in the form of dermatitis herpetiformes. However, this patient's histologic features are not consistent with celiac disease. (C) Crohn disease may also have similar presenting symptoms. However, these histologic findings are not characteristic of Crohn disease. (D) Hartnup disease is an autosomal recessive metabolic disorder affecting the absorption of nonpolar amino acids. Symptoms usually present in infancy. This patient's symptoms are not consistent with this disorder.

21 A 33-year-old woman presents to her primary care physician with nausea, vomiting, chronic diarrhea, and frequent abdominal pain following meals. She reports that she has been to many physicians in the past but has not yet been successful in controlling her symptoms. Laboratory studies show positive antiendomysial antibodies. Which of the following is unlikely to be a complication of this disease?

(A) Anemia
(B) Increased risk of miscarriage
(C) Lymphoma of the small intestine
(D) Sarcoma of the small intestine
(E) Subfertility

The answer is D: Sarcoma of the small intestine. Celiac disease is a chronic diarrheal disease characterized by intestinal malabsorption. It is caused by ingestion of gluten-containing foods. Common presenting complaints include diarrhea, cramps, abdominal pain, flatulence and distention, and other gastrointestinal complaints. Additionally, patients with celiac sprue are at increased risk for many complications of their disease including lymphomas and adenocarcinomas of the small intestine, short stature and stunted growth, subfertility, anemia, osteopenia, and seizure disorders. Women of childbearing age also have a higher rate of miscarriage than the general female population. However, sarcoma of the small bowel does not occur at increased rates in patients with celiac disease.

(A) Anemia is a common problem in patients with celiac sprue and may be a result of vitamin and/or mineral malabsorption or chronic inflammation. (B) Women with celiac disease that are of childbearing age are at increased risk of having miscarriages. (C) Patients with celiac disease are at increased risk of intestinal lymphomas. (E) Numerous studies have shown that both men and women with celiac disease may suffer from fertility problems.

 22 A 24-year-old man presents to his physician with an 8-month history of diarrhea, malaise, recurrent abdominal pain, and occasional fevers. On physical examination, there is tenderness to palpation of the lower quadrants of the abdomen without rebound or guarding. Oral ulcers are noted on the buccal mucosa. An upper gastrointestinal series shows a 10-cm stenotic segment of the ileum. Laboratory studies show:

Hemoglobin: 12.1 g/dL
Leukocytes: 13,000/mm^3
Albumin: 2.5 g/dL
C-reactive protein: elevated

The patient undergoes surgery with resection of the involved segment of small bowel. What is the most likely diagnosis?

(A) Adenocarcinoma of the small intestine
(B) Celiac disease
(C) Crohn disease
(D) Gastritis
(E) Ulcerative colitis

The answer is C: Crohn disease. This patient is most likely suffering from Crohn disease. Common symptoms of Crohn disease include nonbloody diarrhea, abdominal pain and cramping, fatigue, malaise, and low-grade fevers. The most common section of bowel affected by Crohn disease is the terminal ileum. Strictures may form and manifest as stenotic bowel on imaging.

(A) Adenocarcinoma of the colon is unlikely considering the patient's age and clinical picture. (B) Celiac disease is associated with ingestion of gluten-containing foods and may have a similar presentation to Crohn disease. However, this patient's clinical picture including imaging and oral ulcers is more characteristic of Crohn disease. (D) Although gastritis presents with gastrointestinal symptoms, it is more often acute in nature and would not have this patient's oral ulcer or imaging findings. (E) Ulcerative colitis shares many of the same features of Crohn disease and is also an inflammatory bowel disease. However, the ileum is not involved in inflammatory bowel with the exception of so called "backwash ileitis."

  A 45-year-old man presents with a 3-month history of epigastric pain. He describes the pain as dull, achy, and intermittent that will occasionally wake him up at night. The pain does not radiate and has not changed in character since the onset. He admits that the pain is exacerbated by coffee intake but reports that eating seems to temporarily help the pain. He denies weight loss, vomiting, fever, chills, or gross blood in his stools. He does not drink alcohol or smoke. On physical examination, there is mild epigastric tenderness with palpation. There is no rebound or guarding. What is the most likely diagnosis?

(A) Crohn disease
(B) Duodenal ulcer
(C) Esophageal spasm
(D) Gastric ulcer
(E) Pancreatitis

The answer is B: Duodenal ulcer. This patient is most likely suffering from a duodenal ulcer. Duodenal ulcers are the most common location of peptic ulcers in the gastrointestinal tract. Epigastric pain is the most common complaint in patients with peptic ulcer disease and is characterized by a gnawing or burning sensation that occurs after meals. This patient's nighttime pain is a common complaint in duodenal ulcers and characteristically occurs several hours after meals. Most patients with duodenal ulcers have a combination of decreased duodenal bicarbonate secretion and increased gastric acid secretion. Upper endoscopy is the preferred diagnostic test in evaluation of patients with peptic ulcer disease. Additionally, testing for *Heliobacter pylori* is an essential part of the workup since it has been found to be a major cause of duodenal ulcers.

(A) Crohn disease is a form of inflammatory bowel disease that can affect any part of the gastrointestinal tract from mouth to anus. There are numerous manifestations of Crohn disease that may include both gastrointestinal in nature and extraintestinal. Biopsy with histologic examination is important for confirming the diagnosis. This patient's symptoms are not consistent with a diagnosis of Crohn disease. (C) Esophageal spasms are abnormal contractions of the esophageal muscle that may cause impairment in swallowing. Common symptoms include difficulty swallowing and chest pain. This patient's symptoms are not consistent with a diagnosis of esophageal spasms. (D) Gastric ulcers may appear similar to duodenal ulcers but are less common. They too are associated with infection with *H. pylori*. Signs and symptoms that suggest gastric ulcer over duodenal ulcer include pain immediately after eating and pain made worse with food. This patient's symptoms are more suggestive of a duodenal ulcer since there is delayed and nocturnal pain temporarily relieved by food intake. (E) Although epigastric pain does occur in pancreatitis, it usually radiates to the back and also occurs with food intake. This patient's symptoms are more characteristic of peptic ulcer disease than pancreatitis.

 A 3-day-old neonate that was initially feeding well after birth presents with bilious vomiting, abdominal distention, and irritability. On examination, the patient has a palpable right upper quadrant mass and the abdomen appears distended. A barium enema reveals an acute tapering of bowel with a "bird's beak" appearance and proximal dilation of small bowel. The infant is diagnosed with a midgut volvulus and emergently taken to the operating room. During the operation, it is noted that there is a 2-cm segment of dusky small bowel. The volvulus is repaired and blood flow restored to the area. Unfortunately, the viability of the bowel segment cannot be determined intraoperatively. Which of the following is the next best step in management?

(A) Close the patient and closely monitor for signs of peritonitis
(B) Close the patient and provide nasogastric suction, antibiotics, and continued intravenous support
(C) Close the patient, provide support, and repeat examination of the bowel in 12 to 36 hours
(D) Remove the entire small bowel
(E) Remove the portion of small bowel

The answer is C: Close the patient, provide support, and repeat examination of the bowel in 12 to 36 hours. This patient has questionable viability of a segment of small bowel. During surgery, if ischemic bowel is present these segments should be removed. If the viability of the bowel cannot be determined, a second operation may be necessary to reassess the viability of bowel. This surgery is typically performed 12 to 36 hours after the initial surgery.

(A) Although the patient should be closely monitored for signs of peritonitis, failure to remove ischemic portions of bowel would greatly increase this patient's chance of mortality. Thus, a second operation is necessary at this point. (B) The initial management of suspected volvulus involves nasogastric suction, antibiotics, and intravenous support. Although this will continue to be important postoperatively, the bowel in this patient will need to be reexamined. (D) Removing the entire small bowel is unnecessary and would most likely result in death or long-term morbidity for the infant. (E) Removing the portion of small bowel before viability is determined could result in the infant having short bowel syndrome. Short bowel syndrome is a dreaded and unfortunate complication when significant portions of bowel are removed. A better approach would be to reexamine the small bowel with repeat surgery.

25 A 35-year-old woman with a recent diagnosis of valvular heart disease complains of flushing, vague abdominal pain, and watery diarrhea. A carcinoid tumor is suspected. Which of the following is the best initial test for diagnosis?

(A) 24-Hour urine test for 5-HIAA
(B) Abdominal ultrasound
(C) Computed tomography imaging of the head
(D) Measurement of serum niacin levels
(E) Radionucleotide scan with octreotide

The answer is A: 24-Hour urine test for 5-HIAA. Although carcinoid tumors of the intestine are often asymptomatic, they may present with symptoms such as those described in this patient. Additional signs may include facial telangiectasias, rashes (from niacin deficiency), wheezing, and edema. The initial workup for carcinoid tumors involves a 24-hour urine test for urinary levels of 5-HIAA, a metabolite of tryptophan metabolism. The levels are usually greatly increased in patients with carcinoid tumors. Additional testing may include noncontrast CT imaging of the abdomen, which is the imaging modality of choice due to the vascularity of the tumors.

(B) Abdominal ultrasounds may have limited use in tumors of size less than 1 cm, but are generally not useful in the diagnosis of carcinoid tumors. (C) Although CT imaging of the abdomen would be useful as an additional test to identify the location of the tumor, the head is a very unlikely location for this tumor. (D) Although niacin levels may be diminished in carcinoid tumors since it is involved in the metabolism of serotonin, low levels of niacin are very nonspecific for the diagnosis of carcinoid tumors. (E) A radionucleotide scan (OctreoScan) may be useful in the diagnosis of carcinoid tumors when other imaging modalities have failed to localize the tumor.

7

Colon, Rectum, and Anus

---

1 A 52-year-old man with a history of intermittent rectal bleeding presents to his primary care physician for evaluation. His father and mother have a history of colorectal polyps. His mother was recently diagnosed with colon cancer. The physician recommends colonoscopy, but the patient refuses and instead only wants to have a barium enema because he is claustrophobic and has fears of being able to withstand being in the CT scanner. Which of the following statements are true regarding barium enema and its ability to detect colorectal pathology?

(A) Abnormal findings can be observed
(B) Diagnosis and therapy are possible
(C) Evaluates the entire colon
(D) Reaches where 60% to 70% of polyps occur

The answer is C: Evaluates the entire colon. Barium enema does evaluate the entire colon and is complementary to flexible sigmoidoscopy. However, any abnormal finding needs to be evaluated with colonoscopy. Thus, colonoscopy would be the better test to perform in this patient.

(A) Abnormal findings need to be further evaluated with colonoscopy. (B) Diagnosis is possible with barium enema but therapy can only be performed with colonoscopy and biopsy/fulgeration. (D) Flexible sigmoidoscopy can be used to reach an area where 60% to 70% of colon polyps and cancers occur.

---

2 A 56-year-old man presents to a local health fair sponsored by a religious organization in an effort to promote public health screening for common diseases. For a $4.00 fee, patients can receive fecal occult blood testing and a digital rectal examination performed by a physician who has graciously donates his time. Which of the following statements is true regarding this screening process?

(A) Digital rectal examination will find 50% of tumors are palpable
(B) Fecal occult blood testing has good sensitivity
(C) Fecal occult blood testing has good specificity
(D) Positive fecal occult blood testing necessitates barium enema
(E) Positive predictive value for fecal occult blood testing is 20%

The answer is E: Positive predictive value for fecal occult blood testing is 20%. Fecal occult blood testing has poor sensitivity and specificity. The positive predictive value of this test is about 20%. All patients with a positive fecal occult blood test need to have a colonoscopy.

(A) Digital rectal examination will find 10% of tumors are palpable. (B) Fecal occult blood testing has poor sensitivity. (C) Fecal occult blood testing has poor specificity. (D) Positive fecal occult blood testing necessitates colonoscopy.

3 Regarding risk factors for colorectal carcinoma, which of the following patients would portend the most significant risk, and, thus, would warrant screening with colonoscopy?

(A) 27-year-old man with a family history of colon polyps in his 50-year-old father
(B) 29-year-old man with Crohn disease diagnosed 5 years ago
(C) 40-year-old man with intermittent rectal bleeding after bowel movements
(D) 55-year-old man with ulcerative colitis diagnosed at age 15
(E) 70-year-old man with internal and external hemorrhoids

The answer is D: 55-year-old man with ulcerative colitis diagnosed at age 15. Regarding risk factors for colorectal cancer, everyone over the age of 50 is at risk. However, patients with ulcerative colitis are at increased risk and that risk is 12% to 20% after 30 years of diagnosis. Thus, such patients should be screened with periodic colonoscopy.

(A) This patient is at low risk for colorectal cancer at his age. (B) This patient is at increased risk for colorectal cancer but less than that for a patient with ulcerative colitis. (C) This patient is at low risk for colon cancer because he is under 50 years of age. (E) Although this patient is above age 50 and is at risk for developing colon cancer, he is at lower risk than the patient with a 30-year history of ulcerative colitis.

4 A 35-year-old woman with a history of multiple hamartomas scattered throughout the gastrointestinal tract presents to her primary care physician for follow-up. The physical examination picture is shown in *Figure 7-1*.

There are also pigmented spots on the palmar surfaces of her hands. This patient is at risk for which of the following medical problems?

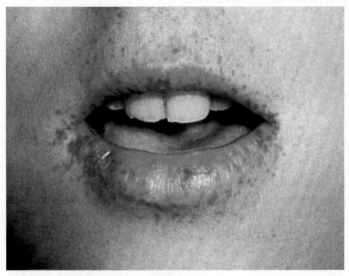

Figure 7-1

(A) Brain cancer
(B) Breast cancer
(C) Skin cancer
(D) Thyroid cancer
(E) Uterine cancer

The answer is B: Breast cancer. This patient has Peutz-Jeghers syndrome. This condition is characterized by single or multiple hamartomas that can be scattered throughout the GI tract in small bowel, colon, and stomach. Pigmented spots around the lips, oral mucosa, face, and palmar surfaces are also common. There is a slightly increased risk of various carcinomas such as stomach, ovary, breast, cervix, and lung.

(A) Peutz-Jeghers syndrome does not have an increased risk of brain cancer. (C) Peutz-Jeghers syndrome does not have an increased risk of skin cancer. (D) Peutz-Jeghers syndrome does not have an increased risk of thyroid cancer. (E) Peutz-Jeghers syndrome does not have an increased risk of uterine cancer.

5) A 57-year-old man with a history of vague left lower quadrant pain, bloating and alternating constipation, and diarrhea presents to his primary care physician for follow-up. Physical examination is noncontributory. Barium enema reveals multiple sigmoid diverticuli. What is the most likely explanation for these findings?

(A) Aperistaltic segment
(B) High fiber diet
(C) Increased intraluminal pressure
(D) Mass lesion in the rectum
(E) Polyposis coli

The answer is C: Increased intraluminal pressure. This patient likely has diverticulosis. This is caused by increased intraluminal pressure which causes the inner layer of the colon to bulge through this area of weakness in the colon wall. Low fiber diet, positive family history, and increase in age are considered to be risk factors.

(A) Aperistaltic segment is not thought to be an etiologic factor in development of diverticulosis. (B) Low fiber diet can cause constipation which can increase intraluminal pressures. (D) The barium enema did not reveal evidence of a mass lesion. (E) The barium enema did not reveal evidence of colon polyps.

---

 6 A 68-year-old man with a history of vague left lower quadrant pain, bloating and alternating constipation, and diarrhea presents to his primary care physician for follow-up. He has a known history of diverticulosis. Most recently, he complains of passing air through his penis as well as fecal matter. Further, he has had four urinary tract infections in the last 6 months. What is the most appropriate next step in the management of this patient?

(A) Anoscopy
(B) Digital rectal examination
(C) CT scan of the abdomen and pelvis
(D) Rigid sigmoidoscopy
(E) Ultrasound

The answer is C: CT scan of the abdomen and pelvis. This patient with known diverticulosis now has diverticulitis with evidence of a colovesical fistula. Typical features include passage of air with urination, passage of fecal matter with urination, and recurrent urinary tract infections. The best test to diagnose this is CT scan of the abdomen and pelvis.

(A) Anoscopy will not evaluate the sigmoid colon and will miss identification of the fistula. (B) Digital rectal examination, while important in the general physical examination, will miss this lesion. (D) Sigmoidoscopy may only show erythema but not the fistula tract unless it is large. (E) Ultrasound will not identify a colovesical fistula.

---

 7 A 26-year-old woman complains of a 6-month history of bloody diarrhea, abdominal pain, and intermittent fevers. She has a history of irritable bowel syndrome but has had a worsening of her symptoms during the above time period. Her past medical history is unremarkable. Physical examination reveals abdominal distension. Bowel sounds are present in all quadrants. Rectal examination reveals multiple anal fissures. What is the most appropriate diagnostic testing for this patient?

(A) Anoscopy
(B) Colonoscopy
(C) Flexible sigmoidoscopy
(D) Rigid sigmoidoscopy
(E) No further diagnostic testing is required for this patient

The answer is B: Colonoscopy. This patient likely has ulcerative colitis. Colonoscopy may reveal thickened, friable mucosa. Fissures and pseudopolyps may also be present. This disease almost always involves the rectum and extends backward toward the cecum to varying degrees.

(A) Anoscopy is a limited procedure and will not allow visualization of the entire colon. (C) Flexible sigmoidoscopy will allow visualization of the rectum and sigmoid colon but will miss higher levels of the colon. (D) For reasons described above, rigid sigmoidoscopy will miss lesions at higher levels on the colon, such as the ascending colon or cecum. (E) This patient requires further testing to establish a definitive diagnosis.

 8 A 71-year-old woman presents to her primary care physician complaining of rectal bleeding. She had some mild left-sided abdominal cramps but subsided within a few minutes. She has never had a prior episode of rectal bleeding. Physical examination reveals mild left lower quadrant abdominal pain without evidence of guarding or rebound tenderness. Rectal examination reveals no fresh blood in the rectal vault. Colonoscopy reveals several outpouchings of the sigmoid colon wall without evidence of bleeding or perforation. The remainder of the colonoscopy is within normal limits. White blood cell count is normal. What is the most appropriate treatment for this patient?

(A) Antibiotic therapy
(B) Left hemicolectomy
(C) Right hemicolectomy
(D) Subtotal colectomy
(E) Watchful waiting

The answer is E: Watchful waiting. This patient has diverticulosis. This is due to the presence of outpouchings in the wall of the colon that occur where the arterial supply penetrates the bowel wall. For the patient who stops bleeding and is asymptomatic requires no further treatment.

(A) Intravenous antibiotic therapy is not required in this patient as there is no evidence of infection. (B) Elective colectomy is not recommended at the first episode. Thus, left hemicolectomy is not required. (C) Elective colectomy is not recommended at the first episode. (D) Elective colectomy is not recommended at the first episode. Thus, right hemicolectomy is not required.

9 An 85-year-old man is brought to the emergency department because of acute abdominal pain and progressive abdominal distention. He is a resident of a local nursing home. He has not been eating because of progressive nausea. Abdominal radiographs are shown in *Figure 7-2*.

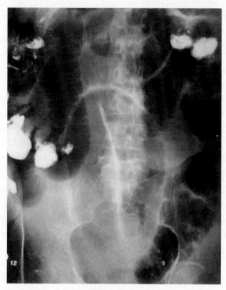

Figure 7-2

What is the initial treatment for this patient?

(A) Gastrograffin enema
(B) High fiber diet
(C) Lactulose
(D) Rectal tube decompression
(E) Surgical resection

The answer is D: Rectal tube decompression. This patient has sigmoid volvulus. The centrally located sigmoid loop is outlined by trapped air as shown in the radiograph. This condition can be reduced with a rectal tube, which is the treatment of choice. In addition, one can consider decompression with enema

(A) Gastrograffin enema is not a treatment of sigmoid volvulus. (B) High fiber diet has no role in the treatment of volvulus. (C) Lactulose is unlikely to be of benefit in the management of this patient. (E) Cecal calculus is treated with surgical intervention.

A 41-year-old woman with Crohn disease has undergone multiple surgical procedures. She has undergone an ileostomy recently but still has evidence of some distal jejunal disease. Her current medications include prednisone and aminosalycyclic acid. Which of the following effects of prolonged therapy with glucocortecoids are possible for this patient?

(A) Antibody production
(B) Collagen formation
(C) Fibroblast dysfunction
(D) Inflammatory cell migration
(E) Wound healing

The answer is C: **Fibroblast dysfunction.** This patient would be expected to have fibroblast dysfunction. Patients with inflammatory bowel disease may require treatment with exogenous corticosteroids. These agents suppress the immune system and impair inflammatory cell migration.

(A) Antibody production is impaired. This is appropriate in Crohn disease. (B) Other effects of corticosteroids include impaired wound healing. Collagen formation will not occur normally. (D) Inflammatory cell migration is not a significant effect of glucocortecoids. (E) Wound healing is a less common effect of glucocortecoids.

 A 36-year-old woman with recurrent gastrointestinal bleeding presents to her primary care physician with another bout of bleeding. The differential diagnosis for her condition includes angiodysplasia and diverticular disease. Which of the following features would favor the diagnosis of colonic diverticulosis?

(A) Bleeding is brisk
(B) Bleeding occurs due to colonic wall weakness
(C) Bleeding is sudden
(D) Bleeding is self-limiting
(E) Submucosal colonic wall degeneration occurs in the sigmoid colon

The answer is B: **Bleeding occurs due to the colonic wall weakness.** In both diverticular disease and angiodysplasia, bleeding is brisk, sudden, and often self-limiting. This does not differentiate between these conditions. However, in patients with colonic diverticulosis, bleeding occurs when a blood vessel breaks as it passes through the weakened wall of the diverticulum.

(A) Bleeding is brisk in both conditions. (C) Bleeding is sudden in both angiodysplasia and diverticular disease. (D) Bleeding is self-limiting in both angiodysplasia and diverticular disease. (E) Submucosal colonic wall degeneration occurs in the cecum and ascending colon in patients with colonic angiodysplasia.

12 A 41-year-old man with a history of intermittent rectal bleeding presents to his primary care physician for evaluation. He has never been treated for this condition before. Physical examination of the heart, lungs, and abdomen is unremarkable. Which of the following management steps is likely to be least cost-effective in the search for the cause of bleeding in this patient?

(A) Anorectal examination
(B) Anoscopy
(C) Bleeding scan
(D) Colonoscopy
(E) Proctosigmoidoscopy

The answer is C: Bleeding scan. This patient has intermittent lower gastrointestinal bleeding. A careful history, physical examination, and diagnostic evaluation of the lower GI tract are recommended. Bleeding scan is costly and will not likely provide further information as to the source of bleeding. Thus, it is not recommended in this patient as a first-line management step.

(A) Anorectal examination may provide the source of bleeding in this patient and may reveal the presence of fissure, fistula, or external hemorrhoids. (B) Anoscopy is a cost-effective diagnostic test and may reveal any of the above pathologies. (D) Colonoscopy would evaluate the entire lower GI tract from anus to cecum. (E) Proctosigmoidoscopy may reveal the presence of fissure, fistula, internal or external hemorrhoids, as well as any other inflammatory or neoplastic lesion of the rectum and sigmoid colon.

13 A 57-year-old man has recurrent lower gastrointestinal bleeding. Colonoscopy is performed and fails to localize the source of bleeding. His most recent hematocrit is 24% after 3 units of packed red blood cells. Selective visceral arteriography is considered by the treating physician. Advantages of this procedure include:

(A) Embolization procedure must be done separately
(B) Noninvasive test
(C) Precise localization of bleeding
(D) Works well for bleeding <0.1 mL/min

The answer is C: Precise localization of bleeding. Selective visceral arteriography localizes bleeding more precisely. It can be used for therapeutic embolization at the same time as the diagnostic procedure. It is an invasive test and requires a higher rate of bleeding (>0.5 mL/min).

(A) Embolization can be done at the same time as the diagnostic procedure. (B) This is an invasive test. (D) Technitium-99 sulfur colloid isotope scan works well for bleeding <0.1 mL/min.

14 A 57-year-old man with known diverticulosis with bouts of diverticulitis is hospitalized on the medical service because of recurrent left lower quadrant pain. CT scan is performed and reveals the presence of diverticulosis with a 2-cm area of inflammatory mass without evidence of fluid within the mass. What is the most likely diagnosis?

(A) Acute diverticulitis
(B) Diverticular abscess
(C) Diverticular phlegmon
(D) Sigmoid colon carcinoma
(E) Transsigmoidal fistulization

The answer is C: Diverticular phlegmon. This patient has a diverticular phlegmon. This is the local response to diverticular inflammation and can lead to the formation of an inflammatory mass. This is the definition of a phlegmon. The mass is not fluid filled. Treatment involves bowel rest and intravenous antibiotics.

(A) A diverticulum may become inflamed when a fecalith obstructs its neck. (B) An abscess suggests a fluid collection. Phlegmon does not have a fluid collection only a mass of inflammatory tissue. (D) The CT scan does not reveal evidence of colorectal carcinoma. (E) The CT scan does not reveal evidence of fistulization. Peridiverticular abscess may erode into adjacent viscera which can form a fistula.

 15 A 63-year-old man with recurrent diverticular disease presents to the emergency department with left lower quadrant, fever, chills, nausea, and vomiting for 3 days. Physical examination reveals tenderness in the left lower quadrant without evidence of guarding or rebound tenderness. CT scan is performed and reveals the presence of diverticulosis and diverticulitis with a 2-cm area of inflammatory mass without evidence of fluid within the mass. What is the most appropriate treatment for this patient?

(A) Antibiotics, bowel rest, and intravenous fluids
(B) CT guided percutaneous drainage
(C) Open drainage of abscess
(D) Surgical resection with end colostomy
(E) Watchful waiting

The answer is A: Antibiotics, bowel rest, and intravenous fluids. This patient has a diverticular phlegmon. This is the local response to diverticular inflammation and can lead to the formation of an inflammatory mass. This is the definition of a phlegmon. The mass is not fluid filled. Treatment involves bowel rest and intravenous antibiotics.

(B) CT-guided drainage is appropriate for the treatment of diverticular abscess. (C) This patient does not have a fluid collection suggestive of a diverticular abscess. (D) There is no reason to perform surgical resection with colostomy given the CT findings above. This patient should respond well to antibiotics, bowel rest, and intravenous fluids. (E) Watchful waiting is inappropriate for this patient with a diverticular phlegmon. The patient would benefit from antibiotics, bowel rest, and intravenous fluids.

---

 16 A 36-year-old woman with ulcerative colitis presents to her physician for a follow-up visit. She has been treated with corticosteroid enemas and sulfasalazine. Physical examination of the heart, lungs, and abdomen is unremarkable. Examination of the lower limbs reveals the presence of red, tender papules. What is the most likely reason for this finding?

(A) Coagulopathy
(B) Clubbing
(C) Erythema nodosum
(D) Scleritis
(E) Uveitis

The answer is C: **Erythema nodosum.** This patient has ulcerative colitis and demonstrates some extraintestinal features of the disease. Erythema nodosum is a dermatologic manifestation which is characterized by symmetric, red, tender papules on the extensor surface of the limbs.

(A) Coagulopathy and thromboembolism are vascular complications of ulcerative colitis. (B) Clubbing is another dermatologic manifestation of this condition. (D) Scleritis is an ocular manifestation of this condition. (E) Uveitis is an ocular manifestation of this condition.

---

 17 A 28-year-old woman with ulcerative colitis presents to her physician for a follow-up visit. She has been treated with corticosteroid enemas and sulfasalazine. She now complains of worsening diarrhea. Her latest erythrocyte sedimentation rate is within normal limits. The rationale behind the use of antidiarrheal agents in this patient would include which of the following?

(A) Induce remission of ulcerative colitis
(B) Prevent sigmoid colon cancer development
(C) Prevent rectal cancer development
(D) Prevent disease recurrence
(E) Reduce diarrheal episodes

The answer is E: **Reduce diarrheal episodes.** Antidiarrheal agents may be used in patients with inflammatory bowel disease to reduce bowel frequency. They do not affect the course of the disease. Bowel rest and total parenteral nutrition are indicated for patients with severe diarrheal disease.

(A) Antidiarrheal agents do not induce remission of ulcerative colitis. (B) Antidiarrheal agents do not prevent sigmoid colon cancer development. (C) Antidiarrheal agents do not prevent rectal cancer development. (D) Antidiarrheal agents do not prevent disease recurrence.

---

18 A 74-year-old man with a history of recurrent anal canal fistulas presents with the same complaint of anorectal pain and drainage. Physical examination reveals an extrasphincteric anorectal fistula. He has never had anoscopy performed. Which of the following diagnostic considerations would be pertinent in this patient?

(A) Anorectal carcinoma
(B) External hemorrhoids
(C) Internal hemorrhoids
(D) Pilonidal sinus
(E) Thrombosed external hemorrhoid

The answer is A: Anorectal carcinoma. This patient has a history of recurrent anal canal fistulas. It is important to know that low rectal or anal canal carcinomas may present as fistulas. In a patient with recurrent fistulas, this diagnosis most be considered and ruled out.

(B) External hemorrhoids are unlikely in this patient and were not noted in the physical examination findings for this patient. (C) Internal hemorrhoids may be felt on digital rectal examination. (D) Pilonidal sinus may present as a pit in the intergluteal fold. (E) Thrombosed external hemorrhoids would be easily visible on anal canal examination.

---

19 A 54-year-old man is in the operating room undergoing repair of an extrasphincteric fistula-in-ano. He has no prior surgical history. His current medical problems include hypertension, diabetes mellitus, recurrent sinusitis, and irritable bowel syndrome. Principles of surgical management of this condition include which of the following?

(A) Avoidance of tract guide in fistula tract
(B) Elimination of primary opening of fistula tract
(C) Intravenous corticosteroids preoperatively
(D) Partial unroofing of fistula tract
(E) Washout of the rectal canal with antibiotic irrigation

The answer is B: Elimination of primary opening of fistula tract. Principles of surgical repair of fistula include unroofing of the fistula, elimination of the primary opening of the fistula tract, and establishing adequate drainage. It is prudent to open the entire fistula tract with a guide in place.

(A) It is prudent to place a tract guide in the fistula tract. (C) Intravenous corticosteroids are not recommended in fistula repair. (D) Complete unroofing of the fistula tract is recommended. (E) Washout of the rectal canal with antibiotic irrigation is not required as part of fistula repair.

20 A 37-year-old hirsute man presents to the ambulatory care clinic complaining of anal pain for 2 weeks. On physical examination of the sacrococcygeal area, he is found to have a hair follicle that appears inflamed. The area is tender to palpation. Should a sinus tract be associated with this lesion, which direction would it be expected to run?

(A) Caudad
(B) Cephalad
(C) Lateral
(D) Medial
(E) Ventral

The answer is B: **Cephalad.** This patient has a pilonidal sinus. This occurs in hirsute patients in their third decade of life. Physical examination reveals an infected hair follicle. The area is tender to palpation. Sinus tracts usually run cephalad in greater than 90% of cases.

(A) Sinus tracts rarely run caudad in patients with pilonidal sinus. (C) Sinus tracts do not run laterally in this condition. (D) Sinus tracts do not run medially in patients with pilonidal sinus. (E) Sinus tracts do not appear ventrally.

21 A 24-year-old man complains of skin flushing, chronic watery diarrhea with cramps, and difficulty with breathing. He presents to the emergency department for evaluation. Physical examination reveals a cardiac murmur and diffuse wheeze bilaterally heard most at the bronchi. Should he be found to have a gastrointestinal source for this problem, which of the following locations would be most likely?

(A) Appendix
(B) Cecum
(C) Descending colon
(D) Jejunum
(E) Sigmoid colon

The answer is A: **Appendix.** This patient likely has carcinoid tumor. The most frequent location is in the appendix. Clinical manifestations include cutaneous flushing, watery diarrhea with abdominal cramps, bronchospasm, and valvular lesions of the right side of the heart. This is more common in young patients such as the one presented in this question.

(B) Cecum is not the most common location for carcinoid tumors. (C) Descending colon is a common location for colorectal carcinoma. (D) Approximately 30% of carcinoids localize to the small intestine. (E) The sigmoid colon is a common location for colorectal cancer and diverticular disease.

22 A 39-year-old woman with longstanding Crohn disease of the ileum and cecum undergoes robotic small bowel resection with extracorporeal anastomosis. The surgical specimen is sent to pathology for further analysis. Which of the following features would be noted upon histologic study of the specimen?

(A) Continuous involvement of the specimen with disease
(B) Ectopic colonic mucosa
(C) Mucosal involvement with inflammation
(D) Submucosal edema with elevation of surviving mucosa
(E) Thinning of the affected bowel segment with widening of the lumen

The answer is D: **Submucosal edema with elevation of surviving mucosa.** Patients with Crohn disease have characteristic pathologic findings. There is chronic inflammation of all layers of the intestinal wall. The involved segment is thickened with narrowing of the lumen. There is submucosal edema with elevation of the surviving mucosa producing a cobblestone appearance. There are skip lesions with segments of normal intestinal mucosa between the affected regions.

(A) There are skip lesions of normal mucosa in between diseased bowel segments. (B) Ectopic colonic mucosa is found in Meckel diverticulum. (C) Mucosal involvement with inflammation is found in ulcerative colitis. (E) The affected bowel is thickened with all layers of the intestinal wall involved and the lumen is narrowed.

 23 A 72-year-old woman with a history of atrial fibrillation presents to the emergency department with severe abdominal pain for the past 2 hours. She has a history of mild Alzheimer dementia but speaks clearly and communicates well despite her disease. The pain is most severe in the lower quadrants, particularly the left. It started abruptly with nausea and vomiting. Physical examination reveals minimal pain to palpation, no rebound tenderness, and blood in the rectal vault on digital rectal examination. What is the most likely diagnosis?

(A) Acute appendicitis
(B) Crohn disease
(C) Diverticulitis
(D) Mesenteric ischemia
(E) Ulcerative colitis

The answer is D: **Mesenteric ischemia.** Acute mesenteric ischemia occurs when the vascular supply to the intestines, usually the superior mesenteric artery, is compromised causing bowel infarction. It commonly presents with severe abdominal pain that is out of proportion to the abdominal examination.

This patient most likely had an arterial embolism from his underlying atrial fibrillation. An angiography is the best test to confirm the diagnosis.

(A) Appendicitis typically presents with right lower quadrant pain that radiates from the umbilicus. Rebound tenderness is commonly positive. (B) Crohn disease is a chronic disease that usually presents with abdominal pain and diarrhea. The pain on examination would be similar to the subjective pain described by the patient. (C) Diverticulitis is common in older individuals and often presents with left lower quadrant pain when there is a flare. However, the abdominal examination will also be positive for left lower quadrant pain. (E) Ulcerative colitis commonly presents with abdominal pain and bloody diarrhea. The pain on examination would be similar to the subjective pain described by the patient.

 24 An 86-year-old woman with Alzheimer dementia in a nursing home develops acute onset of colicky abdominal pain, nausea, and vomiting. She is poorly communicative due to the severity of the Alzheimer disease. She is brought to the emergency department for evaluation. Physical examination reveals significant left lower quadrant tenderness. Plain films of the abdomen reveal a dilated sigmoid colon. Barium enema reveals narrowing of the colon at a point of twisting. What is the most appropriate next step in the management of this patient?

(A) Decompression via sigmoidoscopy
(B) Intravenous ampicillin and gentamicin
(C) Intravenous methylprednisilone
(D) Laparoscopic sigmoid resection
(E) Peripheral parenteral nutrition via cephalic vein

The answer is A: Decompression via sigmoidoscopy. This patient has evidence of colonic volvulus. Specifically, the sigmoid colon has twisted around its mesentery. Patients often present with colicky abdominal pain. The typical patient is elderly and nursing homebound. Treatment involves nonoperative reduction via decompression with sigmoidoscopy.

(B) This volvulus must first be decompressed which is successful in 70% of cases. (C) Corticosteroids are not indicated in the management of sigmoid volvulus. (D) Sigmoid resection is not the first-line treatment in this condition. Decompression should be tried first. (E) Peripheral parenteral nutrition is not a first-line treatment for sigmoid volvulus. Further, it will only provide nutritional support and not treat the obstruction.

 25 A 52-year-old woman with a history of recurrent cellulitis of her right foot has been receiving an oral cephalosporin several times/day for the last 30 days. She began to take the medication up to 6 times/day because she felt that her symptoms were not improving. She presents to the emergency department for further evaluation and treatment. She complains of profuse watery diarrhea without blood or mucus and has crampy abdominal pain. Abdominal x-ray studies do not reveal any abdominal free air. *Clostridium difficile* toxin studies are sent to the laboratory and results are not yet available. What is the next step in the management of this patient?

(A) Change antibiotic to ampicillin
(B) Change antibiotic to clindamycin
(C) Corticosteroids, enema
(D) Corticosteroids, oral
(E) Discontinue cephalosporin

The answer is E: **Discontinue cephalosporin.** This patient has evidence of pseudomembranous colitis. This is an antibiotic-associated colitis where the antibiotic kills organisms that inhibit growth of *C. difficile*. The treatment is to immediately stop the offending antibiotic which in this case is the cephalosporin.

(A) Ampicillin is also implicated in causing pseudomembranous colitis, so this choice would worsen the current condition. (B) Clindamycin is a classic cause of pseudomembranous colitis and should also be avoided in this patient. (C) Corticosteroids are not indicated in the management of pseudomembranous colitis. (D) Corticosteroids are not indicated in the management of pseudomembranous colitis.

Hepatobiliary

1   A 65-year-old woman with liver cirrhosis is readmitted for symptomatic jaundice. On a complete metabolic panel, her total bilirubin level is 10.2 mg/dL. Her urine is found to contain an elevated level of urobilinogen as well. Name the correct pathway for bilirubin from the bloodstream into the urine.

(A) Serum bound bilirubin → Hepatic bound bilirubin → Hepatic conjugated bilirubin → Bile conjugated bilirubin → GI tract conjugated urobilinogen → GI tract free urobilinogen → Serum free urobilinogen → Urine free urobilinogen

(B) Serum bound bilirubin → Hepatic free bilirubin → Hepatic conjugated bilirubin → Bile conjugated bilirubin → GI tract conjugated bilirubin → GI tract free bilirubin → GI tract free urobilinogen → Serum free urobilinogen → Urine free urobilinogen

(C) Serum bound bilirubin → Hepatic free bilirubin → Hepatic conjugated bilirubin → Bile free bilirubin → GI tract free bilirubin → GI tract conjugated bilirubin → GI tract free urobilinogen → Serum free urobilinogen → Urine free urobilinogen

(D) Serum free bilirubin → Hepatic free bilirubin → Hepatic conjugated bilirubin → Bile conjugated bilirubin → GI tract conjugated bilirubin → GI tract free bilirubin → GI tract free urobilinogen → Serum free urobilinogen → Urine free urobilinogen

(E) Serum bound bilirubin → Hepatic free bilirubin → Hepatic conjugated bilirubin → Bile conjugated bilirubin → GI tract conjugated bilirubin → GI tract free bilirubin → GI tract conjugated urobilinogen → Serum free urobilinogen → Urine free urobilinogen

The answer is B: **Serum bound bilirubin → Hepatic free bilirubin → Hepatic conjugated bilirubin → Bile conjugated bilirubin → GI tract conjugated bilirubin → GI tract free bilirubin → GI tract free urobilinogen → Serum free urobilinogen → Urine free urobilinogen.**

Bilirubin is derived from the breakdown of hemoglobin. It then travels in the bloodstream bound to albumin, and enters the liver where it is conjugated to glucuronic acid. The glucuronidated bilirubin is secreted within the bile into the GI tract. Enteric bacteria deconjugate the bilirubin to urobilinogen. Most urobilinogen is further oxidized and reabsorbed into the enterohepatic circulation. Some of this reabsorbed urobilinogen is filtered into the urine, which gives urine its yellow color.

(A) Bilirubin is unbound from albumin when it enters the liver. (C) Bilirubin remains conjugated with glucuronic acid when it is secreted into the bile from the hepatocytes. (D) Bilirubin does not exist in an unbound form in the serum. (E) Urobilinogen is not reconjugated in the GI tract.

 2 A 45-year-old man with a history of cholecystitis who recently had a cholecystectomy presents to the emergency department with a 4-day history of shaking chills and a fever. He also complains of abdominal pain, which has been worsening. His body temperature is 39.1°C, and he has lost 5 kg since his surgery. On examination, he appears lethargic, and has tenderness in his right upper quadrant (RUQ) to palpation with no rebound tenderness. MRI is obtained and a representative image is shown in *Figure 8-1*.

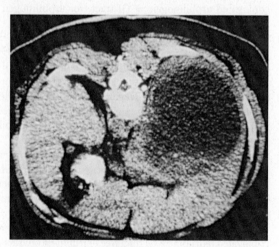

Figure 8-1

What is the treatment of choice?

(A) Surgical resection and antibiotics
(B) Percutaneous drainage only
(C) Antibiotics only
(D) Surgical resection
(E) Percutaneous drainage and antibiotics

The answer is E: **Percutaneous drainage and antibiotics.** Pyogenic liver abscesses mostly originate from infections of the GI or biliary tracts. Often patients have a recent history of an intraabdominal infection (appendicitis, cholecystitis, diverticulitis, infected pancreatitis/pancreatic abscess, and perinephric abscess. Patients present with fever, malaise, rigors, RUQ pain. 50% of patients have positive blood cultures. Diagnosis can be made by CT or MRI scan with 93% accuracy. The MRI shows a fluid-filled collection within the liver. The treatment of choice is percutaneous drainage with selective antibiotics.

(A) Surgery is not a treatment for pyogenic liver abscess. (B) Percutaneous drainage is the first step in treatment, but antibiotics are also required for adequate treatment. (C) Antibiotics alone are never the treatment for any bacterial abscess. (D) Surgery is not a treatment for pyogenic liver abscess.

---

3 A 55-year-old woman with a history of IV drug abuse presents to the emergency department with new onset vaginal bleeding. The patient has not seen a physician in many years, but says she stopped having periods "a few years ago." She described a 5-day history of "off and on bleeding down there," and started using pads again, up to 3 a day. She has a body temperature of 36.9°C, heart rate 95 beats/min, and blood pressure 134/72 mmHg. On examination, she is found to have more noticeable veins around her umbilicus. On pelvic examination, her cervix appears normal, but her vaginal mucosa appears bloody and friable. Blood tests are obtained, and she is found to have a hemoglobin level of 8.4 mg/dL, a platelet count of 190,000, and normal electrolyte levels. Her prothrombin time (PT) is 25 seconds, and her aspartate aminotransferase (AST) and alanine aminotransferase (ALT) are within normal limits. What is the next best step in the management of this patient?

(A) Vaginal packing, to be left in for at least 72 hours
(B) Vitamin K IM
(C) 1-unit pRBCs and vitamin K IM
(D) 1-unit FFP and vitamin K IM
(E) 1-unit pRBCs and 1-unit platelets

The answer is D: **1-unit FFP and vitamin K IM.** This patient's history of IV drug abuse along with an episode of acute bleeding with elevated PT indicates the presence of hepatic dysfunction secondary to chronic viral hepatitis. The most common etiology of cirrhosis in the United States is chronic hepatitis C infection. Initially, hepatitis can be detected by an elevated AST and ALT, but as the disease progresses these values can normalize with the aggregate loss of hepatocytes. At this stage, a prolonged PT/INR and low albumin are seen, which reflects a decrease in hepatic synthetic function. In fact, the presence of a prolonged PT which is refractory to vitamin K administration is the most specific indicator of decreased hepatic synthetic function. In any patient with mucosal bleeding and an elevated PT, the treatment of choice is fresh frozen plasma (FFP) and vitamin K. FFP contains clotting factors for immediate hemostasis, as vitamin K takes 5 to 7 days to boost the production of clotting factors 2, 7, 9, and 10.

(A) Vaginal packing may be used acutely to stop gross bleeding, but leaving it in more than 24 hours increases the risk of staph toxic shock. (B) Vitamin K does not help in the treatment of acute hemorrhage secondary to prolonged PT. (C) Blood transfusion is not indicated for patients with hemoglobin over 7.0 mg/dL (outside of the setting of large gross hemorrhaging). Again, vitamin K does not help in the management of hemorrhage with prolonged PT. (E) This patient does not require either a RBC or platelet transfusion.

 4 A 45-year-old man presents to his primary care physician with a new complaint of right shoulder pain. He denies any trauma or change in activity. He also states that he has been getting sweaty at night, and actually thinks he lost 10 pounds in the last month. He works as a salesman, and has traveled to many countries over the years, sometimes returning with traveler's diarrhea. He currently has a body temperature of 38.1°C, heart rate 96 beats/min, blood pressure 129/84 mmHg. On examination, he has a soft abdomen, which is tender to deep palpation in the RUQ. He has hepatomegaly. A RUQ ultrasound is obtained, which shows a solitary, space occupying echogenic lesion in the right hepatic lobe. What is the initial treatment of choice?

(A) Metronidazole
(B) Percutaneous drainage
(C) Mebendazole
(D) Surgical excision
(E) Broad-spectrum antibiotics IV

The answer is A: Metronidazole PO. Amebic liver abscess is the most common complication of invasive amebiasis, which is caused by the protozoan *Entamoeba histolytica*. It is a common cause of dysentery, especially in poorer communities in the tropics. This patient's international travel puts him at risk of acquiring this infection. The parasites penetrate the bowel, progress to the portal vein, and then end up forming an abscess in the liver. These are seen as space-occupying echogenicities on ultrasound. The first-line treatment is oral metronidazole for 10 days.

(B) Percutaneous drainage is indicated in the case where antibiotic treatment fails to clear the infection. It is not a part of initial therapy. (C) Mebendazole is the treatment for hydatid cysts. (D) Surgical excision is not indicated for amebic abscesses. (E) Broad-spectrum antibiotics IV are not used to treat amebic liver abscesses.

 5 A 32-year-old woman who recently emigrated from Nicaragua presents to the emergency department with new onset abdominal pain.

The pain is constant and located in the RUQ. On examination, her abdomen is soft, tender to palpation in the RUQ, and hepatomegaly with a palpable mass. A RUQ ultrasound is obtained which shows a multiple small cysts within a large cystic mass with a hyperechoic rim. What is the treatment of choice?

(A) Percutaneous aspiration
(B) Mebendazole
(C) Metronidazole
(D) Focused radiation
(E) Embolization

The answer is B: Mebendazole PO. Hytadid cysts are caused by Echinococcal tapeworms, which are commonly found in dogs, especially in Central and South America. These fluid-filled structures are often asymptomatic, and are most commonly located in the liver. They also can present with RUQ pain and hepatomegaly. Serology specific for echinococcal antigens is positive in 90% of cases. These cysts often have calcified walls and several smaller daughter cysts within. Diagnosis can be made with aid of RUQ ultrasound or abdominal CT scan. Treatment of cysts involves antihelminthic therapy (mebendazole, praziquantel, or albendazole).

(A) Hytadid cysts should not be aspirated. Aspiration runs the risk of spillage causing an anaphylactic reaction, as well as spillage can cause spread of the parasite and development of new cysts. (C) Metronidazole is the treatment of choice of an amebic liver abscess, not a hytadid cyst. (D) Radiation has no role in the treatment of hytadid cysts. (E) Embolization can be used in the case of a hemorrhaging adenoma, but not for a hytadid cyst.

6 A 34-year-old woman presents to you as a referral for a 3-cm solitary liver lesion on ultrasound. She was previously evaluated by her PCP for abdominal pain, who ordered a RUQ ultrasound for suspected cholelithiasis. She is otherwise healthy, only taking synthroid for hypothyroidism and an oral contraceptive. On examination, her abdomen is soft, nondistended, nontender, with no palpable masses. Her PCP also ordered a complete blood count (CBC), serum electrolytes (BMP), and alfafetoprotein (AFP), which were unremarkable. She is very concerned about the ultrasound finding, as she looked it up online and found several links about cancer. You order her an abdominal MRI which is shown in *Figures 8-2A and B*.

What is the best course of management for this lesion?

(A) Observation with a repeat ultrasound in 6 months
(B) Discontinuation of oral contraceptives
(C) Embolization
(D) Obtain a percutaneous biopsy of the adenoma
(E) Surgical excision

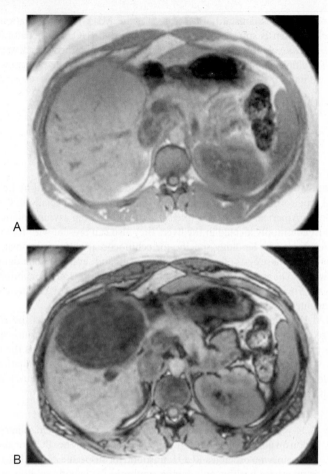

Figure 8-2

The answer is B: Discontinuation of oral contraceptives. Hepatic adenomas are solid lesions seen primarily in women of childbearing age. It is more likely in women with history of oral contraceptive or high-dose estrogen use. About half of cases will present with RUQ abdominal pain due to local compression. Rarely, they can present with hemorrhage into the tumor, and even present as hypotension and shock from intraperitoneal bleeding. Smaller adenomas can be observed, but adenomas often will regress with the cessation of oral contraceptives.

(A) Observation with follow-up ultrasounds is appropriate for asymptomatic tumors under 5 cm, yet for this patient discontinuing oral contraceptive pills (OCPs) is a better choice. (C) Embolization can be performed in the case of an exsanguinating adenoma, which this patient is not experiencing. (D) Hepatic adenomas are vascular structures which should not be biopsied as it can cause heavy bleeding. (E) Surgery is indicated for adenomas over 5 cm in size, presence of an adenoma with an increasing alfafetoprotein (AFP), or an adenoma with irregular borders—as these findings are indicative of malignant transformation.

7 A 29-year-old woman is referred for a solitary liver lesion incidentally found on a CT scan. The patient recently had a bout of acute abdominal pain and was evaluated in the emergency department where the scan was obtained. She is presently asymptomatic. Her abdominal is soft and non-tender on examination, with no masses palpated. Her most recent liver function tests were within the normal range. According to the radiology report, the lesion shows a classic stellate scar pattern. What is the diagnosis?

(A) Cavernous hemangioma
(B) Hepatic adenoma
(C) Focal nodular hyperplasia
(D) Hepatocellular carcinoma
(E) Fibrolamellar carcinoma

The answer is C: **Focal nodular hyperplasia.** Focal nodular hyperplasias are nonneoplastic solid tumors characterized by the "central stellate scar" pattern, which is a central fibrous scar with radiating septa. They are often lobulated and are sharply demarcated from normal liver. They are usually ~5 cm in size. These lesions are often asymptomatic, and no abnormalities are found on physical examination or on liver function tests. Diagnosis is made with CT or MRI finding this classic central scar in a solid liver tumor. These lesions do not need to be treated, unless they are very symptomatic.

(A) Cavernous hemangiomas do not have a stellate pattern, and appear very vascular on MRI, with high T2 signal density. (B) Hepatic adenomas are solid hepatic tumors which lack a stellate pattern. (D) Hepatocellular carcinoma are neoplastic encapsulated tumors which can vary in its appearance, from small and uniform, to larger and mosaic with hemorrhage or necrosis. (E) Fibrola-mellar carcinoma is a rare hepatic neoplasm which can resemble FNH, but it enhances more homogenously with contrast and on MRI is hypointense on T2.

8 A 3-month-old infant presents to the emergency department with new onset jaundice. The child previously had been gaining weight and breastfeeding well. He, however, developed jaundice over the past week. He appears "fussy," and has a body temperature of 37.4°C. On examination, his abdomen is firm and distended. A serum liver profile is obtained which shows a total bilirubin of 14.1, and a direct bilirubin of 12.0. aspartate aminotransferase (AST) and ALT are mildly elevated. A CT scan is obtained, which is shown in *Figure 8-3*.

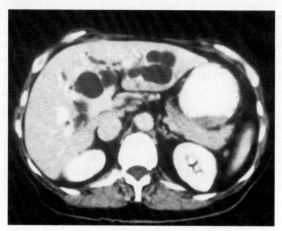

Figure 8-3

What is the treatment of choice?

(A) UV phototherapy
(B) Switch from breast to hydrolyzed formula feeding
(C) Hepaticojejunostomy with excision of the cystic structures
(D) ERCP
(E) Observation

The answer is C: Hepaticojejunostomy with excision of the cystic structures. Cholechodal cyst is a cystic dilatation of the common bile duct or the biliary tree. Most of them present in the first year of life, with symptoms such as jaundice, fever, or abdominal distension. The cystic nature of the common bile duct is not known, but may be due to an anomalous pancreaticobiliary ductal system, allowing for the reflux of pancreatic enzymes into the developing biliary tract. The abnormal dilation of the CBD can be detected on abdominal CT. The treatment of choice is surgical—a radical excision of all cystic parts of the biliary tract with hepaticojejunostomy.

(A) UV phototherapy is the treatment for physiologic jaundice in a neonate, where limited hepatic function in the newborn leads to an unconjugated hyperbilirubinemia. (B) Switching to a hydrolyzed formula is indicated in infants with potential milk allergies. It has no role in this patient. (D) endoscopic retrograde cholangiopancreatography (ERCP) is an indicated procedure for choledocolithiasis in order to rapidly decompress the biliary tree. It has no role in this patient. (E) Observation is indicated in the situation of breastfeeding jaundice, where time and increased feeding can resolve the jaundice.

---

9 A 67-year-old man returns to clinic for continued management of chronic hepatitis C. He has no new complaints, other than "my belly has been really big, as usual." His abdomen is soft, protuberant, non-tender, with an observable fluid wave. His periumbilical veins are very noticeable, as well as a few "spider-like" red lesions on his trunk. His most recent blood tests show a normal aspartate aminotransferase (AST) and ALT, but prolonged PT and albumin of 1.5 mg/dL. After reading more about his condition, he is concerned about the possibility of "throwing up blood." What is the best next step to prevent this?

(A) Start a high protein diet
(B) Start propranolol
(C) Start vasopressin
(D) Start octreotide
(E) Undergo a TIPS procedure

The answer is B: Start propranolol. This patient is known to have chronic hepatitis C, along with multiple physical findings of portal hypertension. In addition, his labs indicate he has advanced cirrhosis, as his AST and ALT have normalized due to compound cellular loss. In patients with cirrhosis, the best way to prevent esophageal variceal rupture is daily β-blockade, with a medication like propranolol.

(A) A high protein diet would not prevent esophageal varices, but may help his albumin somewhat. (C) Vasopressin is used in the acute management of an esophageal variceal rupture via vasoconstriction of splanchnic vasculature. It has no role in prevention. (D) Octreotide is a synthetic somatostatin analogue, which is also used in the acute management of esophageal variceal rupture. (E) Transjugular intrahepatic portosystemic shunting (TIPS) is an invasive procedure that is reserved for patients with a severely acute or refractory esophageal variceal hemorrhage.

10) A 58-year-old man with a history of chronic liver disease and a history of hematemesis is evaluated for an acute mental status change. He is disoriented and unable to give a history. His caretaker denies that any trauma or intoxication has occurred. On examination, he appears older than his stated age, with apparent caput medusae on his protuberant abdomen. His blood is found to have elevated serum ammonia. You are evaluating him for a portal systemic shunt to decrease the sequelae of portal hypertension. What is the maximum portal system pressure intended to prevent bleeding complications?

(A) 12 mmHg
(B) 15 mmHg
(C) 10 mmHg
(D) 8 mmHg
(E) 20 mmHg

The answer is A: 12 mmHg. Portal hypertension arises from an increase in the intrahepatic vascular resistance, leading to an increase in the portal system's blood pressure. This increased pressure leads to the increase in collateral flow to the systemic venous circulation, leading to the development of esophageal varices, hemorrhoids, and caput medusae. First-line treatment for the prevention of variceal rupture is a nonselective β-blocker or a nitrate. In the case of severe or refractory variceal rupture, portal systemic shunting procedures can be done to decrease the pressure in the portal system. The goal is to decrease the portal pressure to be 12 mmHg or less.

(B) The target maximum portal pressure is 12, not 15 mmHg. (C) The target maximum portal pressure is 12, not 10 mmHg. (D) The target maximum portal pressure is 12, not 8 mmHg. (E) The target maximum portal pressure is 12, not 20 mmHg.

---

11   A 40-year-old Thai woman with end-stage liver disease returns to your clinic with recurrent symptoms of portal hypertension. She is fatigued, and unhappy with the size of her "huge belly." On examination, she is jaundiced, her abdomen is distended with a fluid wave, and some red skin lesions are also prominent. She is on lactulose therapy for encephalopathy secondary to hyperammonemia. She has a history of two episodes of hematemesis from bleeding esophageal varices in the last few years. Her most recent blood tests show a total bilirubin of 35 mg/dL, serum albumin of 2.5 g/dL, and INR of 1.90. What is the best treatment to maximize her long-term survival?

(A) Propranolol
(B) Transjugular intrahepatic portosystemic shunt
(C) Liver transplant
(D) Interferon-α
(E) Distal splenorenal shunt

The answer is C: Liver transplant. This patient has signs and symptoms of liver failure (jaundice, has ascites, has spider angiomata, has esophageal varices). The best course of management of liver failure depends on the patient's age, Child-Pugh score, and history of variceal hemorrhage. Based on her young age, her Childs Class C disease (based on her bilirubin, albumin, INR, refractory ascites, and moderate hepatic encephalopathy), and her history of esophageal variceal hemorrhage, she would best benefit from a liver transplant.

(A) Propranolol therapy decreases the risk of esophageal variceal hemorrhage, therefore decreasing mortality. However this patient's liver failure makes transplant a better treatment. (B) A TIPS procedure is great for decreasing the risk of esophageal variceal hemorrhage, but again does not address the liver failure this patient has. (D) Interferon-α is used as a treatment for chronic hepatitis B. It has no role in the treatment of liver failure (although this patient may have hepatitis B based on her nationality). (E) A DSRS procedure is also for portal hypertension and decreasing the risk of esophageal variceal rupture. It is sometimes used to preserve central venous anatomy for a later transplant.

12 A 48-year-old Bulgarian man presents to your clinic with a complaint of feeling "run down." He is not sure when it started, but gradually he has felt more fatigued and has dropped some weight. He admits he feels puzzled, as his stomach is much larger than it used to be. On abdominal examination, his abdomen is soft, protuberant, with a palpable fluid wave. His blood tests reveal an elevated alfa-fetoprotein (AFP), although his aspartate aminotransferase (AST) and ALT are not elevated. He obtains an abdominal MRI which is shown in *Figures 8-4A and B.*

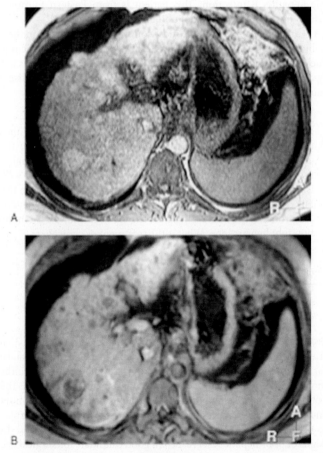

Figure 8-4

What is the most likely cause of this mass?

(A) Chronic hepatitis C
(B) Chronic hepatitis A
(C) Nonalcoholic steatohepatitis (NASH)
(D) Wilson disease
(E) Chronic hepatitis B

The answer is E: Chronic hepatitis B. This patient has hallmarks of liver malignancy: fatigue, weight loss, abdominal swelling. He has an elevated α-fetoprotein, which is associated with hepatocellular carcinoma. In addition, his abdominal MRI shows a single liver mass. There are many causes of hepatocellular carcinoma (HCC), but the most common worldwide is chronic hepatitis B infection. This patient is from Eastern Europe, where hepatitis B immunizations are not ubiquitous.

(A) Chronic hepatitis C is the most common cause of HCC in the United States, but not worldwide. (B) Hepatitis A does not cause a chronic infection, nor does it cause HCC. (C) NASH is a cause of cirrhosis, but it does not commonly cause HCC. (D) Wilson disease is a cause of chronic liver disease, but does not commonly cause HCC.

---

(13) A 50-year-old man returns for a follow-up appointment for the evaluation of an abdominal mass. He continues to have pain in the right upper part of his abdomen. He also complains of some malaise, but thinks he may be not sleeping well. He appears anxious, but well nourished. On abdominal examination, there is a palpable mass in the RUQ. His complete blood count (CBC) is normal, but he does have an alfa-fetoprotein (AFP) on 450 ng/mL. The CT scan shows a 3-cm tumor in the right hepatic lobe. What is the treatment of choice?

(A) Surgical wedge resection
(B) Liver transplant
(C) Chemotherapy
(D) Microwave ablation
(E) External beam radiation

The answer is A: Surgical wedge resection. This patient has a 3-cm liver tumor with an elevated AFP, which point to hepatocellular carcinoma. Hepatocellular carcinoma is almost always caused by chronic liver disease. The most common etiology in the United States is chronic hepatitis C infection. The treatment of hepatocellular carcinoma (HCC) depends on the size of the tumor and the amount of hepatic reserve after surgical resection. In any case, surgical excision is the optimal therapy. Since this patient has a small tumor and does not have signs of poor hepatic reserve, he is a good candidate for surgical excision.

(B) Liver transplantation can also be considered in his patient, as it can be curative of HCC for smaller tumors; but it is second line to excision due to side effects of transplant. (C) Chemotherapy is used adjuvantly or neoadjuvantly to surgical excision; chemotherapy alone does not improve survival. (D) Microwave ablation is used to provide local control or palliation in patients that have poor hepatic reserve and cannot undergo surgical excision. (E) Radiation has no role for the treatment of HCC.

14 A 65-year-old woman presents to her primary care physician with new complaints of fatigue and unintentional weight loss. She is unsure of when her fatigue started, and claims to have lost 10 pounds in the last 6 months. On examination, she appears thin and pale. Her lungs are clear to auscultation bilaterally. Her abdomen is soft, nondistended, and nontender to palpation. She undergoes a rectal examination, and is found to have positive stool occult. Recent lab tests reveal Hb of 9.4 mg/dL. She has never had a colonoscopy, and declines getting one. She is sent for an abdominal CT scan which reveals a tumor in the proximal ascending colon, as well as two small liver masses in the superior right lobe. What is the best initial treatment for the liver masses?

(A) Cryoablation
(B) Multidrug systemic chemotherapy
(C) Surgical excision
(D) External beam radiation
(E) Hepatic artery chemotherapy infusion

The answer is C: Surgical excision. This patient presents with fatigue secondary to malignancy and anemia from occult blood loss in the stool. Her weight loss is also a common symptom of malignancy. From the CT scan, it seems that the primary tumor is colonic in origin, and there are two liver lesions which are most likely metastasis from the colon. The treatment of liver metastatic lesions depends on the location, size, and number of lesions. For this patient, she has a small number of lesions, which are small in size, and are localized in a favorable location for surgical resection. Therefore surgical excision is the best treatment for her liver metastases.

(A) Cryoablation is reserved for palliation and destruction of active disease in that region. However, it does not improve long-term survival. (B) Multidrug systemic chemotherapy is first line for unresectable tumors. It has an important role in both adjuvant and neoadjuvant therapy of colorectal liver metastases. (D) External beam radiation also can be used for local control of active cancer, but it is also for unresectable disease. (E) Hepatic artery chemotherapy infusion is reserved for unresectable liver metastases.

15 A 57-year-old woman presents to the emergency department with severe abdominal pain of 2 hours duration. It began 30 minutes after she had a large burger with fries for dinner. She also complains of feeling very bloated, which she claims to have regularly after eating. She is afebrile, and her abdomen is benign on examination. A RUQ ultrasound is obtained, which reveals several stones in the gallbladder. The arterial supply to gallbladder is via the cystic artery, which is a branch off of which artery?

(A) Common hepatic artery
(B) Proper hepatic artery
(C) Left hepatic artery
(D) Gastroduodenal artery
(E) Right hepatic artery

The answer is E: **Right hepatic artery.** The blood supply to the gallbladder originally comes through the common hepatic artery off of the celiac trunk (which has three initial branches: left gastric artery, splenic artery, and common hepatic artery). Continuing toward the gallbladder, the common hepatic artery branches into the proper hepatic artery (its other branches are the gastroduodenal artery and the right gastric artery). The proper hepatic artery then travels with the portal vein and the common bile duct toward the liver. It then bifurcates to give rise to the right and left hepatic arteries. The cystic artery is a branch off of the right hepatic artery.

(A) The common hepatic artery branches into proper hepatic artery, the gastroduodenal artery, and the right gastric artery. (B) The proper hepatic artery gives rise to the right and left hepatic arteries. (C) The left hepatic artery supplies the left lobe of the liver—it does not give rise to the cystic artery. (D) The gastroduodenal artery gives rise to the right gastroepiploic artery, the superior pancreaticoduodenal artery, and the supraduodenal artery.

---

 16 A 52-year-old man calls his family physician in the evening complaining of new abdominal pain. The patient just had a large chicken dinner, after which the pain came on pretty quick. The patient also complains of bloating. The patient says his body temperature is 99.2°F. The physician tells the man to go to the emergency department if he develops a fever or the pain gets worse, as he is worried about the patient developing an inflamed gallbladder. What hormone is responsible for gallbladder contraction that causes this patient's symptoms?

(A) Secretin
(B) Cholecystokinin
(C) Somatostatin
(D) Gastrin
(E) Vasoactive intestinal peptide

The answer is B: **Cholecystokinin.** The function of the gallbladder is the storage and concentration of bile (via absorption of water and solute). It also aids in the delivery of bile, which emulsifies fats to aid in the digestion of lipids.

The gallbladder contracts when stimulated by the arrival of fatty contents into the duodenum. Gallbladder contractility is controlled by both hormones and the autonomic nervous system. The main hormone that stimulates gallbladder contraction is cholecystokinin.

(A) Secretin acts to increase the amount of water and bicarbonate released from the pancreas and bile duct epithelium in order to buffer the acidic gastric contents. (C) Somatostatin acts to decrease the rate of gastric emptying and the release of many GI hormones. (D) Gastrin acts to increase the amount of HCl secreted by the gastric parietal cells. (E) VIP acts to increase the amount of water and electrolytes secreted into the intestinal lumen. It also actually induces relaxation, not contraction, of the gallbladder.

 A 49-year-old woman presents to her primary care physician with a chief complaint of abdominal pain. Upon further questioning, it is revealed that this patient's pain is mostly in the right upper portion of her abdomen, and that it is worse after big meals. The physician orders a RUQ ultrasound, which shows several gallstones. Which comorbid condition increases the likelihood that these are black pigment stones?

(A) Biliary dysmotility
(B) Hemolytic anemia
(C) Chronic parasitic infections
(D) Hypocalcemia
(E) Anemia of chronic disease

The answer is B: **Hemolytic anemia.** Gallstones form from the precipitation of bile solutes to form solid aggregates. There are two main types of gallstones: cholesterol stones and pigment stones. 70% to 80% of all gallstones are cholesterol stones, and the remaining 20% to 30% of stones are pigment stones. There are two types of pigment stones: black and brown. Black pigment stones consist of calcium bilirubinate and calcium palmitate. They are frequently small and multiple. Two risk factors for the development of black pigment stones are cirrhosis and hemolytic anemia.

(A) Biliary dysmotility is a risk factor for the formation of all types of gallstones, and does not increase the likelihood of black pigment stones. (C) Chronic parasitic infection increases the chance of forming brown pigment stones. (D) Hypocalcemia is not associated with an increased chance of developing gallstones. (E) Anemia of chronic disease is not associated with the formation of gallstones.

 A 48-year-old woman presents to emergency department with a 2-hour history of nausea and abdominal pain. She has felt this pain before, but never this bad. Previous pain episodes occurred in the evening, especially on Sunday nights after going to a steakhouse. During these episodes, she also has felt bloated and occasionally nauseous. The pain usually remits after a few hours. She currently is afebrile and in no acute distress. On examination, her abdomen is mildly distended, and she exhibits some tenderness to palpation. Her complete blood count (CBC) reveals a WBC count of 9,400/μL and a hematocrit of 42. A RUQ ultrasound reveals the presence of gallstones. What is the best next step in the management of this patient?

(A) Percutaneous cholecystostomy
(B) Endoscopic retrograde cholangiopancreatography (ERCP)
(C) Prescribe motrin and phenergen
(D) Laproscopic cholecystectomy
(E) Open cholecystectomy

The answer is C: **Prescribe motrin and phenergen.** This patient has a history of episodic postprandial pain RUQ pain along with the presence of gallstones. Although this patient is having symptoms, the patient is afebrile and has a normal WBC count. This indicates that the patient most likely does not have cholecystitis, but instead symptomatic cholelithiasis. The initial treatment for symptomatic cholelithiasis is supportive, with NSAIDs and antiemetics. A cholecystectomy is indicated, but is not required urgently. It can be performed at a later time.

(A) A cholecystostomy is performed in the case of cholecystitis in a poor surgical candidate. (B) ERCP is a minimally invasive procedure performed to visualize the anatomy of the pancreatic duct and biliary tree. In the case of a gallstone obstructing the common bile duct, a sphincterotomy and stone removal can be performed to decompress the biliary tree. (D) A laproscopic cholecystectomy is indicated in the treatment of cholelithiasis, but it does not need to be performed emergently and instead as an outpatient. (E) An open cholecystectomy may be performed, but again immediate surgery is not required in the case of cholelithiasis.

19. A 53-year-old man presents to the emergency department with a 4-hour history of intense abdominal pain. The pain came on quickly and was colicky at first. The pain is now more constant in the upper abdomen. In addition, he complains of nausea and some right shoulder soreness, which he thinks is due to his golf game. His is febrile, with a body temperature of 38.7°C, and is persistently tachycardic. On examination, he appears in some distress. His abdomen is distended and tender to palpation, especially in the right upper quadrant. His labs show that he has a WBC count of 15,100/μL. A RUQ ultrasound is obtained which shows a thickening of the gallbladder wall and the presence of gallstones. Despite the potential danger, the patient decided to sign out against medical advice. Three days later, he returns to the emergency department with continued abdominal pain. What is the best next step in management?

(A) Urgent cholecystectomy
(B) Conservative medical therapy only
(C) Urgent cholecystostomy
(D) Endoscopic retrograde cholangiopancreatography
(E) Conservative medical therapy followed by elective cholecystectomy

The answer is E: **Conservative medical therapy followed by elective cholecystectomy.** Acute cholecystitis is an inflammation of the gallbladder usually secondary to occlusion of the cystic duct by a gallstone. This can lead to secondary infection by gram-negative bacteria, most commonly *E. coli*. Patients present with RUQ pain and fever. Patients may also have an elevated WBC count. Diagnosis can be made by RUQ ultrasound or HIDA scan. Surgical management of cholecystitis is recommended within 3 days of the initial inflammatory response. If symptoms have been present for more than 3 days prior to presentation, conservative medical management with IV fluids and antibiotics is recommended initially, followed by an elective cholecystectomy 4 to 6 weeks later.

(A) Early cholecystectomy is recommended if patients present within 3 days of the onset of symptoms. (B) Conservative medical therapy is the first step in management, but later elective surgery is also recommended. (D) Cholecystostomy is recommended for poor surgical candidates. (E) ERCP is indicated for obstruction of the common bile duct or pancreatic duct, and is not a treatment for cholecystitis.

 20 A 58-year-old man follows up with his general surgeon with another episode of abdominal pain related to gallstones. His abdominal pain is episodic, especially after a large meal. The pain is nonradiating and is located in the right upper abdomen. He is afebrile, and his abdomen is mildly tender to palpation. The surgeon recommends an elective cholecystectomy. What is/are the advantage/s of a laproscopic cholecystectomy over an open cholecystectomy?

(A) Shorter hospital stay and decreased mortality
(B) Shorter hospital stay and decreased morbidity
(C) Decreased morbidity and decreased mortality
(D) Shorter hospital stay only
(E) Decreased mortality only

The answer is B: **Shorter hospital stay and decreased morbidity.** The treatment of symptomatic cholecystitis is an elective cholecystectomy. There are two main types of cholecystectomy: laproscopic and open. The advantages of laproscopic cholecystectomy are shorter hospital stay and decreased morbidity. The hospital stay is shortened as the procedure is less invasive. The morbidity is decreased as the surgical sounds are smaller.

(A) There is no mortality benefit from the laproscopic approach. (C) There is no mortality benefit from the laproscopic approach. (D) There is a shortened hospital stay, but also a decrease in morbidity. (E) There is no mortality benefit from the laproscopic approach.

21 A 61-year-old woman presents to the emergency department with acute abdominal pain and general malaise. She has been experiencing fevers with shaking chills for the past 12 hours, in addition to her constant abdominal pain. Vital signs are as follows: body temperature is 38.9°C, heart rate 113 beats/min, blood pressure 105/60 mmHg, and respiratory rate of 19 breaths/min. She appears anxious. Her eyes are sunken and her mucous membranes appear dry. Her abdomen is distended, guarded, and tender to palpation in the upper abdomen. Her labs show an elevated WBC count, as well as a lactic acid of 2.4 mmol/L. CT scan is obtained and reveals air in the bladder with thickening of the gall bladder wall and pericholecystic fluid. What is the next most appropriate step in the management of this patient?

(A) Laparoscopic cholecystectomy
(B) Percutaneous cholecystostomy
(C) Intravenous fluid bolus
(D) Broad-spectrum antibiotics
(E) Endoscopic retrograde cholangiopancreatography (ERCP)

The answer is C: Intravenous fluid bolus. Emphysematous cholecystitis is caused by an infection by gas forming bacteria (*E. coli*, *Enterococcus*, *Klebsiella*, or *Clostridia* sp.). These patients are commonly diabetic, and present with RUQ pain and sepsis. The treatment of emphysematous cholecystitis first is IV fluids. These are required to replenish any dehydration and more importantly address the sepsis.

(A) Laparoscopic cholecystectomy is indicated to remove the source of the infection, but the sepsis needs to be addressed first with IV fluids. (B) Percutaneous cholecystostomy is indicated for poor surgical candidates to decompress the gallbladder initially, to be followed by a cholecystectomy in 4 to 6 weeks. (D) Broad-spectrum antibiotics are also imperative in the treatment of emphysematous cholecystitis, but IV fluids should be started first. (E) ERCP can be used to assess for blockage of the common bile duct, but it is to follow the acute treatment of sepsis with IV fluids.

22 A 47-year-old man is brought to the emergency department with new onset somnolence. He was previously healthy, but over the last few days became progressively fatigued. He developed upper abdominal "cramping" over this time, which has been worsening in severity. His wife said he had a body temperature of 101.2°F before she brought him in. His body temperature is 38.7°C, heart rate is 104 beats/min, and blood pressure is 103/53 mmHg. On examination, he appears somnolent and jaundiced. His abdomen is guarded and nondistended. He grimaces when his upper abdomen is palpated, especially on the right side. His complete blood count (CBC) shows a WBC count of 15.2 and a serum hematocrit (HCT) of 41. A hepatic profile (CPM) is obtained, showing a total bilirubin of 8.2 mg/dL and alkaline phosphatase of 350 U/L. What is the best treatment for this condition?

(A) Intravenous fluids and antibiotics
(B) Intravenous fluids, antibiotics, and laparoscopic cholecystectomy
(C) Intravenous fluids, antibiotics, and open cholecystectomy
(D) Intravenous fluids, antibiotics, and endoscopic retrograde cholangiopancreatography
(E) Intravenous fluids and endoscopic retrograde cholangiopancreatography

The answer is D: **Intravenous fluids, antibiotics, and endoscopic retrograde cholangiopancreatography.** Ascending cholangitis is a bacterial infection of the biliary ductal system, due to ductal obstruction leading to increased bacteria in the bile. Causes of cholangitis include choledocholithiasis, benign stricture, or tumors. The classic presentation of ascending cholangitis is *Charcot triad* (fever, RUQ pain, and jaundice). In severe presentations, the addition of mental status change and hypotension yields *Reynolds pentad*. Initial management involves fluids resuscitation and empiric IV antibiotics. The next step is decompression of the biliary tree, which is achieved with either percutaneous transhepatic cholangiography or endoscopic retrograde cholangiopancreatography. In the case of choledocholithiasis, cholecystectomy is indicated once the patient is stabilized to prevent recurrence.

(A) Intravenous fluids and antibiotics alone will not address the built-up pressure in the biliary tree. (B) Cholecystectomy is not indicated for the acute treatment of cholangitis; endoscopic retrograde cholangiopancreatography (ERCP) or percutaneous transhepatic cholangiography (PTHC) is preferred over surgical intervention. (C) Cholecystectomy is not indicated for the acute treatment of cholangitis; ERCP or PTHC is preferred over surgical intervention. (E) Empiric intravenous antibiotics are indicated to treat the infection in the biliary tree, especially in this case where the patient presents with sepsis.

---

 23 A 41-year-old man presents to his primary care physician with recent weight loss. He has lost 10 pounds in the last 2 months, which he finds strange as "my bowels haven't flared up in 4 years." He also complains of some pruritus, which has come on rather insidiously. On review of systems, he declines any fevers, pain, SOB, or N/V/D. But he does recall that he has been feeling "tired lately." He is afebrile and his vital signs are stable. On physical examination, he appears healthy and in no distress. He does not appear jaundiced, but there is some mild scleral icterus.

The rest of his physical examination is unremarkable. Blood tests are ordered, which reveal an unremarkable complete blood count (CBC). But his basic metabolic profile reveals an elevated alkaline phosphatase and a total bilirubin of 4.7. Based on his history of inflammatory bowel disease, he obtains a magnetic resonance cholangiopancreatography to evaluate him for possible primary sclerosing cholangitis. What anatomic finding on magnetic resonance cholangiopancreatography (MRCP) is characteristic of this condition?

(A) Bile duct has alternating areas of dilation and stricture, appearing beaded
(B) Proximal bile duct is dilated and distal bile duct is narrow
(C) Dilation of common bile duct and pancreatic duct (double duct sign)
(D) Dilated common bile duct with filling defects within the duct
(E) Ectasia of pancreatic duct branches

The answer is A: Bile duct has alternating areas of dilation and stricture, appearing beaded. Primary sclerosing cholangitis is a chronic progressive cholestatic disease. It is an autoimmune inflammatory process which targets the intrahepatic and extrahepatic bile ducts leading to strictures. It is associated with inflammatory bowel disease, with 85% having ulcerative colitis and 15% having Crohn disease. Men are affected more than women, with peak incidence in the fourth decade of life. Patients present with signs/symptoms of biliary obstruction, jaundice, pruritus, weight loss, and fatigue. Diagnosis is based on the presence of cholestasis as well as cirrhosis noted on liver biopsy. Endoscopic retrograde cholangiopancreatography (ERCP) or magnetic resonance cholangiopancreatography (MRCP) can be performed, which show the characteristic beaded appearance of the bile ducts due to areas of strictures and dilatation.

(B) Proximal dilation is associated with a single stricture, obstructing stone, or tumor. (C) Double duct sign is highly suggestive of a tumor at the head of the pancreas. (D) Dilated common duct with filling defects is associated with choledocholithiasis, with the filling defects representing the stones. (E) Ectasia of branches of the pancreatic duct is associated with chronic pancreatitis.

24 A 64-year-old woman presents to her physician with chronic upper abdominal pain. The pain has increased over the last 2 weeks. She has lost 20 pounds unintentionally in the last 3 months. Physical examination reveals a palpable abdominal mass in the right upper quadrant. Her labs are unremarkable. An abdominal CT scan reveals a mass in the gallbladder without evidence of lymphadenopathy. An open cholecystectomy is performed, and the gallbladder is sent for frozen section. The results show gallbladder adenocarcinoma, with tumor invasion into the perimuscular fibrous tissue. What is the next step in treatment of this patient?

(A) No further treatment required

(B) Biopsy of the sentinel lymph node

(C) Extended resection of adjacent liver tissue with a 2-cm margin with lymphadenectomy

(D) Extended resection of adjacent liver tissue with a 1-cm margin only

(E) Extended resection of adjacent liver tissue with a 1-cm margin with lymphadenectomy

The answer is C: Extended resection of adjacent liver tissue with a 2-cm margin with lymphadenectomy. Gallbladder cancer is 90% adeno-carcinoma, and is more common in women, especially those with a history of gallstones. Other risk factors include Native American heritage, gallstones >2.5 cm, porcelain gallbladder, choledocho cysts, primary sclerosing chol-angitis, and cholecystoenteric fistula. At diagnosis, 25% are localized to the gallbladder, 25% have regional lymph node or organ metastasis, and 40% already have distant metastasis. Patients present with RUQ pain, often appear-ing similar to other biliary conditions. Other symptoms include weight loss, jaundice, and a RUQ abdominal mass (Courvoisier sign). Diagnosis can be made with RUQ ultrasound or abdominal CT. Management depends on the stage of the cancer. If the cancer is into the muscle or beyond, an additional resection with a 2-cm margin in the adjacent tissue is indicated with a regional lymphadenectomy.

(A) If the cancer is localized to the gallbladder (remains submucosal with no muscular invasion), open cholecystectomy is all that is required. (B) There is no role for a biopsy of Calot node in the management of gallbladder cancer. (D) In the case of the cancer spreading into the muscle of the gallbladder, a 2-cm margin is indicated, not 1 cm. In addition, a regional lymphadenectomy is also indicated. (E) In the case of the cancer spreading into the muscle of the gallbladder, a 2-cm margin is indicated, not 1 cm.

25 A 57-year-old woman presents to the emergency department with jaundice. She was previously healthy, but over the last months became progressively jaundiced. She developed upper abdominal cramping over the past 2 weeks, which has been worsening in sever-ity. She took her body temperature at home today, and found it to be 102°F. Her vital signs are as follows: body temperature is 38.9°C, heart rate is 91 beats/min, and blood pressure is 123/73 mmHg. She appears anxious. Her abdomen is soft and nondistended, but she is tender and guards when her upper abdomen is palpated, especially on the right side. Her complete blood count (CBC) shows a WBC count of 10.2 and a serum hematocrit (HCT) of 41. A basic meta-bolic profile is obtained, showing a total bilirubin of 6.2 mg/dL and alkaline phosphatase of 290 U/L. What is the initial diagnostic test of choice?

(A) Right upper quadrant ultrasound
(B) Abdominal CT scan
(C) Endoscopic retrograde cholangiopancreatography
(D) Magnetic resonance cholangiopancreatography (MRCP)
(E) Hepatobiliary iminodiacetic acid scan

The answer is B: Abdominal CT scan. The patient is presenting with a cholangiocarcinoma, which is a cancer originating in the biliary tree. It is more likely in patients with history of biliary stasis, infection, stones, and chronic inflammation—which can be due to conditions like primary sclerosing cholangitis, choledocho cysts, hepatolithiasis, and biliary enteric fistulae. Cholangiocarcinoma is classified based on location: intrahepatic, perihilar, and distal. Most patients present with jaundice, pruritus, fever, and abdominal pain. For diagnosis, abdominal CT is the initial test of choice for visualization of the dilated bile ducts, regional lymph nodes, and vascular anatomy.

(A) RUQ ultrasound is the initial test of choice for gallstones and cholecystitis. (C) ERCP may be used to further evaluate the patency of the pancreatic duct and biliary tree, but a CT scan is less invasive and evaluates the organ parenchyma. (D) MRCP may be used to evaluate the ductal patency, but is not the best initial test. (E) HIDA scan is a good initial test for cholecystitis, not cholangiocarcinoma.

1. A 53-year-old woman with tubular carcinoma undergoes a modified radical mastectomy. Which of the following structures are part of the border of axillary lymph node dissection?

   (A) Axillary vein and trapezius
   (B) Latissimus dorsi and deltoid muscles
   (C) Pectoralis major and latissimus dorsi muscles
   (D) Pectoralis minor and external oblique muscles
   (E) Rectus abdominis and pectoralis minor

The answer is C: Pectoralis major and latissimus dorsi muscles. A modified radical mastectomy differs from a radical mastectomy in that the former spares the pectoralis major muscle and is performed in patients whose tumors do not invade the muscle. Both types involve lymph node dissection. The borders of the axillary lymph nodes are the axillary vein (apex), latissimus dorsi muscle (lateral), pectoralis major muscle (medial), and the fifth to sixth ribs (inferior).

(A) The axillary vein is the apical border of axillary node dissection. However, the trapezius muscle lies too far posterior to be of use in defining axillary borders. (B) The latissimus dorsi muscle is the lateral border of axillary node dissection. The superior border is the axillary vein, not the deltoid muscle. (D) Neither the pectoralis minor (which lies deep to the pectoralis major) nor the external oblique muscles (too far inferiorly) form borders for axillary lymph node dissection. (E) The rectus abdominis is too inferior to serve as a lateral border in axillary dissection. The pectoralis minor lies deep to the pectoralis major and is not one of the borders.

2. A previously healthy 30-year-old woman comes to the clinic complaining of nipple discharge. Which of the following characteristics of the discharge as would be gained from her history and physical would most concerning for malignancy?

(A) Bilateral discharge
(B) Green in color
(C) Occurs spontaneously
(D) Occurs with stimulation
(E) White in color

The answer is C: Occurs spontaneously. Most nipple discharge is benign in nature, but certain characteristics aid in differentiating discharge due to benign processes from those due to malignancy. Benign discharge is usually bilateral; clear, white, or green in color; and occurs with stimulation/palpation rather than spontaneously. Characteristics more concerning for malignancy include unilateral discharge, bloody discharge, and discharge that occurs spontaneously.

(A) Discharge that manifests bilaterally is more likely to be benign. Unilateral discharge is more concerning for malignancy. (B) Discharge that is green, white, or clear is more likely benign. Bloody discharge is more likely malignant. (D) Discharge that occurs with stimulation is more likely benign. Spontaneous discharge is more likely malignant. (E) Discharge that is green, white, or clear is more likely benign. Bloody discharge is more likely malignant.

3 A 45-year-old woman presents to her primary care physician complaining of a new breast mass discovered on self-examination. Which of the following would be the best screening test to evaluate this patient's mass?

(A) Fine-needle aspiration (FNA)
(B) Mammogram
(C) MRI
(D) Ultrasound
(E) No evaluation is necessary; a mass in a woman of this age is most likely cancer and should be removed as soon as possible

The answer is D: Ultrasound. Evaluation of the breasts is best done starting with a history and physical. If a mass is felt on physical examination, an ultrasound would be the best next step to determine the nature of the mass, that is, whether it is solid or cystic. Once visualized on ultrasound, a mass can be biopsied with FNA. Mammograms are a useful screening tool in otherwise asymptomatic patients, starting with a baseline at age 40. Because this woman has already found a mass, the best next step would be ultrasonography.

(A) FNA is performed once the mass has been visualized and characterized by ultrasound. Cystic masses can be therapeutically drained in this manner while FNA can be used to extract cells for cytology testing. (B) Mammograms are a useful screening tool in otherwise asymptomatic patients, starting with a baseline at age 40. Because this woman has already found a mass, the best next step would be ultrasonography. (C) MRIs are more useful for examining tumor extent in a patient known to have breast cancer and can be used to differentiate between recurrent tumor and postsurgical scar following operation. A patient with a mass of unknown significance would be best first evaluated by ultrasonography and FNA. (E) Although regular mammograms are recommended starting in patients at age 40, most breast masses are still benign. In any case, further evaluation can save a patient from unnecessary surgery.

---

 4 A 52-year-old woman with invasive breast cancer is undergoing a modified radical mastectomy. Lymph nodes behind (deep to) the pectoralis minor muscle are found to contain cancer. Lymph nodes medial to the pectoralis minor muscle are clear. This corresponds to invasion at which level of the axillary chain?

(A) Level 1
(B) Level 2
(C) Level 3
(D) Level 4
(E) More information is needed

The answer is B: **Level 2.** As in other areas of the body, lymphatic drainage follows venous drainage. The route of lymphatic drainage from the breast is through the axillary chain. This is divided into three levels as follows: level 1 corresponds to lymphatics lateral to the pectoralis minor muscle, level 2 corresponds to lymphatics behind (deep to) the pectoralis minor muscle, and level 3 corresponds to lymphatics medial to the pectoralis minor muscle. There is no level 4.

(A) Level 1 corresponds to lymphatics located lateral to the pectoralis minor muscle. The nodes in this patient, deep to her pectoralis minor muscle, would be in level 2. (C) Level 3 corresponds to lymphatics located medial to the pectoralis minor muscle. The nodes in this patient, deep to her pectoralis minor muscle, would be in level 2. (D) There is no level 4 in the axillary chain. The nodes in this patient, deep to her pectoralis minor muscle, would be in level 2. (E) The axillary chain is divided into three levels corresponding to areas medial, deep, and lateral to the pectoralis minor muscle. The nodes in this patient, deep to her pectoralis minor muscle, would be in level 2.

---

 5 A 33-year-old woman discovers a lump on her right breast while showering. Which quadrant is the most common site for breast cancer?

(A) Lower inner
(B) Lower outer
(C) Upper inner
(D) Upper outer
(E) All sites are roughly equally affected

The answer is D: Upper outer. The breast is divided into four segments: the upper and lower inner and upper and lower outer quadrants. Breast cancer can arise in any of these quadrants, but most cancers arise from the upper outer quadrant. This is likely due simply to the relatively larger proportion of breast tissue contained in this quadrant (it includes the axillary tail of Spence) and not due to any cellular differences in the resident tissue.

(A) The most common site for breast cancer is the upper outer quadrant, likely because it contains relatively more breast tissue than the other quadrants. (B) The most common site for breast cancer is the upper outer quadrant, likely because it contains relatively more breast tissue than the other quadrants. (C) The most common site for breast cancer is the upper outer quadrant, likely because it contains relatively more breast tissue than the other quadrants. (E) The most common site for breast cancer is the upper outer quadrant, likely because it contains relatively more breast tissue than the other quadrants.

---

 6 A 27-year-old G_1P_1 woman has been breastfeeding her 2-week-old son. Her left breast becomes red, swollen, tender, and warm over two days. Her right breast is unaffected. On physical examination, multiple small, tender lumps can be palpated in the left breast. The same milky discharge can be expressed from both nipples. Which of the following would be part of her treatment?

(A) Stop breastfeeding from the left side
(B) Surgical drainage
(C) Ultrasound of left breast
(D) Urgent mammogram
(E) Use of a pump if breastfeeding becomes too painful

The answer is E: Use of a pump if breastfeeding becomes too painful. Mastitis is caused by a bacterial infection (usually *Staphylococcus* or *Streptococcus* species) of the breast. These infections commonly occur during lactation as bacteria enter through breaks in the skin in and around the nipple. Treatment involves antibiotics to cover *Streptococcus* and *Staphylococcus* given for 10 to 14 days. Importantly, the breast ducts should continue to be drained either by normal breastfeeding or pumping so that the milk produced does not serve as a growth medium for the bacteria.

(A) Breastfeeding should continue as long as can be tolerated. If breastfeeding becomes too painful, a pump should be used to keep the milk draining. (B) Surgical drainage would be considered in the case of an abscess. An abscess would be less likely than mastitis in the setting of an entire breast affected (red, swollen, and tender) for only 2 days. An abscess can form in a patient with untreated mastitis. (C) Ultrasound imaging is used to evaluate suspicious lesions of the breast. The lumps palpated on this patient's examination are consistent with clogged ducts and do not warrant further investigation. (D) A mammogram would be helpful if cancer was suspected. This patient's acute presentation is more consistent with mastitis, which is treated with continued drainage and antibiotics.

 7 A 34-year-old woman presents with a painful left breast of 18 hours' duration. The pain is localized along a narrow path underneath her left breast. Physical examination reveals a visible, palpable, tender cord approximately 12 cm in length. An image of the patient is shown in *Figure 9-1*.

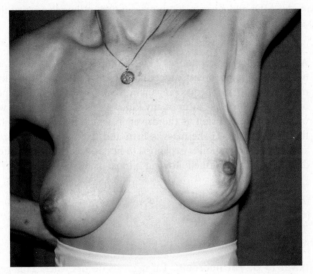

Figure 9-1

Which of the following would be the best treatment for this patient?

(A) Antibiotics
(B) IVIG
(C) NSAIDs
(D) Surgical excision
(E) Thrombolytics

The answer is C: **NSAIDs.** Mondor disease is a superficial thrombophlebitis; specifically, it affects the thoracoepigastric vein. The resulting clot can be palpated as a cord running under the skin along the course of the vein. The condition requires no treatment, but NSAIDs and a warm compress can hasten resolution and relieve some of the pain associated with Mondor disease. The image of this patient reveals retraction of the lateral portion of the breast which crosses to the midline at the inferior areolar margin and is accompanied by a palpable cord.

(A) Antibiotics would be useful in mastitis and as part of the treatment of an abscess. Mondor disease is thrombotic, however, and patients with this condition would not benefit from antibiotic use. (B) IVIG is used in treatment of some immune deficiencies, autoimmune diseases, and some acute infections. Mondor disease is thrombotic in nature and patients with this condition would not likely benefit from IVIG. (D) Surgery is indicated for abscesses and sinus tracts, but is not necessary in the treatment of Mondor disease. NSAIDs and a warm compress can hasten the recovery of this self-limited condition. (E) Although Mondor disease is thrombotic in nature, thrombolytics are not necessary. NSAIDs and a warm compress can hasten the recovery of this self-limited condition.

---

8 A 58-year-old woman notices a small lump in her right breast. A close friend of hers has breast cancer and she is concerned that the lump may be malignant. She has no pain or nipple discharge and no personal or family history of cancer of any kind. A few weeks ago, she was in a motor vehicle collision as the driver in which her right breast struck the steering wheel. The mass is firm and fixed. The need for biopsy and further evaluation is explained to her as well as a short differential diagnosis. Which of the following is most likely the cause of her lump?

(A) Cyst
(B) Fat necrosis
(C) Fibroadenoma
(D) Intraductal papilloma
(E) Phyllodes tumor

The answer is B: Fat necrosis. Fat necrosis occurs when damage to the adipose tissue of the breast (as from trauma or radiation) leads to a breakdown of the triglycerides into fatty acids and glycerol which then complex with calcium to form a hardened, calcified mass that may mimic cancer. Diagnosis is ascertained by biopsy and is the most likely etiology of the lump in this patient with a recent history of breast trauma.

(A) Cysts are a common finding in breasts, but have a rubbery consistency and are generally mobile on examination. A firm, fixed breast mass following trauma is likely due to fat necrosis although further investigation is warranted. (C) Fibroadenomas are also common findings in breasts, though usually found in younger women. They are more firm than cysts, but also have a rubbery texture and are generally mobile. A firm, fixed breast mass following trauma is likely due to fat necrosis although further investigation is warranted. (D) Intraductal papilloma is a tumor of the breast that usually presents with ipsilateral nipple discharge. A firm, fixed breast mass following trauma is likely due to fat necrosis although further investigation is warranted. (E) Phyllodes tumors resemble giant fibroadenomas but are more cellular. A firm, fixed breast mass following trauma is likely due to fat necrosis although further investigation is warranted.

9 A 43-year-old woman presents with a palpable mass in the lower inner quadrant of her left breast. Ultrasound shows a fluid-filled cyst. Fine needle aspiration (FNA) demonstrates a nonbloody greenish fluid. Which of the following would be an appropriate next step for the management of this cyst?

(A) Aspiration
(B) Excision
(C) Irradiation
(D) Warm compress
(E) No intervention indicated

The answer is A: Aspiration. Breast cysts are common findings and are mostly benign. A mass is determined to be cystic (rather than solid) with ultrasound. After a mass is shown to be cystic via ultrasound, FNA is used to examine the characteristics of the fluid. Simple cysts are benign, are characterized by clear or green fluid, and require only aspiration of the fluid as treatment. Milk-filled cysts (galactoceles) are also benign and would likewise be treated with aspiration. A cyst with bloody fluid raises concern for malignancy and may require excision.

(B) Excision is reserved for cysts containing bloody fluid. A simple cyst with green or clear fluid is benign and can be treated by aspiration drainage. (C) This patient likely has a benign, simple cyst based on the results of the FNA. Irradiation is not useful in the treatment of simple cysts but is sometimes used in treating breast cancer. (D) This patient likely has a benign, simple cyst based on the results of the FNA. Warm compresses are not useful in the treatment of such cysts but may be helpful in a patient with mastitis or a venous thrombus (Mondor disease). (E) A simple cyst such as that found in this patient would best be treated by aspiration to drain its contents.

10 A 27-year-old G_0P_0 woman complains of bilateral breast pain. Both breasts are equally affected and the pain is reportedly worse right before her menses. She consistently uses condoms for contraception. Which of the following would be the best next step in the management of this patient's likely condition?

(A) Antibiotics
(B) Evening primrose oil
(C) Gabapentin
(D) Supportive bra and analgesics
(E) Tamoxifen

The answer is D: Supportive bra and analgesics. Cyclic breast pain is a pain that follows the same monthly pattern as a woman's menstrual cycle. As in the patient in the question stem, cyclic pain is often worse just before menses. Physical examination and mammography should be included in the workup to rule out cancer. The pain is usually bilateral and treatment involves a supportive bra and analgesics such as acetaminophen if the pain is severe.

(A) The bilateral cyclic pain seen in this patient is not likely due to infection. Infectious mastitis is usually unilateral and noncyclical. Antibiotics are unnecessary and not indicated in the management of cyclical breast pain. (B) Evening primrose oil has not been shown to have benefit over placebo in decreasing either cyclic or noncyclic breast pain. (C) Gabapentin is used in the treatment of neuropathic pain, but this patient's pain is not likely neuropathic. Cyclic breast pain is best treated with supportive bras and analgesics. (E) Tamoxifen has been shown to reduce cyclic breast pain, but its use is limited due to concerns for its increased risk of endometrial cancer.

11 A 57-year-old woman is found to have a left upper outer quadrant breast mass on routine mammography. Fine needle aspiration (FNA) reveals invasive tubular carcinoma. Her paternal grandmother died of breast cancer at age 82. Which genetic abnormality is most likely to be found in this patient?

(A) BRCA-1 mutation
(B) BRCA-2 mutation
(C) p53 mutation
(D) PTEN mutation
(E) This patient likely has none of these mutations

The answer is E: **This patient likely has none of these mutations.** Although specific hereditary mutations that lead to the development of breast cancer are known to exist, most breast cancers, including hereditary types, involve unknown genetic mutations. This patient has a weak family history of breast cancer—only one grandmother who died of breast cancer at an advanced age—and may or may not have inherited a genetic mutation from her grandmother that lead to breast cancer in herself. Regardless, the most likely case is that her cancer came about due to a mutation in some unknown gene rather than those specific genes listed.

(A) Between 60% and 80% of women with the BRCA-1 mutation will develop breast cancer during their lives, but most breast cancers are due to mutations in as yet unknown genes. (B) Between 30% and 80% of women with the BRCA-2 mutation will develop breast cancer during their lives, but most breast cancers are due to mutations in as yet unknown genes. (C) p53 mutations have been implicated in some cases of breast cancer, but most breast cancers are due to mutations in as yet unknown genes. (D) PTEN mutations have been implicated in some cases of breast cancer, but most breast cancers are due to mutations in as yet unknown genes.

12 A 23-year-old woman requests breast cancer susceptibility testing when her mother is diagnosed with breast cancer at age 48. Her maternal grandmother died of breast cancer at age 61. Susceptibility testing reveals a mutation in BRCA-1. What is her approximate lifetime risk of developing breast cancer?

(A) 5% to 20%
(B) 20% to 40%
(C) 40% to 60%
(D) 60% to 80%
(E) 80% to 100%

The answer is D: 60% to 80%. Most genetic mutations leading to development of breast cancer, including heritable mutations, are in unknown genes. However, a few well-documented mutations exist that have been shown to strongly predispose carriers to breast cancer. Included in these is the BRCA-1 mutation. This gene codes for a DNA repair enzyme. Mutation of this gene confers a 60% to 80% lifetime risk of breast cancer on carriers.

(A) The lifetime breast cancer risk is 60% to 80% for the BRCA-1 mutation. (B) The lifetime breast cancer risk is 60% to 80% for the BRCA-1 mutation. (C) The lifetime breast cancer risk is 60% to 80% for the BRCA-1 mutation. (E) The lifetime breast cancer risk is 60% to 80% for the BRCA-1 mutation.

---

13 A 59-year-old Caucasian woman has recently been diagnosed with breast cancer. She has been married for 32 years and lives in an affluent neighborhood. She has two children, the first of which was born when she was 19. Her age at first menses was 16 and her current BMI is 22 kg/m². Which of the following is one of her risk factors for breast cancer?

(A) Age at first pregnancy
(B) Age at menarche
(C) High socioeconomic status
(D) Marriage status
(E) Thin body habitus

The answer is C: High socioeconomic status. A number of risk factors exist that contribute to the development of breast cancer. Having a personal history of breast cancer or a family history of premenopausal bilateral breast cancer quadruples the risk. Having any first-degree relative who has breast cancer, having endometrial or ovarian cancer, being obese, being older than 30 at time of first pregnancy, and being of high socioeconomic status confer a 2 to 4× risk of developing breast cancer. Being single and Caucasian and having early menarche and late menopause each increases the risk of developing breast cancer by up to 2×.

(A) Her age at first pregnancy was 19, which puts her at lower risk for breast cancer. Being over 30 at first pregnancy confers a relative risk 2 to 4× above baseline. (B) Her age of 16 at menarche is well above the average of 12 to 13 years. Early menarche, on the other hand, confers a 2 to 4× relative risk of developing breast cancer. (D) Being married puts a woman at low risk for breast cancer. Being single confers up to a 2× relative risk. (E) Obesity carries a 2 to 4× relative risk increase over baseline for developing breast cancer. Having a thin body habitus lowers the risk of breast cancer.

14 A 57-year-old woman comes to the clinic complaining of 2 months of progressively worsening itchiness and pain over her left nipple and areola. Physical examination shows scaly skin and a straw-colored discharge from her left nipple. Microscopic examination of biopsy tissue reveals vacuolated cells. A picture of the affected nipple is shown in *Figure 9-2*.

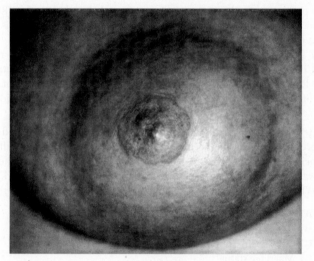

Figure 9-2

What would be the best treatment for her suspected condition?

(A) Mastectomy
(B) Oral corticosteroid
(C) Radiation
(D) Topical corticosteroid cream
(E) Use more supportive bra

The answer is A: Mastectomy. This patient most likely has Paget disease of the breast based on her history and physical examination findings (red, pruritic, eczematous skin over the nipple and areola) and the microscopic examination of her biopsy (vacuolated cells). These are all seen in Paget disease. Paget disease of the breast is a rare type of breast cancer affecting primarily the nipple-areolar complex. The picture of the nipple shows eczema and flattening of the surrounding tissue. Evaluation includes a mammogram to look for a mass. Standard treatment is mastectomy.

(B) Corticosteroids may be useful in treating eczema from atopic dermatitis or contact dermatitis, but this patient's eczema with vacuolated cells on microscopic examination suggests instead Paget disease of the breast. The standard treatment is mastectomy. (C) This patient's eczema with vacuolated cells on microscopic examination suggests Paget disease of the breast. The standard treatment is mastectomy. Radiation may be used in breast cancer patients when there is chest wall involvement or high-risk patients following mastectomy. (D) Corticosteroids may be useful in treating eczema from atopic dermatitis or contact dermatitis, but this patient's eczema with vacuolated cells on microscopic examination suggests instead Paget disease of the breast. The standard treatment is mastectomy. (E) This patient's eczema with vacuolated cells on microscopic examination suggests Paget disease of the breast. The standard treatment is mastectomy.

---

15 A 36-year-old woman with a family history of breast cancer presents for a routine breast examination. She reports having felt no masses on self-breast examination. No masses are felt in the breast proper on either side, but the patient shies away and will not allow the examiner to palpate her axillae stating, "It tickles too much." What is the best next step?

(A) Encourage the patient to check her axillae at home
(B) Explain the importance of checking the axillae
(C) Halt the examination since no distal masses were felt
(D) Order a mammogram instead
(E) Perform an MRI

The answer is B: **Explain the importance of checking the axillae.** The breast examination involves checking the breasts for symmetry, nipple retraction and drainage, palpation for masses, and palpation of the axillae and supraclavicular region for adenopathy. This type of screening is important, especially given this patient's family history of breast cancer. Although no masses are reported and none are felt in the initial examination, the importance of checking the axillae should be impressed upon this patient's mind. Many women do not realize that 2% of patients with cancer initially present with enlarged axillary nodes in the absence of palpable breast masses.

(A) This patient reports performing self-breast examination and she should be encouraged to check her own axillae as part of this examination. However, the self-breast examination is not an adequate replacement for the clinical breast examination and her axillae should be checked during this visit. (C) Although no masses are reported and none are felt in the initial examination, the importance of checking the axillae should be impressed upon this patient's mind. Many women do not realize that 2% of patients with cancer initially present with enlarged axillary nodes in the absence of palpable breast masses. (D) A mammogram may be helpful but is not a replacement for the clinical breast examination. A mammogram may not visualize every breast mass and would not visualize enlarged axillary nodes. (E) MRIs are not used for breast cancer screening because of their low specificity. The importance of checking the axillae should be explained to this patient so she can make an informed decision regarding the examination.

---

16 A 50-year-old woman undergoes a routine mammogram that reveals a suspicious mass in her left breast. A fine-needle biopsy is performed on the mass to investigate its makeup. Which of the following types of breast cancer is considered invasive?

(A) DCIS
(B) LCIS
(C) Paget disease
(D) Tubular carcinoma
(E) None of these lesions are considered invasive

The answer is D: Tubular carcinoma. The breast is subject to a variety of cancers, some of which are considered noninvasive and others invasive. Noninvasive cancers include ductal carcinoma *in situ* (DCIS), lobular carcinoma *in situ* (LCIS), and Paget disease of the breast (although Paget disease may involve an invasive component). Cancers considered invasive include tubular carcinoma, colloid/mucinous carcinoma, papillary carcinoma, medullary cancer, invasive lobular cancer, and inflammatory cancer. The treatment of the noninvasive types is directed at preventing evolution to an invasive type.

(A) DCIS is not invasive (as the name *in situ* suggests). The only type considered invasive of those listed is tubular carcinoma. (B) LCIS is not invasive (as the name *in situ* suggests). The only type considered invasive of those listed is tubular carcinoma. (C) Paget disease is not considered an invasive type of breast cancer, although some presentations may involve an invasive component. (E) Tubular carcinoma of the breast is considered invasive. It is one of the more favorable histologic types of invasive breast cancer.

---

17 A 62-year-old woman presents to her primary care physician complaining of redness, pain, and swelling in her right breast. She has not seen a physician for at least 20 years. The skin of the lower outer quadrant of her right breast is dimpled, swollen, and red. These findings likely represent which type of breast cancer?

(A) Inflammatory breast cancer
(B) Invasive lobular carcinoma
(C) Mucinous carcinoma
(D) Papillary carcinoma
(E) Tubular carcinoma

The answer is A: Inflammatory breast cancer. The appearance of the skin over her right breast suggests blockage of subdermal lymphatics. The dimpled and swollen appearance is termed peau d'orange, meaning "orange skin" because of its resemblance to the fruit. This pattern is seen in inflammatory breast cancer. Inflammatory signs, of course, are also seen, for example the redness and pain in the same area. This is a histologic type with a poor prognosis.

(B) Invasive lobular carcinoma involves small malignant cells infiltrating around benign ducts. This type of cancer does not generally cause a blockage of lymphatic ducts to lead to the peau d'orange appearance. (C) Mucinous carcinoma is characterized by invasive, malignant cells that produce mucous, forming a jelly-like tumor. This type of cancer does not generally cause a blockage of lymphatic ducts to lead to the peau d'orange appearance. (D) Papillary carcinoma, also known as intraductal papilloma, is the most common cause of bloody discharge in women aged 20 to 40. This type of cancer does not generally cause a blockage of lymphatic ducts to lead to the peau d'orange appearance as inflammatory breast cancer does. (E) Tubular carcinoma is so named for the tubules formed by the malignant cells visible under microscopy. It does not generally cause a blockage of lymphatic ducts to lead to the peau d'orange appearance as occurs in inflammatory breast cancer.

 18 A 59-year-old woman complains of a painless, hard lump in her right breast that she first noticed a week ago. She admits that she does not perform self-breast examinations and has not had a breast examination or mammogram in almost 8 years. Which of the following is a common site for breast cancer metastases?

(A) Breast cancer is not known to metastasize
(B) Gonads
(C) Kidney
(D) Lung
(E) Spleen

The answer is D: Lung. Breast cancer, like many other cancer types, is staged using the TNM system. "T" stands for tumor size, "N" refers to nodal involvement of the ipsilateral axillary nodes and ipsilateral internal mammary nodes, and "M" stands for distant metastases, including ipsilateral supraclavicular nodes. Common sites for metastasis of breast cancer include lungs, liver, bone, brain, and adrenal glands.

(A) Breast cancer is known to metastasize regularly if not caught early. Common sites of metastasis include lungs, liver, bone, brain, and adrenal glands. Spread to the ipsilateral supraclavicular lymph nodes is also considered metastatic. (B) The gonads are not a common site for metastatic spread of breast cancer. Common sites include the lungs, liver, bone, brain, and adrenal glands. (C) The kidneys are not a common site for metastatic spread of breast cancer. Common sites include the lungs, liver, bone, brain, and adrenal glands.

(E) The spleen is not a common site for metastatic spread of breast cancer. Common sites include the lungs, liver, bone, brain, and adrenal glands.

 19 A 65-year-old woman presents to the clinic following the discovery of a suspicious mass on routine mammogram. She has a variety of questions, including further workup and possible treatment options. Which of the following is a benefit of mastectomy over breast conservation surgery?

(A) Decreased damage to lymphatics
(B) Decreased infections
(C) Decreased recurrence
(D) Increased survival
(E) There is no difference in these outcomes between mastectomy and breast conservation

The answer is C: Decreased recurrence. Treatment for breast cancer can include surgery, chemotherapy, radiation therapy, and/or hormonal therapy. Surgical options include breast conservation surgeries and mastectomies. Breast conservation involves a local lumpectomy to remove the tumor followed by sentinel lymph node biopsy and possibly axillary lymphadenectomy. Mastectomy may be radical, modified radical, and skin-sparing. The only major difference between mastectomy and breast conservation is that mastectomy carries a lower risk of recurrence.

(A) There is no significant difference in damage to lymphatics between these two surgical options. The only major difference between mastectomy and breast conservation is that mastectomy carries a lower risk of recurrence. (B) There is no significant difference in infections between these two surgical options. The only major difference between mastectomy and breast conservation is that mastectomy carries a lower risk of recurrence. (D) There is no significant difference in survival between these two surgical options. The only major difference between mastectomy and breast conservation is that mastectomy carries a lower risk of recurrence. (E) The major difference between mastectomy and breast conservation is that mastectomy carries a lower risk of recurrence.

 20 A 60-year-old woman presents to the clinic following the discovery of a suspicious mass on routine mammogram. She has a variety of questions, including further workup and possible treatment options. Which of the following chemotherapeutic regimens is commonly used in the treatment of breast cancer?

(A) Bleomycin, etoposide, cisplatin
(B) Cyclophosphamide, methotrexate, fluorouracil
(C) Doxorubicin, cisplatin
(D) Gemcitabine, cisplatin
(E) None of these

The answer is B: Cyclophosphamide, methotrexate, fluorouracil.
Chemotherapy for breast cancer is used in the treatment of patients with positive lymph nodes, tumors greater than 1 cm, and estrogen receptor/progesterone receptor-negative patients (hormone insensitive tumors). Chemotherapy is also used in patients with metastases or recurrence. Common chemotherapeutic agents for breast cancer include cyclophosphamide, methotrexate, fluorouracil, and adriamycin. Side effects of these drugs include hair loss, myelosuppression, and cardiac toxicity (from adriamycin).

(A) Bleomycin, etoposide, and cisplatin are commonly used in the treatment of testicular germ cell tumors. This regimen is not used in the treatment of breast cancer. (C) Doxorubicin and cisplatin are used in the treatment of osteosarcoma. This regimen is not used in the treatment of breast cancer. (D) Gemcitabine and cisplatin are used in the treatment of metastatic bladder cancer. This regimen is not used in the treatment of breast cancer. (E) Common chemotherapeutic agents for breast cancer include cyclophosphamide, methotrexate, fluorouracil, and adriamycin.

 21. A 63-year-old African American woman undergoes mammography to investigate a mass discovered on breast examination in the upper outer quadrant of her left breast. She has a variety of questions, including further workup and possible treatment options. Which of the following patients with breast cancer would be the best candidate for hormonal therapy?

(A) A 31-year-old whose mother, maternal grandmother, and aunt all developed breast cancer
(B) A 55-year-old man with no family history of breast cancer
(C) A 59-year-old woman with an ER/PR-positive tumor
(D) A 60-year-old woman with BRCA-1 mutation
(E) A 60-year-old woman with BRCA-2 mutation

The answer is C: A 59-year-old woman with an ER/PR positive tumor. Hormone therapy in breast cancer works for those tumors with estrogen receptor/progesterone receptor (ER/PR)-positive cells. Patients with these tumor types have better outcomes in general, and for postmenopausal women hormone therapy is as effective as chemotherapy in treating ER/PR-positive breast cancer. Hormone therapy works by blocking the growth that natural hormones would cause in the cancer cells either by blocking estrogen receptors (tamoxifen and raloxifene) or by inhibiting excess estrogen synthesis (aromatase inhibitors such as anastrozole).

(A) Heritable breast cancers are not necessarily good candidates for hormone therapy. Response to hormone therapy can be predicted only by the presence or absence or hormone receptors on tumor cells. (B) Men with breast cancer are not necessarily good candidates for hormone therapy. Response to hormone therapy can be predicted only by the presence or absence or hormone receptors on tumor cells. (D) Patients with the BRCA-1 mutation are not necessarily good candidates for hormone therapy. Response to hormone therapy can be predicted only by the presence or absence or hormone receptors on tumor cells. (E) Patients with the BRCA-2 mutation are not necessarily good candidates for hormone therapy. Response to hormone therapy can be predicted only by the presence or absence or hormone receptors on tumor cells.

22 A 65-year-old man complains of a lump that has been growing larger over the past few months. He presents to his primary care physician for further evaluation. He has a prior medical history of hypertension, diabetes mellitus, basal cell carcinoma, and gastroesophageal reflux disorder. His prior surgical history is notable for excision of basal cell carcinoma lesions, right inguinal hernia repair, and open cholecystectomy. Which of the following features, if found, would suggest benign disease such as gynecomastia rather than cancer?

(A) Fixation of mass to the chest wall
(B) Pain on palpation
(C) Ulceration
(D) Unilateral lesion
(E) All of the above suggest cancer

The answer is B: Pain on palpation. Men can develop breast cancer, but it is both a small percentage of all cancers in men (<1%) and a small percentage of total breast cancers (also <1%). Workup is the same as that in women, including clinical examination, mammography, and fine needle aspiration (FNA). Features that suggest cancer rather than a benign etiology for a breast mass in a man include unilateral lesions (although gynecomastia is commonly unilateral, breast cancer is almost exclusively unilateral), painless lesions, fixed lesions (to the chest wall or to the skin), and ulceration. Gynecomastia generally produces tenderness.

(A) Fixation of the mass to the skin or to the chest wall suggests malignancy rather than gynecomastia or some other benign disease. (C) Ulceration is often seen in cancer. Gynecomastia and other benign conditions would generally not cause ulceration. (D) Gynecomastia may present unilaterally, but breast cancer in men is almost exclusively unilateral. Bilateral lesions would suggest gynecomastia rather than cancer. (E) All of the responses are suggestive of cancer except pain on palpation. Pain or tenderness is more likely due to a benign lesion. Breast cancer lesions are generally painless.

23 A 15-year-old young man complains of bilateral, tender breast enlargement first noticed 5 months ago. He is a football player for his high school team and sometimes complains of anterior chest pressure over his breasts when he wears shoulder pads after games and practices.

He has no prior medical or surgical history. He is originally concerned that he may be developing breast cancer, but is reassured by explanations that gynecomastia is much more likely. Which of the following would be the best treatment if he indeed has gynecomastia?

(A) Chemotherapy
(B) Duct drainage with FNA
(C) Hormone therapy
(D) Simple mastectomy
(E) Watchful waiting, no intervention is necessary

The answer is E: Watchful waiting, no intervention is necessary. Gynecomastia is common, occurring in 60% to 70% of early teenage boys (12 to 15 years old). In this age group, the condition is benign and almost always regresses spontaneously. Less commonly it can occur in older men as well. Causes in older men include certain medications, alcohol abuse, marijuana abuse, and cirrhosis. Mastectomy can be performed if the gynecomastia is severe or distressing to the patient.

(A) Gynecomastia in a man of this age (15 years) is common and benign and generally requires no treatment. Chemotherapy is used in the treatment of breast cancer in patients with positive lymph nodes or metastases. (B) Gynecomastia is not caused by blocked ducts, but by the abnormal development in men of normal, female-appearing breast tissue. Most cases resolve spontaneously and require no treatment. (C) Hormone therapy is useful in patients with estrogen receptor/progesterone receptor-positive tumors. This patient most likely has gynecomastia, which requires no treatment at his age. (D) Simple mastectomy can be performed if the gynecomastia is distressing to the patient or becomes very large.

 A 74-year-old woman who underwent a right modified radical mastectomy 10 years previously for breast cancer presents to her physician with a hard mass on her right anterior chest. On physical examination, a 0.8 cm × 0.6 cm lump is found in the midclavicular line at the level of the third rib of her right chest. The lump is firmly adherent to her chest wall. Which of the following would be the best next course of action?

(A) Chemotherapy
(B) Hormone therapy with leutinizing hormone releasing hormone (LHRH) agonist
(C) Radiation therapy to axillary lymph nodes
(D) Surgical removal of the lump and right pectoralis major muscle
(E) Watchful waiting, no intervention is necessary

The answer is C: Radiation therapy to axillary lymph nodes. The standard treatment for recurrence of breast cancer that involves the chest wall after a mastectomy is radiation therapy. Prognosis is worse for patients with recurrent disease within 2 years vs. those with recurrence after 5 years. The recurrence is usually in the same quadrant as the original disease. Ten percent of patients with recurrence will also have metastatic disease.

(A) Chemotherapy would be a good choice for a patient known to harbor distant metastases. This patient, with apparently localized chest wall involvement, would best be treated with radiation therapy. (B) Hormone therapy would be a good choice for a patient who was originally treated with hormone therapy and had good response. This patient was treated with mastectomy and now has recurrence in the chest wall. She would best be treated with radiation therapy. (D) The best treatment for recurrence involving the chest wall after mastectomy is radiation therapy. (E) The best treatment for recurrence involving the chest wall after mastectomy is radiation therapy.

---

 25 A 47-year-old woman presents to her physician for a complete physical examination required for her new job and insurance policy. She notes that she has gained 5 pounds in the last month from her baseline weight of 150 lbs. During the examination, a right breast mass is noted in the upper outer quadrant. Mammography followed by FNA confirms malignancy. Which of the following is the best prognostic indicator for this patient?

(A) Axillary node status
(B) Cellular appearance on FNA
(C) Findings on mammography
(D) Percent weight change in past 3 months
(E) Tumor size

The answer is A: Axillary node status. Cancer staging is done to predict a patient's prognosis and to direct treatment methods. Clinical staging involves the physical examination and mammogram and possibly additional tests in the setting of metastasis. Pathologic staging is based on the TNM (tumor, node, metastasis) system. Parameters such as tumor size, tumor extent, axillary node status, and metastases are evaluated. Of these, axillary node status bears the highest correlation with survival and has the best prognostic value.

(B) Cellular appearance on FNA is useful in the sense that findings direct possible further interventions such as excisional biopsy for samples with cellular atypia. The FNA biopsy is not as useful as the axillary node status for predicting outcome. (C) Mammography is useful to evaluate whether a mass found on examination has benign or malignant features. Findings on mammography do not correlate with outcome nearly as well as axillary node status. (D) Weight changes have not been shown to accurately predict outcomes in breast cancer as axillary node status does. Axillary node status would be the best prognostic indicator in this patient. (E) Poor prognostic features of the tumor itself include swelling around the tumor, dimpling, or fixation of the tumor to the chest wall or skin. Axillary node status, however, is still the best predictor of survival.

Gynecological Disorders

1 A 42-year-old man presents to his primary care physician complaining of a small painless ulcer on the glans penis. He states that 3 weeks ago, he had unprotected sexual intercourse with a woman and then developed a small papule 2 weeks later which became ulcerated. He denies fever, chills, sweats, or weight loss. He has a history of anaphylaxis to penicillin. Physical examination reveals a 2-cm painless ulcer on the ventral surface of the glans penis. The urethra is not involved. Examination of fluid extracted from the ulcer by dark field microscopy reveals treponemes and the venereal disease research laboratory (VRDL) is positive at 1:64. What is the most appropriate treatment for this patient?

(A) Amphotericin B
(B) Chloramphenicol
(C) Clarithromycin
(D) Doxycycline
(E) Gentamicin

The answer is D: Doxycycline. This patient has primary syphilis as suggested by the presence of a chancre. The best treatment is a one-time dose of intramuscular penicillin. However, this patient has a history of anaphylaxis to penicillin. For this patient, treatment with doxycycline for 2 weeks is acceptable.

(A) Amphotericin is appropriate for fungal infections. (B) Chloramphenicol is rarely used today because of the risk of pancytopenia. (C) Clarithromycin is not a firstline therapy for syphilis. (E) Gentamicin is useful for the treatment of gram-negative infections.

2 A 19-year-old man complains of a thick yellow urethral discharge and dysuria for 1 day. He has had multiple sexual partners during the past 3 months. His last unprotected intercourse was 5 days ago. Physical examination of the heart, lungs, and abdomen are unremarkable.

The phallus is uncircumcised, and the testes are descended bilaterally. Yellow discharge is present at the meatus. What is the most likely etiologic agent?

(A) *Chlamydia trachomatis*
(B) *Mycoplasma hominis*
(C) *Neisseria gonorrhoeae*
(D) *Trichomonas vaginalis*
(E) *Ureaplasma urealyticum*

The answer is C: *Neisseria gonorrhoeae*. The findings described for the adolescent in this case are most compatible with sexually acquired urethritis caused by *Neisseria gonorrhoeae*. Typically, severe dysuria and copious purulent discharge develop in the male 2 to 6 days after exposure. Approximately 20% of men will develop the urethritis syndrome following a single sexual contact with an infected partner.

(A) *Chlamydia trachomatis* is more common in young adults over the age of 20 years. (B) *Mycoplasma hominis* is an unlikely cause of urethritis. (D) *Trichomonas vaginalis* typically occurs in women. (E) *Ureaplasma urealyticum* is more common in young adults over the age of 20 years and is unlikely to cause purulent urethritis.

3. A 24-year-old woman who is 16 weeks' pregnant presents to her obstetrician for a routine prenatal examination. She has a prior medical history of sickle cell anemia and family history of diabetes mellitus. Physical examination of the heart, lungs, and abdomen is within normal limits. Fetal heart tones are audible with Doppler ultrasonography. Urinalysis reveals +2 bacteria and leukocyte esterase. What is the most likely pathogen?

(A) *Escherichia coli*
(B) *Group B streptococci*
(C) *Klebsiella pneumoniae*
(D) *Pseudomonas aeruginosa*
(E) *Proteus mirabilis*

The answer is A: *Escherichia coli*. The prevalence of asymptomatic bacteriuria in pregnant women ranges from 2% to 7%. This risk is doubled in women with sickle cell anemia. Other risk factors include low socioeconomic status and diabetes mellitus. *Escherichia coli* is most commonly found in this condition.

(B) *Group B streptococci* is less frequently associated with asymptomatic bacteriuria in pregnancy. (C) *Klebsiella pneumoniae* is the second most common cause of asymptomatic bacteriuria in pregnancy. (D) *Pseudomonas aeruginosa* is less commonly associated with asymptomatic bacteriuria in pregnancy. (E) *Proteus mirabilis* is the third most common cause of asymptomatic bacteriuria in pregnancy.

4   A 78-year-old woman presents to her family physician complaining of dysuria. She has no prior medical or surgical history. Female pelvic examination reveals protrusion of the uterus into the vagina to the hymenal ring. There is also a grade I cystocele and rectocele. There is no urethral hypermobility. Stress incontinence in lithotomy is not observed. What is the most likely explanation for these findings?

(A) Age-related laxity of the broad and round ovarian ligaments
(B) Endometrial hyperplasia
(C) Fecal impaction of the sigmoid colon
(D) Nulliparity
(E) Tear in the urogenital diaphragm

The answer is A: **Age-related laxity of the broad and round ovarian ligaments.** A common result of normal aging is the increased laxity of the broad round ovarian and cardinal ligaments, usually combined with loss of tone in myofascial structures such as the urogenital diaphragm. This results in uterine prolapse into the vagina, most commonly presenting as dysuria. A tear in the diaphragm can also cause uterine prolapse but is less common and is usually accompanied by symptoms of incontinence.

(B) Endometrial hyperplasia occurs due to unopposed estrogen effects on the endometrium lining the uterus. This increases the patient's risks for endometrial cancer. (C) Fecal impaction of the sigmoid colon would not lead to uterine prolapse. (D) Nulliparity has been associated with an increased risk of breast cancer. (E) A tear in the urogenital diaphragm could cause bladder prolapse.

5   A 70-year-old woman presents to her family physician complaining of a constant bloody vaginal discharge, which she has had for 3 months. Physical examination reveals a mass on the posterior wall of the vaginal fornix. A biopsy of the mass is obtained, and the pathology report suggests potentially metastatic squamous cell carcinoma of the vagina. Considering the location of the lesion, to which lymph nodes are the malignant cells most likely to metastasize first?

(A) Deep inguinal
(B) External iliac
(C) Internal iliac
(D) Superficial inguinal
(E) Superficial internal pudendal

The answer is C: **Internal iliac.** Lymph from the lower 25% of the vagina (below the hymen) drains downward to the perineum, where it is received by the superficial inguinal lymph nodes. The upper three-quarters of the vagina, on the other hand, drain upward to the internal iliac nodes. Since the fornix lies adjacent to the cervix, it is classified as lying within the upper three-quarters of the vagina.

(A) This deep inguinal nodes receive lymphatics after the superficial nodes. (B) The external iliac nodes receive lymphatics after the duperficial and deep nodes. (D) This answer is incorrect. (E) This answer is incorrect.

 6 Which of the following poses the greatest risk of malignancy in an otherwise healthy 30-year-old woman?

   (A) Adenomyosis
   (B) Immature teratoma
   (C) Infection with HPV type II
   (D) Leiomyoma
   (E) Mature teratoma

The answer is B: Immature teratoma. Immature teratoma is usually a malignant tumor in women, as opposed to mature teratoma, which is usually benign. This is, however, reversed for men, in whom mature teratomas are more likely to be malignant.

(A) Adenomyosis is a benign extension of endometrial glands and stroma into the myometrium, most often causing uterine enlargement. (C) Human papillomavirus (HPV) type II is a benign strain of HPV. (D) Leimyomas, or fibroids, are extremely common benign tumors of the uterus. They may very rarely transform into leiomyosarcomas. (E) Mature teratomas in women are commonly benign.

 7 A 28-year-old woman presents to her primary care physician complaining of abdominal bloating coincident with her menses. Her physician notes a nodular texture of the uterus on bimanual examination, and ultrasound shows several asymmetric masses within and radiating from the uterine corpus on the left. Serum pregnancy test results are negative. What is the most likely explanation for this finding?

   (A) Adenomyosis
   (B) Endometrial hyperplasia
   (C) Endometriosis
   (D) Leiomyoma
   (E) Molar pregnancy

The answer is D: Leiomyoma. Leiomyomas, otherwise known as fibroids, are the most common benign tumors of the uterus. They are also commonly estrogen responsive, causing them to enlarge in a cyclic pattern. When they are severe, they may cause mass effects in the abdomen, such as bloating.

(A) Adenomyosis also commonly causes uterine enlargement, but this is usually bilateral and nonnodular. (B) The same is true for endometrial hyperplasia, which also rarely reaches the size of leiomyomas or adenomyosis. (C) Endometriosis can result in chocolate cysts, but these rarely reach the size needed to cause mass effects. (E) A molar pregnancy could also result in an asymmetric abdominal mass, but in this case the pregnancy test would have been positive.

 A 72-year-old nulliparous woman develops scant vaginal bleeding in the absence of any other symptoms. She presents to her primary care physician for further evaluation. Pelvic and bimanual examinations are unremarkable. Urinalysis reveals trace blood; however, the Pap test shows a finding of adenocarcinoma. Which of the following is most closely associated with this finding?

(A) Adenomyosis
(B) Chronic use of oral contraceptives
(C) Endometriosis
(D) Endometrial hyperplasia
(E) Leiomyoma

The answer is D: Endometrial hyperplasia. Any bleeding in a postmenopausal woman should be assumed to be adenocarcinoma due to endometrial hyperplasia until proven otherwise. Endometrial hyperplasia itself results from excessive estrogen stimulation over time; sources of this stimulation include obesity, nulliparity, anovulatory cycles, and estrogen supplementation.

(A) In adenomyosis, ectopic endometrium is located in the myometrium. During menstruation, increased pain with or without bleeding will occur. It is not associated with adenocarcinoma. (B) Estrogen-progestin combined oral contraceptive pills have not been shown to increase the risk of cancer, and in fact, have been shown to decrease the risk of endometrial and breast cancer. (C) In endometriosis, endometrium is deposited outside of the uterine cavity. Patients usually present with severe pelvic pain. It is not associated with adenocarcinoma. (E) Leiomyomas, commonly known as uterine fibroids, are benign tumors of the uterus smooth muscle. They are not associated with adenocarcinoma.

 A 29-year-old nulliparous woman presents to her physician complaining of noncyclic vaginal bleeding and mild but persistent abdominal cramping. She has no other complaints and her past medical history is significant only for allergic rhinitis. She is not currently taking any medications. The physician is concerned about the possibility of a uterine mass, so a rectal examination is performed. What structure will most likely be compressed by palpation during this examination?

(A) Ischiorectal fossa
(B) Pouch of Douglas
(C) Supralevator space
(D) Urinary bladder
(E) Vesicouterine pouch

The answer is B: Pouch of Douglas. Palpation within the rectum anteriorly against the uterus impinges upon the rectouterine pouch, also known as the Pouch of Douglas. The Pouch of Douglas must be inspected when trying to detect for endometriosis.

(A) The ischiorectal fossa lies lateral and inferior to the Pouch of Douglas. (C) The supralevator space lies lateral and superior to the Pouch of Douglas. (D) The urinary bladder is located at the anterior aspect of the uterus. (E) The vesicouterine pouch lies between the two.

---

10 A 4-day-old neonate is brought to the emergency department with bleeding from the umbilical stump and his gastrointestinal tract. He was delivered at home and never received prenatal or perinatal care. His mother says that he is being exclusively breastfed, but has had difficulty feeding since birth. His mother has a history of smoking and alcohol use during pregnancy. Physical examination shows active mucosal bleeding and several bruises. Laboratory studies show a normal platelet count and fibrinogen levels. The prothrombin time is prolonged. Which of the following interventions could have prevented this illness?

(A) Administration of anti-D immunoglobulin
(B) Maternal alcohol abstinence
(C) Maternal smoking cessation
(D) Intramuscular injection of vitamin K
(E) Prenatal folic acid

The answer is D: Intramuscular injection of vitamin K. This infant is presenting with hemorrhagic disease of the newborn secondary to vitamin K deficiency. Vitamin K is routinely given to infants during perinatal care. Infants are prone to vitamin K deficiency as a result of inadequate vitamin K in breast milk and lack of gut flora. Vitamin K-dependent clotting factors include factors II, VII, IX, and X, protein C, and protein S. Laboratory studies consistent with vitamin K deficiency include a prolonged prothrombin time and normal partial thromboplastin time. Treatment is administration of vitamin K, which should reverse the symptoms.

(A) Anti-D immunoglobulin (Rhogam) is useful in preventing hemolytic disease of the newborn. It is given to the mother to prevent antibody formation. Giving the immunoglobulin to the baby is not indicated. (B) Maternal alcohol consumption puts the infant at risk for fetal alcohol syndrome. Fetal alcohol syndrome is characterized by micrognathia, midfacial hypoplasia, smooth philtrim, short palpable fissures, and a thin upper lip. Maternal alcohol consumption is not a known risk factor for vitamin K deficiency. (C) Maternal smoking cessation is not known to prevent hemorrhagic disease of the newborn. (D) Prenatal folic acid is used to prevent neural tube defects. It is not effective in preventing hemorrhagic disease of the newborn.

CHAPTER

11

Endocrine Surgery

1 A 34-year-old woman who is 2 days post-op for a thyroidectomy complains of a change in her voice. She says "it sounds like I have a frog in my throat!" What is the most likely etiology of her complaint?

(A) Laryngospasm
(B) Lacerated superior laryngeal nerve
(C) Neuropraxia of recurrent laryngeal nerve
(D) Vagus nerve damage
(E) Post-op acid reflux

The answer is C: Neuropraxia of recurrent laryngeal nerve. One of the risks of thyroidectomy is damage to the recurrent laryngeal nerve, which courses very close to the gland. The recurrent laryngeal nerve is a branch of the vagus nerve (also known as cranial nerve X), which supplies motor function to the majority of the laryngeal muscles. Unilateral nerve damage most commonly presents as hoarseness. Due to its close proximity to the thyroid gland, surgeons are very careful to correctly identify and protect this nerve. However, even if they identify and avoid the nerve, there is a possibility that mere manipulation of the nerve can cause neuropraxia, which is a temporary dysfunction of the nerve, leaving the patient transiently hoarse. The patient's normal voice usually returns within a few weeks.

(A) Laryngospasm is an uncontrolled contraction of the vocal chords that partially obstructs the patient's airway. It is a complication that can occur acutely after extubation. (B) The superior laryngeal nerve is a branch of the vagus nerve that supplies the cricothyroid muscle. This muscle acts to produce higher pitch, and damage to it leaves patients with a more monotone voice. (D) The vagus nerve courses much more lateral than what is regularly dissected in a thyroidectomy, and thus is extremely unlikely to be damaged. (E) Acid reflux can be more prominent in patients that just had surgery, and it presents as epigastric burning, chronic nighttime cough, and trouble swallowing.

2) A 41-year-old woman presents to the clinic complaining of "increased nerves" and weight loss. On further questioning, she reveals that she has been feeling her heart racing often, and needs to bring an extra shirt with her as she seems to sweat through her clothing unusually quickly. She recently lost 10 pounds, which she was not trying to do. On examination, she has a fine tremor, and a large mass in the front of her neck that moves when she swallows. She also has large eyes which appear to be "popping out." An image of the patient is shown in *Figure 11-1*.

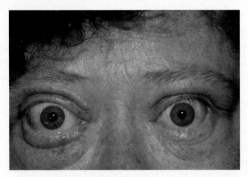

Figure 11-1

What is the definite treatment of choice for this condition?

(A) Subtotal thyroidectomy
(B) Total thyroidectomy
(C) Propranolol
(D) ^{131}I radioablation
(E) Methimazole

The answer is D: ^{131}I radioablation. Graves disease is a disorder of the thyroid gland that manifests with a goiter, exophthalmos, and a hyperthyroid state. The mechanism of this disorder is autoimmune: the body produces auto-antibodies called thyroid-stimulating immunoglobulins (TSIs). These antibodies bind to thyroid stimulating hormone (TSH) receptors on the thyroid follicular cells, which leads to an increased production and secretion of thyroid hormone into the bloodstream. The TSIs also interact with fibroblasts in the orbital soft tissues, which lead to inflammation and edema that pushes the eyeball forward. The treatment of Graves disease ranges from antithyroid medications, to radioactive iodine (RAI) treatment, to surgical removal of the gland. RAI is an effective treatment for Graves disease, as the entire gland is hypermetabolic and uptakes iodine at a supranormal rate. The entire gland is then subjected to radiation, which destroys it.

(A) Subtotal thyroidectomy is used for treatment of a single toxic thyroid adenoma. It will not effectively treat Graves disease, where the entire gland has excessive hormone secretion. (B) Total thyroidectomy is a third-line treatment for Graves disease behind RAI due to its increased risk of complications. (C) Propranolol is an effective treatment of the acute hyperthyroid state, as many of the symptoms of hyperthyroidism are mediated by the sympathetic nervous system. It is not a definitive treatment for Graves disease. (E) Methimazole is an antithyroid medication that is first-line treatment for Grave disease. However, it is not a definite treatment, and a one-time radioablation treatment is preferable over taking this medication for life.

3 A 28-year-old woman is seen in the clinic for a routine physical examination. She has no complaints. On examination, you notice a nodule when palpating her thyroid. What is the best next step?

(A) Fine-needle aspiration (FNA)
(B) Ultrasound
(C) CT scan
(D) Sestamibi scan
(E) RAI scan

The answer is A: Fine-needle aspiration (FNA). Over 95% of thyroid nodules are benign, but it is recommended to further evaluate thyroid nodules found on examination. Of the tests to evaluate a thyroid nodule, FNA is the most effective and cost-effective test. FNA allows for a direct sampling of the tissue for pathologic analysis. It is minimally invasive, not requiring any anesthesia, and the false negative rate is only 5%. If the results of the FNA are either indeterminate or inadequate, the recommendation is to first repeat the FNA, which can be done with ultrasound guidance.

(B) Ultrasound is also used to evaluate thyroid nodules. It is second-line diagnostic study to an FNA, and often both are used to accurately establish the diagnosis. (C) CT scans are not used for the evaluation of a simple thyroid nodule. (D) Sestamibi scan is a test used to evaluate for parathyroid hyperactivity. It has no role in the evaluation of the thyroid nodule. (E) RAI scans use ^{123}I to evaluate the amount of activity the gland is undergoing by looking at how readily it takes up iodine from the blood. It can show a thyroid nodule to be "hot" and thus is used for patients with symptoms of hyperthyroidism.

4 A 54-year-old man returns to the clinic for a follow-up of a thyroid nodule. The patient has no complaints. At the last visit, a fine needle aspiration (FNA) was performed, and the results are still pending. When reviewing his labs, you notice that he has an elevated serum calcitonin. He also recalled having an uncle who died from thyroid cancer. What other cancer type needs to be evaluated for?

(A) Craniopharyngioma
(B) Insulinoma
(C) Prolactinoma
(D) Gastrinoma
(E) Pheochromocytoma

The answer is E: Pheochromocytoma. The combination of a thyroid nodule with an elevated serum calcitonin indicates the presence of medullary thyroid carcinoma. This malignancy can be seen as a part of multiple endocrine neoplasia IIA or IIB. The other malignancy seen in both IIA and IIB is pheochromocytoma. This tumor usually arises from the adrenal medulla, but 10% are extra-adrenal. It is diagnosed by history (episodic palpitations, tachycardia, flushing, sense of impending doom), elevated vanylmandelic acid (VMA) and total metanephrines on a 24-hour urine assay, and CT scan to localize the tumor. The other finding in MEN IIA is parathyroid hyperplasia, while the other findings for multiple endocrine neoplasia (MEN) IIB are marfanoid habitus and mucosal neuromas.

(A) Craniopharyngioma is a nonendocrine tumor of the pituitary gland's embryonic tissue (rests of epithelium derived from Rathke pouch). It is not associated with MEN or medullary carcinoma of the thyroid (MTC) syndromes. (B) Insulinoma is a tumor derived from pancreatic β cells which secretes insulin. It is associated with MEN I, which has manifestations from the "3 Ps" (pancreas, pituitary, and parathyroid). (C) Prolactinoma is the most common pituitary tumor, which produces high levels of prolactin. It can be associated with MEN I. (D) Gastrinoma is a pancreatic tumor that produces gastrin, causing Zollinger-Ellison syndrome. It can be associated with MEN I.

5 A 61-year-old man returns to the clinic for a follow-up of a biopsy of a nodule in his thyroid. He has no complaints, other than the "large, ugly lump" in his neck. The result from his thyroid biopsy shows "atypical cells with capsular and vascular invasion." What is the initial treatment?

(A) Subtotal thyroidectomy
(B) Radioiodine ablation
(C) Thyroidectomy
(D) Methimazole
(E) Systemic chemotherapy

The answer is C: Thyroidectomy. The presentation of an asymptomatic thyroid nodule is common with thyroid cancers. The most common of these is the papillary type. The second most common is follicular type, which has the pathologic characteristics of capsular invasion and vascular invasion. The treatment for follicular thyroid carcinoma is a total thyroidectomy followed up radioiodine ablation. The patient should be monitored for recurrence with serial physical examinations, ultrasounds, and RAI reuptake scans if at moderate to high risk of recurrence.

(A) Subtotal thyroidectomy has been used for the treatment of thyroid cancer localized to just one lobe of the gland. However, it limits the use of thyroglobulin as a tumor marker and the use of RAI to monitor for any recurrence. (B) RAI is also used in the treatment of follicular thyroid carcinoma, but after surgery to remove the cancer. (D) Methimazole is an antithyroid medication used in the treatment of hyperthyroidism. It has no role in thyroid cancer, which does not produce thyroid hormone. (E) Systemic chemotherapy is used for metastatic thyroid cancer. Surgical excision is indicated for this localized malignancy.

 6 A 30-year-old man presents to the ED for "nervousness and my heart is racing." He has a 3-month history of intermittent palpitations, 8-pound unintentional weight loss, and thinning hair. Physical examination reveals a hard nodule in the anterior portion of his neck, which elevates with swallowing. His thyroid stimulating hormone (TSH) is found to be 0.1 mIU/L. Which artery directly gives rise to the inferior thyroid artery?

(A) External carotid artery
(B) Subclavian artery
(C) Transverse cervical artery
(D) Thyrocervical trunk
(E) Parathyroid artery

The answer is D: Thyrocervical trunk. The thyroid gland is supplied by two arteries bilaterally: the inferior and superior thyroid arteries. The superior thyroid artery is the first branch of the external carotid artery and courses alongside the superior laryngeal nerve. The inferior thyroid artery is a branch of the thyrocervical trunk, which comes off of the subclavian artery. It courses superiorly alongside the recurrent laryngeal nerve.

(A) The external carotid artery gives risk to the superior thyroid artery, not the inferior. (B) The subclavian artery gives rise indirectly to the inferior thyroid artery, but through the thyrocervical trunk, which is the direct source of the inferior thyroid artery. (C) The transverse cervical artery is another artery that comes off of the thyrocervical trunk. (E) This is a distractor, as there is no such structure; the parathyroid gland gets its blood supply from the inferior thyroid artery.

 7 A 61-year-old man returns to the clinic for a follow-up of a thyroid nodule. The patient has no complaints. At the last visit, a fine needle aspiration (FNA) was performed, and the results are still pending. On physical examination, you find a 1-cm nodule on the lateral margin of the left lobe. When reviewing his labs, you notice that he has an elevated serum calcitonin. What is the treatment of choice?

(A) Subtotal thyroidectomy with ipsilateral neck dissection
(B) Total thyroidectomy with ipsilateral neck dissection
(C) Radioiodine ablation
(D) Total thyroidectomy with bilateral neck dissections
(E) Systemic chemotherapy

The answer is B: Total thyroidectomy with ipsilateral neck dissection.
The diagnosis for this patient is medullary thyroid carcinoma (MTC), which presents as a thyroid mass along with an elevated serum calcitonin. It arises from the parafollicular cells of the thyroid, which normally produce calcitonin. This also can be associated with multiple endocrine neoplasia syndromes, which contain the amyloid RET protooncogene. The treatment of choice for MTC is total thyroidectomy with ipsilateral neck dissection, as the cancer is less differentiated and more invasive than other thyroid cancers.

(A) There is no thyroid cancer which is treated in this way. Subtotal thyroidectomy is reserved for smaller, well-differentiated cancers localized to one lobe of the gland. (C) RAI is used as an adjunct to thyroidectomy for papillary and follicular thyroid cancers. It has no role for MTC, as the parafollicular cells do not uptake iodine. (D) This treatment may be used for very extensive MTC which is found in the gland bilaterally. For this patient, it is not required as the tumor is just localized to the left lobe. (E) Systemic chemotherapy is used to treat metastatic disease. In this patient, there is no evidence of metastasis, and surgical resection is the treatment of choice.

---

 8 A 26-year-old man presents to his primary care physician for a follow-up of an elevated calcium level found on routine blood tests. He has a new complaint of hip pain, which he cannot attribute to any trauma or change in behavior. He also complains of some anxiety. When asked about family history, he states that "it seems like many of my family members have trouble with their calcium levels." His repeat Ca level is 11.1 mg/dL, and he has a parathyroid hormone (PTH) of 5 pg/mL (normal is 10 to 60 pg/mL). What is the best next step?

(A) 24-hour urine calcium
(B) Sestamibi scan
(C) Prescribe sensipar
(D) Hemodialysis
(E) Parathyroidectomy

The answer is A: 24-hour urine calcium. This patient has repeatedly elevated calcium levels, alongside a family history of the same, which indicates he has familial hypocalciuric hypercalcemia. He also has symptoms of hypercalcemia (bone pain and psychiatric changes), which can be remembered by the mantra "Renal Stones, Painful Bones, Abdominal Groans, and Psychic Moans." He also has a suppressed PTH level, which indicates that the parathyroid is not the source of the hypercalcemia. Of the choices, a 24-hour urine calcium of <200 mg/day is the best test for diagnosing this condition.

(B) Sestamibi parathyroid scintigraphy is a nuclear medicine study used to assess the activity of the parathyroid glands. It is used to identify parathyroid adenomas or hyperplasia, both of which produce an elevated PTH level. (C) Sensipar is a medication used to treat secondary hyperparathyroidism. This patient has hypoparathyroidism. (D) Hemodialysis is used to treat severe hypercalcemia complicated by renal failure. It is not indicated for this patient. (E) Parathyroidectomy is the treatment of choice for primary hyperparathyroidism refractory to medical management. It is not indicated for this patient.

 9 A 29-year-old woman is 1 day post-op for a thyroidectomy for a benign symptomatic goiter, when she complains of numbness around her mouth. She also complains of occasional leg spasms, which she has never had before. On physical examination, she has a positive Chvostek sign. What is best next test to confirm the diagnosis?

(A) Check vitamin D
(B) Check PTH
(C) Abdominal CT scan
(D) Urinalysis
(E) Check TSH

The answer is B: Check PTH. This patient recently had a thyroidectomy and is complaining of new onset perioral numbness and tetany. She also has a positive Chvostek sign, where tapping on the inferior portion of the zygoma produces facial spasms. These are signs and symptoms of hypocalcemia, which is likely due to inadvertent removal of the parathyroid glands along with the thyroid gland. The best test to confirm this diagnosis is to check a PTH level, which will be undetectable if all four parathyroids were removed.

(A) Hypocalcemia can result from low vitamin D level, although that is much less likely than hypoparathyroidism in this particular patient. (C) An abdominal CT scan could be used to evaluate for pancreatitis, which can cause hypocalcemia. However, this patient lacks the epigastric pain, fever, or nausea/vomiting which would indicate this as the diagnosis. (D) Urinalysis can be used to assess for urinary tract infection, but this will not help with the diagnosis in this patient. (E) TSH will likely be normal or perhaps elevated post-op for a thyroidectomy, depending on the dosing of thyroid hormone replacement. It will not help find the correct diagnosis.

 10 A 67-year-old man presents to the emergency department with a 2-month history of increasing abdominal pain and nausea and vomiting. On examination, his abdomen is soft and nondistended. His lab results show a calcium level of 15.1 mg/dL. Upon further workup of this elevated calcium level, he is found to have a PTH level of 320 pg/mL. What is surgical treatment for his condition?

(A) Parathyroidectomy and ipsilateral lymph node dissection only
(B) Parathyroidectomy only
(C) Parathyrodectomy and thyroidectomy only
(D) Excision, ipsilateral thyroid lobectomy, and ipsilateral lymph node dissection
(E) Parathyroidectomy and radioiodine ablation

The answer is D: **Excision, ipsilateral thyroid lobectomy, and ipsilateral lymph node dissection.** Parathyroid carcinoma is caused by a malignant transformation of parathyroid chief cells. It presents as significant hypercalcemia, which can manifest as "Renal Stones, Painful Bones, Abdominal Groans, and Psychic Moans." Calcium levels are dramatically elevated to levels >14 mg/dL, which is much greater than that seen with simple parathyroid adenomas. There also is significant hyperparathyroidism, with levels 3 to 10 times the normal amount. There is a palpable nodule in half of these patients. The treatment of choice is excision of the parathyroid tissue, along with an ipsilateral thyroid lobectomy and lymph node dissection. Prognosis is poor in these patients.

(A) Excision of the ipsilateral thyroid lobe is also indicated for parathyroid carcinoma. (B) Excision of the ipsilateral thyroid lobe and ipsilateral lymph nodes is indicated for parathyroid carcinoma. (C) An ipsilateral lymph node dissection is also indicated. (E) RAI has no role in the treatment of parathyroid carcinoma, as parathyroid tissue does not uptake iodine. In addition, ipsilateral lymph node and thyroid tissue also must be excised.

 11 A 58-year-old man presents with dull intermittent abdominal pain for the past 3 months. He also complains of new onset back pain that does not remit with rest. On examination, the pain is localized in his lower back on the midline. His labs show a calcium level of 12.0 mg/dL, as well as a Cr of 2.1 mg/dL. What is the best next step?

(A) Furosemide
(B) Alendronate
(C) IV NS bolus
(D) Hemodialysis
(E) Calcitonin

The answer is C: **IV NS bolus.** This patient with new onset back pain, elevated creatinine, and hypercalcemia most likely has multiple myeloma. Multiple myeloma is a monoclonal gammopathy that causes hypercalcemia via direct inflammatory response that lyses the bone. Regardless of the cause, the acute treatment of hypercalcemia is an IV bolus of normal saline.

Once adequately hydrated, other methods can be employed to remove the excess calcium from the body.

(A) Furosemide is the next step in the treatment of hypercalcemia after IV hydration. It is a loop diuretic which inhibits the Na-K-2 Cl cotransporter in the thick ascending limb of the loop of Henle and causes increased Ca loss in the urine. (B) Alendronate is a bisphosphonate, which acts to decrease Ca levels in the blood by inhibiting osteoclastic activity in the bone. It can be used to treat hypercalcemia, but IV NS would come prior. (D) Hemodialysis is used in cases of extreme hypercalemia in the setting of renal failure. It is not required in this patient. (E) Calcitonin can help lower calcium levels by inhibiting bone resorption. As it is used to treat severe hypercalcemia, it has no role in this patient.

 A 31-year-old woman is referred to an endocrinologist for an elevated calcium level found on routine blood tests. She complains of mild depression and some pain in her lower legs. Her current labs show a Ca level of 11.2 mg/dL and a PTH of 95 pg/mL (normal is 10 to 60 pg/mL). She receives the diagnosis of hyperparathyroidism. What is the embryologic source of the inferior parathyroid glands?

(A) Third pharyngeal cleft
(B) Fourth pharyngeal pouch
(C) Fifth pharyngeal arch
(D) Fourth pharyngeal arch
(E) Third pharyngeal pouch

The answer is E: Third pharyngeal pouch. The parathyroid glands originate from the third and fourth pharyngeal pouches, which form in the endodermal side of the pharyngeal arches. Each pouch gives rise to different head or neck structures, which share a common migratory course as the fetus matures. The third pouch gives rise to inferior parathyroid glands and the thymus and is supplied by the glossopharyngeal nerve. The fourth pouch gives rise to the superior parathyroids and the parafollicular cells of the thyroid gland.

(A) The third pharyngeal cleft is the ectodermal side of the pharyngeal arches and contributes to the formation of the cervical sinus. (B) The fourth pharyngeal pouch gives rise to the superior parathyroid glands. (C) The fifth pharyngeal arch only exists transiently during development and does not form and structures. (D) The fourth pharyngeal arch contributes to the superior parathyroids, soft palate muscles, and the cricothyroid muscle.

 A 38-year-old man presents to the emergency department stating "I feel like I'm going to die!" He recalls this has happened to him three times in the past week, each time getting a headache and feeling his heart race really fast. His vitals show a heart rate of 134 beats/min and a blood pressure of 175/105 mmHg. On examination, he appears distressed and diaphoretic. EKG shows sinus tachycardia with no ST segment changes.

Labs show normal complete blood count (CBC), basic metabolic panel (BMP), troponin I, a normal thyroid stimulating hormone (TSH), and elevated free metanephrines. What is the best next step?

(A) Treatment with Esmolol
(B) Treatment with Ativan
(C) Treatment with phenoxybenzamine
(D) Tx with propylthiouracil and propranolol
(E) Abdominal CT scan

The answer is C: Treatment with phenoxybenzamine. This patient presents with classic symptoms and signs for a pheochromocytoma. Pheochromocytoma is a catecholamine-producing tumor which stimulates α- and β-adrenergic receptors to produce effects like tachycardia, hypertension, and diaphoresis. There is a "Rule of 10s": 10% are bilateral, 10% are extra-adrenal, 10% are familial, 10% are malignant, 10% are multiple, and 10% occur in children. The treatment of pheochromocytoma is ultimately surgical excision of the tumor. But initially patients require medical management with α-blockers, like phenoxybenzamine, for cardiovascular stabilization.

(A) Pure β-blockers, such as esmolol, and those without any alpha-blocking properties, must never be used in the case of a pheochromocytoma without first treating with an α-blocker. Pure β-blockade leads to unopposed α-agonism which can cause severe and/or refractory hypertension. (B) Benzodiazepines such as ativan, are used for acute treatment of panic attacks. Panic attacks present similarly to pheochromocytoma, but pheochromocytoma must be ruled out prior to making the diagnosis of panic d/o. (D) Propylthiouracil and propranolol are used for the treatment of thyrotoxicosis, which presents with extreme symptoms of hyperthyroidism (tremor, palpitations, etc.). (E) Abdominal CT scan is the test of choice to localize a pheochromocytoma, with an accuracy of 90% to 95%. A CT scan to locate the tumor should occur after the initial stabilization with α-blockers.

---

14 A 50-year-old woman recently discharged for a COPD exacerbation presents with new lethargy and nonspecific abdominal pain. She has vomited once and feels nauseous. On examination, she is drowsy and only oriented to person. Her blood pressure is 91/45 mmHg, heart rate 132 beats/min, respiratory rate 20 breaths/min, and O_2 saturation 97%. She was being treated with 60-mg prednisone for the past 3 weeks, which she had just finished taking yesterday. Her labs show a sodium of 134, potassium of 5.7, chloride of 101, bicarbonate of 21, and a glucose of 72. What is the best treatment of her condition?

(A) Kayexalate
(B) Fludrocortisone
(C) Omeprazole
(D) Dexamethasone
(E) Ondansetron

The answer is D: Dexamethasone. This patient is in acute adrenal crisis due to her recent course of prednisone for her chronic obstructive pulmonary disease (COPD) exacerbation. She was taking high-dose prednisone for 3 weeks, which suppressed her hypothalamic-pituitary-adrenal axis and effectively shut down her glucocorticoid production. The use of exogenous corticosteroids decreased the amount of adrenocorticotropic hormone (ACTH) released, which led to atrophy of the adrenal cortex as ACTH has trophic effects. When she discontinued the prednisone, her atrophied adrenal cortex was unable to produce a sufficient amount of cortisol, which led to the crisis. This could have been prevented by tapering down the dose of exogenous steroids slowly over 2 to 3 weeks. The treatment of choice is glucocorticoid replacement.

(A) Kayexalate is a resin that binds potassium ions in the gut to remove them from the body. It is used as a more definitive treatment of hyperkalemia. (B) Fludrocortisone is a synthetic mineralocorticoid used to treat hypoaldosteronism, and has no role for acute adrenal crisis. (C) Omeprazole is a proton pump inhibitor used for the treatment of gastroesophageal reflux disease (GERD) or peptic ulcers. It has no role for acute adrenal crisis. (E) Ondansetron is a 5-HT3 receptor antagonist used in the treatment of nausea. It will not treat acute adrenal crisis.

 15 A 58-year-old man is brought into the emergency department by his wife who states "he's been really out of it all day." She states that he has been "run down" all week, and has been drinking "a whole lot of water." She feels that he has been going to the bathroom unusually frequently as well. On physical examination, he appears drowsy and has dry mucous membranes. He has an elevated blood pressure, which is new when compared to his previous visits. His CBC is within normal limits, but his serum electrolytes shows sodium of 150 and a potassium of 3.2. CT scan is obtained and is shown below in *Figure 11-2*.

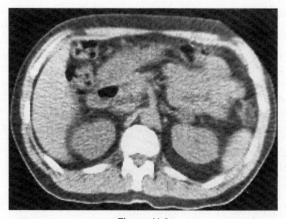

Figure 11-2

What is the diagnostic test of choice?

(A) Plasma aldosterone/renin activity
(B) Blood glucose level
(C) Dexamethasone suppression test
(D) Plasma aldosterone level
(E) Plasma cortisol level

The answer is A: Plasma aldosterone/renin activity. This patient is suffering from an aldosteronoma causing hypertension, dehydration, and hyperkalemia. In normal conditions, low renal tubule sodium leads to increased renin secretion, which increases angiotensin II levels, which then triggers increased aldosterone production. Aldosterone then acts on the kidneys to retain sodium and water to increase intravascular volume. This patient has an overproduction of aldosterone from a benign tumor in his adrenal gland which does not respond to normal feedback loops. This excess aldosterone causes the kidney to retain sodium and water, and waste potassium. The excess sodium and water leads to an increased blood volume which causes hypertension. The test of choice to identify this is an aldosterone/renin ratio, as the aldosterone from the tumor suppresses the renin level. A plasma aldosterone/renin ratio >30 is diagnostic. The CT scan reveals the small adrenal tumor on the left side.

(B) This would be a good screen for diabetes, which can present similarly. For hyperaldosteronism, a blood glucose level has no diagnostic value. (C) Dexamethasone suppression tests are used to diagnose the source of Cushing syndrome. (D) A plasma aldosterone level, although elevated, is not as useful for diagnosing hyperaldosteronism as the aldosterone/renin ratio. (E) A spot plasma cortisol level is not a useful test, as levels fluctuate a lot throughout the day. For the diagnosis of Cushing syndrome, it is better to obtain a 24-hour urinary cortisol.

 16 A 48-year-old woman presents for her annual gynecologic examination. She has a new complaint of weight gain around her neck and shoulders. She also complains of difficulty with peripheral vision, especially having trouble seeing cars in the lane next to her when she is driving. On examination, her skin seems tanner, even though has not "gotten much sun lately." Other findings include she has a thickened amount of tissue on the back of her neck, and she has numerous purplish lines on her belly. She is very upset about these changes, as she cannot explain where they came from. For this patient, what is the expected test result?

(A) Low cortisol with low-dose dexamethasone administered
(B) High ACTH with high-dose dexamethasone administered
(C) Low ACTH with high-dose dexamethasone administered
(D) Low serum glucose
(E) High serum 17-OH progesterone

The answer is B: High ACTH with high-dose dexamethasone administered. This patient has Cushing disease, which is a specific type of Cushing syndrome caused by an adrenocorticotrophic hormone (ACTH)-producing pituitary tumor. The "tunnel vision" this patient is experiencing is due to the mass effect of the tumor compressing the optic chiasm. In Cushing disease, excess ACTH from the pituitary tumor stimulates the adrenal gland to secrete excess cortisol. The tumor lacks any feedback inhibition, and keeps secreting excess ACTH. To delineate between different types of Cushing syndrome, first start with a low-dose dexamethasone suppression test. If cortisol remains elevated, then the patient is subjected to a high-dose dexamethasone suppression test, which suppresses pituitary ACTH production. In Cushing disease, the cortisol level will be low and the ACTH level will be high with high-dose dexamethasone.

(A) In normal individuals, cortisol production is suppressed by low-dose dexamethasone. This result rules out Cushing syndrome. (C) This result occurs in Cushing syndrome caused by a primary adrenal adenoma or hyperplasia, where uncontrolled cortisol production from the adrenals suppresses pituitary ACTH. (D) No matter the specific type, hyperglycemia is seen in all types of Cushing syndrome. (E) Elevated serum 17-hydroxy (OH) progesterone is seen in congenital adrenal hyperplasia. This presents as ambiguous genitalia at birth, precocious puberty, or less commonly as a "salt wasting" syndrome.

 A 68-year-old woman presents to her primary care physician (PCP) for an annual examination. She has no new complaints. She has a 10-year history of sarcoidosis managed with daily oral prednisone. On examination, she has a thickened amount of tissue on the back of her neck, and she has numerous purplish lines on her belly. Her lab results are normal, with the exception of a glucose level of 161. For this patient, what are the likely test results?

(A) High ACTH, high cortisol
(B) Low ACTH, low cortisol
(C) High ACTH, low cortisol
(D) Low ACTH, high cortisol
(E) Normal ACTH, high cortisol

The answer is B: Low ACTH, low cortisol. Exogenous corticosteroids suppress the endogenous production of cortisol. This occurs at the level of the hypothalamus, which decreases the amount of corticotrophin releasing hormine (CRH) release, which in turn decreases the amount of adrenocorticotrophic hormone (ACTH) produced by the anterior pituitary. Adrenocorticotrophic hormone (ACTH) functions to stimulate the zona fasciculata of the adrenal cortex to secrete cortisol, and the lack of ACTH leads to decreased production. ACTH is also a trophic factor for the zona fasciculata, and the lack of ACTH leads to atrophy of the gland. The gland then secretes a decreased amount of cortisol.

(A) These labs would be seen in someone with Cushing disease. (C) These labs would be seen in someone with primary adrenal insufficiency. (D) These labs would be seen in someone with secondary adrenal insufficiency. (E) These labs would be seen in either a normal individual or mild adrenal hyperplasia.

18. A 40-year-old woman presents to emergency department with right upper quadrant (RUQ) pain after eating fried chicken bucket. The patient has no fever, but is very tender in her RUQ to palpation, with no rebound tenderness. She obtains a CT scan which shows moderate cholelithiasis. The scan also reveals a 3-cm mass in the right adrenal gland. Lab testing shows her electrolytes to be normal, as well as an aldosterone/renin ratio, and a cortisol level. What is the best next step to address this incidental finding?

   (A) Adrenalectomy
   (B) 24-hour urine for vanylmandelic acid (VMA)
   (C) Repeat CT scan in 6 months
   (D) Adrenal biopsy
   (E) Repeat CT scan in 1 year

The answer is B: 24-hour urine for vanylmandelic acid (VMA). An incidentaloma is the discovery of an asymptomatic adrenal lesion on imaging done for another indication. Most of these masses are benign, but when found all must be properly monitored. The management consists of an annual physical examination with laboratory studies: serum potassium, aldosterone/renin ratio, cortisol, and a 24-hour urine for vanylmandelic acid (VMA), metanephrines, and normetanephrines. If the mass is under 4 cm and all of these labs are negative (showing the mass to be nonfunctional), then follow-up CT scans should be done every 6 to 12 months. If the mass is stable at 2 years, then no further management is necessary. Indications for surgical resection include if the mass is shown to grow, if the mass is 6 cm or larger, or if the mass is function (no matter the size).

(A) Adrenalectomy would be indicated if the mass were functional, growing, or 6 cm or greater. (C) Before any follow-up is scheduled, a 24-hour urine study for VMA needs to be done to rule out pheochromocytoma. Once shown to be nonfunctional, a follow-up CT scan is to be done in 6 to 12 months. (D) Adrenal biopsy is not recommended for the management of an incidentaloma. (E) See the explanation for answer **C**.

19. A 40-year-old man presents with a 4-month history of erectile dysfunction. He denies any nocturnal erections. On ROS, he admits to having trouble seeing peripherally. His examination is essentially normal, with the exception of excess subcutaneous tissue around his areolas bilaterally. He previously was been healthy, and does not take

any medications. He has an extensive family history of many cancer types, including an uncle with Zollinger-Ellision syndrome. What is the inheritance pattern for this disorder?

(A) Autosomal recessive
(B) X-linked recessive
(C) Mitochondrial
(D) Autosomal dominant
(E) X-linked dominant

The answer is D: Autosomal dominant. The patient has a prolactinoma, which is a tumor of the anterior pituitary gland that secretes the hormone prolactin. The presence of a pituitary tumor along with this family history of multiple cancers including a gastrin-producing pancreatic tumor is consistent with multiple endocrine neoplasia type I. This disorder is caused by a gene mutation in the tumor suppressor gene MEN-I. The mutation is transmitted in an autosomal dominant fashion, where inheritance of one mutated copy leads to the disorder. The formation of neoplasms follows the "two hit" hypothesis, where the first hit is the germline mutation inherited from a parent and present in all cells at birth. And the second hit is a somatic mutation of the remaining wild-type copy of the MEN-I gene, leading to tumor development.

(A) MEN syndromes are not autosomal recessive, where one needs to inherit two mutated copies to have the disorder. (B) MEN syndromes are not X-linked recessive, where the gene is located on the X chromosome and men are affected more often as a result. (C) MEN syndromes are not inherited via mitochondrial DNA, which follows a matriarchal pattern. (E) MEN syndromes are not X-linked dominant, where women are much more likely to be afflicted.

 20 A 38-year-old woman presents with 3-year history of postprandial pain, weight loss, and diarrhea. She has tried several proton pump inhibitors, but none have alleviated her pain. Her abdominal examination showed mild tenderness to palpation in the epigastric region. When asking about her family, the patient states that her sister had "elevated calcium levels that required neck surgery." What test will confirm the diagnosis?

(A) CCK stimulation test
(B) Secretin stimulation test
(C) Somatostatin level
(D) Postprandial gastrin level
(E) Capsule endoscopy

The answer is B: Secretin stimulation test. This patient presents with epigastric pain that is refractory to medical therapy, along with weight loss and diarrhea. This is suspicious for Zollinger-Ellison syndrome, caused by a gastrin-producing pancreatic tumor. Her sister's neck surgery is likely a parathyroidectomy for hyperparathyroidism, which makes MEN-I syndrome possible in this patient. MEN-I syndrome manifests as neoplasms from the "3 Ps" (pancreas, pituitary, and parathyroid), and is associated with a mutation in the tumor suppressor gene MEN-I. To diagnose a gastrinoma, serum gastrin levels are found to be elevated. In cases where gastrin is not substantially elevated, a secretin stimulation test is employed. Secretin is administered IV, which stimulates the release of gastrin. If the measured amount of serum gastrin increases >200 pg/mL, it is considered a positive test.

(A) A CCK stimulation test is used to evaluate the gallbladder's ability to empty its contents, and is not used for the workup of a gastrinoma. (C) Somatostatin's function in the GI tract is to slow down gastric emptying and decrease pancreatic secretions. Serum levels of somatostatin are not used to evaluate gastrinoma. (D) To evaluate for a possible gastrinoma, an elevated fasting serum gastrin level is taken. This test loses its diagnostic value if the blood is drawn postprandially. (E) Capsule endoscopy is used to evaluate the small bowel. It can be used to look for jejunal ulcers, which are virtually pathopneumonic for gastrinoma. In the workup for a gastrinoma, a secretin stimulation test would come before a capsule endoscopy.

12

Pancreas and Spleen

1 A 45-year-old man with a history of alcoholism presents with persistent abdominal pain. He describes the pain as worse after eating. He localizes the pain to the epigastric area with radiation to his back. Additionally he has noticed clay colored stools. His temperature today is 37.1°C, blood pressure 135/80 mmHg, pulse 80 beats/min, and respirations 16 breaths/min. His weight is 15 kg less than his previous measurement 6 months ago. A magnetic resonance cholangiopancreatography (MRCP) is performed by the gastroenterologist and an image is shown in *Figure 12-1*.

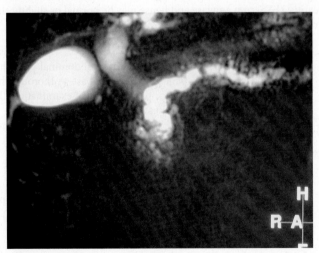

Figure 12-1

Which of the following test results will most likely be found on this patient's workup?

(A) Decreased fecal fat
(B) Granular calcifications on CT imaging
(C) Greatly increased serum CA 19-9
(D) Multiple poorly defined neoplastic lesions on CT imaging
(E) Significantly elevated serum amylase and lipase

The answer is B: **Granular calcifications on CT imaging.** This patient's history and physical signs suggest a diagnosis of chronic pancreatitis. Chronic pancreatitis is a chronic inflammatory state of the pancreas that ultimately leads to impaired pancreatic functions. Common conditions that lead to chronic pancreatitis include alcohol, hereditary, cystic fibrosis, trauma, hypercalcemic states, and certain infections. Patients usually complain of persistent abdominal pain and steatorrhea (indicated by his clay-colored stools) resulting from malabsorption. Weight loss in chronic pancreatitis is usually due to malabsorption. Chronic pancreatitis is associated with an increased risk of pancreatic cancer. Several clues on diagnostic imaging will suggest chronic pancreatitis in this patient. These include among others course granular calcifications (common finding), pancreatic pseudocysts, and peripancreatic fibrosis. The MRCP performed in this case reveals dilation of the pancreatic duct with a stone present as well as branch duct ectasia.

(A) Fecal fat content will be increased in chronic pancreatitis. (C) Although serum CA 19-9 may be mildly elevated in chronic pancreatitis, it is not typically elevated to the same levels as pancreatic cancer. (D) Multiple poorly defined neoplastic lesions on CT imaging suggest pancreatic malignancy rather than pancreatitis. (E) Serum amylase and lipase may be normal or slightly elevated in chronic pancreatitis.

2) A 69-year-old man presents with recurrent abdominal pain that has been diagnosed as acute pancreatitis in the past. A thorough history fails to reveal any risk factors for pancreatitis. On examination, there is mild jaundice. Laboratory studies show:

> Serum amylase: 310 U/L
> Serum lipase: 290 U/L
> Total bilirubin: 3.3 mg/dL
> Direct bilirubin: 1.5 mg/dL

An magnetic resonance cholangiopancreatography (MRCP) was performed and shows two separately draining dorsal and ventral ducts. Which of the following is the most likely diagnosis?

(A) Annular pancreas
(B) Anomalous pancreaticobiliary junction
(C) Choledochal cyst
(D) Hereditary pancreatitis
(E) Pancreatic divisum

The answer is E: Pancreatic divisum. This patient's history and imaging findings suggest pancreatic divisum, a rare congenital disorder of the pancreas in which a single pancreatic duct fails to form. Instead, two ducts (dorsal and ventral ducts) are present. Patients are most often asymptomatic and the congenital anomaly is most commonly found during autopsy. However, pancreatitis symptoms may occur in approximately 1% of patients. The most accurate method of diagnosis is endoscopic retrograde cholangiopancreatography (ERCP). Treatment in symptomatic individuals often will include a sphincterotomy.

(A) Annular pancreas is a congenital disorder of the pancreas in which a ring of pancreatic tissue completely encircles the duodenum. In some cases, the annular pancreas may compress the duodenum and cause bowel obstruction. If symptoms do occur, they are usually a result of partial or complete blockage of the intestine. Several conditions are associated with annular pancreas and include Down syndrome and polyhydramnios. Treatment is surgical with generally excellent outcomes. However, patients with the condition are at increased risk of pancreatic and/or biliary tract cancer. (B) Anomalous pancreaticobiliary junction is a congenital condition in which the pancreatic and bile ducts unite outside the duodenal wall and form a long common channel. The condition may result in acute pancreatitis and is associated with choledochal cysts and biliary tract cancers. Treatment is surgical. This patient's findings are not consistent with this disorder. (C) Choledochal cysts are congenital dilations of the bile ducts. They may occasionally present with intermittent abdominal pain, jaundice, and right upper quadrant masses along with a laboratory finding of direct hyperbilirubinemia. There are multiple subtypes of cysts, and treatment is surgical with a roux-en-Y anastomosis of the biliary duct. There is a slightly increased risk of malignancy (2%) in patients with choledochal cysts. This patient's findings are not consistent with this disorder. (D) Hereditary or familial pancreatitis is a hereditary condition in which there are mutations or substitutions in the trypsinogen (PRSS1) gene. The mechanism of pancreatitis is likely due to increased autoactivation or reduced deactivation of trypsinogen. This patient does not have a family history of pancreatitis, and his imaging findings suggest a different diagnosis.

---

3. A 30-year-old man presents with nausea, vomiting, and severe abdominal pain that has increased in severity over the last day. The patient reports that the pain is worse when he lies on his back. He describes the pain as "stabbing" and "shooting to my back." He denies a history of alcoholism, smoking, or drugs. His past medical history is unremarkable and he is not taking any medications. His temperature is 38.3°C, blood pressure 140/87 mmHg, pulse 110 beats/min, and respirations 20 breaths/min. On examination, there is tenderness and guarding in the epigastric area. Which of the following is the next best step in management?

(A) Abdominal CT scan
(B) ERCP
(C) Nothing by mouth, intravenous hydration, analgesics, and antibiotics
(D) Nothing by mouth, intravenous hydration, and analgesics
(E) Surgery

The answer is D: **Nothing by mouth, intravenous hydration, and analgesics.** This patient is presenting with signs and symptoms of acute pancreatitis. The initial management in patients with mild-to-moderate acute pancreatitis is supportive (keeping the patient nothing by mouth, providing intravenous support, and analgesics for pain relief). Laboratory studies should be sent for confirmation including serum amylase, lipase, liver enzymes, electrolytes, blood urea nitrogen, creatinine, glucose, cholesterol, and triglyceride levels.

(A) Diagnostic imaging is unnecessary in most cases of pancreatitis although it can be used when the diagnosis is in doubt. This patient has a high probability of acute pancreatitis, and although imaging may be obtained, it is not the next best step in management. (B) endoscopic retrograde cholangiopancreatigraphy (ERCP) is useful procedure to evaluate the pancreatic and biliary duct system. However, it is only indicated in patients with acute gallstone pancreatitis and should not be used as a first-line diagnostic tool. (C) Although nothing by mouth, intravenous hydration, and analgesics are important in this patient's management, antibiotics are not needed in most cases of acute pancreatitis. (E) The mainstay of treatment of acute pancreatitis is bowel rest with nothing given by mouth and intravenous fluids. Supplementation with pain medications is appropriate as well. Surgical treatment is not recommended for this condition.

 A 65-year-old man with a history of alcoholism presents with nausea, vomiting, and an acute "stabbing" pain in the epigastric region. He is subsequently diagnosed with acute pancreatitis. Which of the following laboratory findings are included in Ranson criteria at admission?

(A) Age > 45 years
(B) Hematocrit fall > 10%
(C) Leukocytes > 16,000 cells/mm^3
(D) Sequestration of fluids > 6 L
(E) Serum calcium < 8.0 mg/dL

The answer is C: **Leukocytes greater than 16,000 cells/mm^3.** Ranson criteria are a clinical prediction rule that helps estimate the severity and prognosis of an acute pancreatitis. It was originally introduced in 1974. Each criterion is assigned a one-point value. The total points are then added up and used to predict mortality. There are separate criteria for assessment at admission and within 48 hours. For admission, the assessment is as follows:

1. Age greater than 55 years
2. White blood cell count greater than 16,000/mm^3
3. Lactate dehydrogenase greater than 600 U/L
4. AST greater than 120 U/L
5. Glucose greater than 200 mg/dL

For within 48 hours, the assessment is as follows:

1. Serum calcium less than 8.0 mg/dL
2. Hematocrit fall of greater than 10%
3. Hypoxemia (P$_{O2}$ less than 60 mmHg)
4. Blood urea nitrogen (BUN) increase of 5 mg/dL or more after intravenous hydration
5. Base deficit of greater than 4 mEq/L
6. Sequestration of fluids greater than 6 L

If the final score is between 0 and 2, then there is 2% associated mortality. A score between 3 and 4 corresponds to 15% mortality. Score of 5 to 6 is 40% mortality. Finally, a score of 7 to 8 is associated with 100% mortality.

(A) Age greater than 55 years (not 45) is a criterion for admission. (B) A hematocrit fall of greater than 10% is a criterion for within 48 hours rather than at admission. (D) Sequestration of fluids greater than 6 L is a criterion for within 48 hours. (E) Serum calcium less than 8.0 mg/dL is a criterion for within 48 hours.

---

 5 A 50-year-old man presents with an acute onset of epigastric pain following a scorpion bite. The physician suspects an acute pancreatitis and orders laboratory studies and imaging for confirmation. The patient is subsequently admitted and intravenous support initiated. Laboratory studies at admission and at 48 hours after admission return with the following values:

At admission:

Serum sodium: 139 mEq/L
Serum potassium: 3.9 mEq/L
Serum chloride: 103 mEq/L
Serum calcium: 8.5 mg/dL
BUN: 15 mg/dL
Glucose: 250 mg/dL
Hemoglobin: 12.7 g/dL
Hematocrit: 35%
Leukocytes: 17,500/mm^3
Platelets: 300,000/mm^3
Lactate dehydrogenase: 350 U/L
AST: 95 U/L
ALT: 110 U/L
P$_{O2}$: 75 mmHg

At 48 hours:

> Serum sodium: 142 mEq/L
> Serum potassium: 4.0 mEq/L
> Serum chloride: 102 mEq/L
> Serum calcium: 7.9 mg/dL
> BUN: 15 mg/dL
> Glucose: 110 mg/dL
> Hemoglobin: 11.5 g/dL
> Hematocrit: 32%
> Leukocytes: 13,500/mm³
> Platelets: 300,000/mm³
> Lactate dehydrogenase: 150 U/L
> AST: 56 U/L
> ALT: 70 U/L
> P_{O_2}: 75 mmHg
> Fluid sequestration: 3.5 L
> Base deficit: 2 mEq/L

Based on Ranson criteria, which of the following is the patient's estimated mortality?

(A) 2%
(B) 5%
(C) 15%
(D) 40%
(E) 100%

The answer is C: 15%. This patient presenting with an acute pancreatitis obtains three points with Ranson criteria (glucose greater than 200 mg/dL on admission, leukocytes greater than 16,000/mm³ on admission, and serum calcium less than 8.0 mg/dL at 48 hours). With three to four points, the associated mortality according to Ranson criteria is approximately 15%.

(A) 2% mortality is the rate for a score of between 0 and 2. (B) 5% mortality is not associated with a Ranson criteria score. (D) 40% mortality is the rate for a score of 5 or 6. (E) 100% mortality is the rate for a score of 7 or 8.

 6 A 62-year-old black man presents with abdominal pain, fatigue, and 30-lb weight loss over the last 6 months. He describes the abdominal pain as "dull," located in the epigastric region with radiation to the back. He also describes darker than normal urine and light colored stools. His temperature is 36.7°C, blood pressure 135/80 mmHg, pulse 65 beats/min, and respirations 14 breaths/min. The physical examination is remarkable for mild scleral jaundice. The liver edge is smooth and not enlarged. There is a positive Homan sign on the left leg. Which of the following is the next best step in diagnosis?

(A) Computed tomography scan of the abdomen
(B) ERCP
(C) Laboratory studies
(D) MRI of the abdomen
(E) Transcutaneous ultrasound of the abdomen

The answer is A: **Computed tomography scan of the abdomen.**
Although pancreatic cancer typically has a more subtle presentation, patients may sometimes complain of more obvious signs of pancreatic disease such as malabsorption, jaundice, and epigastric pain. Due to low cost and high sensitivity/specificity, the initial test for diagnosis of a suspected pancreatic malignancy is CT imaging.

(B) Endoscopic retrograde cholangiopancreatigraphy (ERCP) is a highly sensitive test for detecting pancreatic or biliary carcinomas. However, it lacks specificity for pancreatic cancers and is much more invasive than CT imaging. (C) Laboratory studies are generally very nonspecific for pancreatic cancer. Patients may present with anemia and this patient most likely has elevated bilirubin associated with obstructive jaundice. Although tumor markers such as CA 19-9 may also be helpful as an adjunct to imaging, there is no standardized role for this test in the workup for pancreatic carcinoma. Studies have shown that CA-19-9 levels greater than 100 U/mL are highly specific for malignancy. (D) Although the role of MRI may be expanding in pancreatic cancer, it continues to be more expensive and no better in the diagnosis of pancreatic malignancy than CT imaging. (E) Although ultrasound is frequently performed before CT imaging when these symptoms are present, the role of ultrasound in the diagnosis of pancreatic malignancies is limited due to overlying gas from the gastrointestinal tract.

 7 A 3-year-old boy presents with failure to thrive and recurrent sinopulmonary infections. His past medical history is also remarkable for several episodes of bowel obstruction. Laboratory studies in the past have shown an increase in sweat chloride levels. Which of the following is the most common pancreatic manifestation that can be expected to develop in this patient?

(A) Endocrine insufficiency
(B) Exocrine insufficiency
(C) Pancreatic malignancy
(D) Type 1 diabetes mellitus
(E) Type 2 diabetes mellitus

The answer is B: **Exocrine insufficiency.** Exocrine failure is the most common and initial manifestation of pancreatic disease in cystic fibrosis and occurs in 85% to 90% of patients. Exocrine functions of the pancreas include bicarbonate and digestive enzyme secretions. Patients with cystic fibrosis will almost always require pancreatic enzyme supplements to help maintain growth and development.

(A) Endocrine insufficiency occurs less commonly (although still substantial) in patients with cystic fibrosis with a rate between 30% and 50%. Endocrine functions include hormone production including secretion of glucagon and insulin. As a result, many patients with cystic fibrosis eventually develop impaired insulin production and diabetes. (C) Although the risk for pancreatic cancer in patients with cystic fibrosis may be increased according to some studies, it is still a rare occurrence since many patients do not have normal lifespans. (D) Although both share impaired insulin production, type 1 diabetes is an autoimmune phenomenon unrelated to cystic fibrosis-induced diabetes. (E) Although type 2 diabetes shares some characteristics of cystic fibrosis-induced diabetes, it is not more common in cystic fibrosis patients.

8 A 63-year-old woman presents to the emergency department with epigastric and left upper quadrant abdominal pain. On further questioning, she reports multiple similar episodes of abdominal pain in the past. Her past medical history is remarkable for a chronic and recurring "skin rash," for which she takes a low-dose topical corticosteroid. She smokes 1 pack per day for the last 20 years. She admits to drinking 1 glass of wine nightly with meals. Her temperature is 37.1°C, blood pressure 130/80 mmHg, pulse 100 beats/min, and respirations 20 breaths/min. On examination, her abdomen is soft and nondistended with significant epigastric tenderness. Laboratory studies show the following:

Serum amylase: 790 U/L
Serum lipase: 2,650 U/L

CT imaging is obtained and a representative image is shown in *Figure 12-2*.

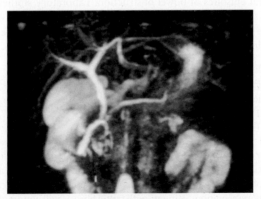

Figure 12-2

Which of the following is the most likely cause of her recurrent abdominal pain?

(A) Alcohol-induced chronic pancreatitis
(B) Annular pancreas
(C) Corticosteroids
(D) Gallstone pancreatitis
(E) Pancreatic carcinoma

The answer is B: Annular pancreas. This patient's CT imaging findings and history of recurrent pancreatitis suggest annular pancreas as the etiology of her abdominal pain. Annular pancreas is an uncommon developmental malformation characterized by a ring of pancreatic tissue that encircles the duodenum. The most common portion surrounded is the descending duodenum, although other portions of the small bowel may be affected. The condition is more prevalent in men and with other developmental syndromes/anomalies such as Down syndrome, congenital heart disease, duodenal atresia, imperforate anus, and others. In most cases, the patients are asymptomatic. If annular pancreas presents in early infancy, it will usually be characterized by symptoms of duodenal obstruction. In adults, a more common way to present is with recurrent pancreatitis.

(A) Although this patient does have a history of alcohol use, the amount is not necessarily excessive. Additionally, the recurrent episodes of acute pancreatitis are better explained by annular pancreas. (C) Although corticosteroids are a known cause of acute pancreatitis, this patient has most likely been using low dose and topical corticosteroids for a long time without problems. Low doses and topical routes are much less likely to cause pancreatitis. (D) This patient's history, examination, and other objective findings are not consistent with gallstone pancreatitis. (E) Although pancreatic carcinoma may be a cause of pancreatitis, this patient's findings are not consistent with a malignancy.

 9 A 35-year-old man suffers a gunshot wound to the mid abdomen. During exploratory surgery, the surgeon finds an injured blood vessel that supplies the pancreas. Which of the following vessels does not supply blood to at least a portion of the pancreas?

(A) Celiac artery
(B) Ileocolic artery
(C) Inferior pancreaticoduodenal artery
(D) Superior pancreaticoduodenal artery
(E) Splenic artery

The answer is B: Ileocolic artery. The pancreas receives its blood supply from several arterial branches. The main blood supply comes from branches of the celiac and superior mesenteric arteries. The pancreatic body and tail receives a majority of its blood supply from the splenic artery. The superior and inferior pancreaticoduodenal arteries supply the head and uncinate processes of the pancreas as well as portions of the duodenum. The ileocolic is the only artery listed above that does at least in part supply the pancreas.

(A) The celiac artery branches into the splenic and common hepatic arteries, which both supply branches to the pancreas. (C) The inferior pancreaticoduodenal artery is a branch of the superior mesenteric artery that supplies the pancreas. (D) The superior pancreaticoduodenal artery is a branch of the common hepatic artery, which originates from the celiac trunk and helps supply the pancreas. (E) The splenic artery arises from the celiac artery and supplies a significant portion of pancreas.

---

10 A 39-year-old woman presents with severe epigastric pain, nausea, and vomiting. She reports that the pain started suddenly and has since started to radiate to her back. Her vitals are within normal limits. Physical examination reveals moderate icterus and a tender epigastric region with light palpation. An abdominal ultrasound shows numerous gallstones within the gallbladder. Laboratory studies reveal the following:

> Serum amylase: 4,100 U/L
> ALT: 235 U/L
> AST: 195 U/L
> Albumin: 3.6 g/dL
> Total bilirubin: 0.5 mg/dL

Which of the following is the best management of this patient?

(A) Corticosteroids
(B) Diagnostic ERCP
(C) Laparoscopic cholecystectomy
(D) Pancreaticoduodenectomy
(E) Platelet-activating factor antagonist

The answer is C: **Laparoscopic cholecystectomy** This patient is most likely experiencing an acute pancreatitis secondary to gallstone obstruction. The initial management is similar to that of an acute pancreatitis of any cause with nothing by mouth, intravenous support, and analgesics for pain relief. However, patients with gallstone pancreatitis should undergo a cholecystectomy prior to discharge. The reason for early cholecystectomy is primarily due to the high rate of recurrent pancreatitis. Another option for patients with gallstone pancreatitis with evidence of ascending cholangitis or symptoms not responding to medical therapy is ERCP with sphincterotomy and stone extraction.

(A) Corticosteroids are contraindicated in the treatment of acute pancreatitis since they may exacerbate the situation. (B) Diagnostic endoscopic retrograde cholangiopancreatigraphy (ERCP) is generally not indicated in acute pancreatitis due to its associated morbidity. However, it may sometimes be used along with sphincterotomy and stone extraction when the pancreatitis is unresponsive to medical therapy or if there is evidence of cholangitis. (D) Pancreaticoduodenectomy (Whipple procedure) is used to treat pancreatic cancer. It does not have a role in the management of routine pancreatitis secondary to gallstone obstruction. (E) Although platelet-activating factor antagonist has been studied in the treatment of acute pancreatitis, a large clinical trial using the platelet-activating factor antagonist lexipafant showed no benefit over current treatment regimens.

---

11 A 41-year-old homeless man presents to the emergency department with worsening epigastric pain for several months. He rates the pain as 6/10 and reports the pain as radiating to his back. He admits to frequently drinking alcohol and has been hospitalized in the past with chronic pancreatitis. Which of the following complications of chronic pancreatitis is this man at the most risk for?

(A) Autoimmune pancreatitis
(B) Biliary stones
(C) Diabetes mellitus
(D) Pancreatic carcinoma
(E) Splenic vein thrombosis

The answer is C: Diabetes mellitus Along with chronic pain and episodes of acute pancreatitis, diabetes mellitus from destruction of pancreatic beta cells is a major complication of chronic pancreatitis. Some studies have estimated the prevalence of glucose intolerance in patients with chronic pancreatitis to be 40% to 70%. Half of these patients will ultimately suffer from insulin-dependent diabetes mellitus. Diabetes secondary to chronic pancreatitis often occurs late in the disease process and is characterized by the low incidence of ketosis and a higher incidence of hypoglycemia.

(A) Although autoimmune pancreatitis may be a cause of chronic pancreatitis, it does not necessarily occur with increased frequency in patients with chronic pancreatitis due to chronic alcohol use. (B) Although biliary stones may occur in patients with chronic pancreatitis secondary to alcohol use, it occurs less frequently than diabetes. However, bile duct strictures do commonly occur with chronic pancreatitis and may result in overt jaundice and cholangitis. (D) Pancreatic cancer is a known complication of chronic pancreatitis, but occurs less frequently than diabetes. (E) Splenic vein thrombosis is a known complication of chronic pancreatitis and occurs due to its close approximation to the pancreas and resulting inflammation of the vein. However, its incidence is much less than diabetes. Complications of splenic vein thrombosis may include the formation of abnormal communicating veins between the stomach and spleen, which may result in massive hemorrhage. The treatment of choice for splenic vein thrombosis secondary to chronic pancreatitis is splenectomy.

12 A 55-year-old man with a long history of chain smoking complains of worsening pruritus. He also reports that over the last several months he has lost 20 kg and his skin has started to have a "yellow" appearance. He denies abdominal pain, nausea, vomiting, or stool changes. His temperature is 36.9°C, blood pressure 135/85 mmHg, pulse 80 beats/min, and respirations 16 breaths/min. His physical examination is remarkable for jaundice and excoriations. Laboratory studies reveal a direct bilirubin of 6.2 mg/dL and a greatly elevated alkaline phosphatase. The remaining laboratory studies are within normal limits. An abdominal ultrasound shows a dilated common bile duct with no gallstones or pancreatic masses visible. An abdominal CT examination shows no further findings. Which of the following is the next best step in management?

(A) Exploratory laparotomy
(B) Observation only
(C) Percutaneous biopsy of the pancreas
(D) Repeat abdominal CT scan in 6 months
(E) Upper gastrointestinal endoscopy with transduodenal ultrasound of the pancreas

The answer is E: Upper gastrointestinal endoscopy with transduodenal ultrasound of the pancreas. This patient's symptoms are concerning for an obstruction of the biliary tract. Additionally, this patient's history of painless jaundice along with a long history of heavy smoking is very concerning for pancreatic cancer as the etiology. Despite abdominal ultrasound and CT imaging, a cause for this patient's symptoms has not yet been identified. The next best step is endoscopic ultrasound, which provides excellent imaging of the pancreatic head and surrounding tissues. Endoscopic studies will also allow a simultaneous endoscopic retrograde cholangiopancreatography if necessary to further evaluate the lesion and provide biopsies.

(A) An exploratory laparotomy is invasive and would be premature at this point as other diagnostic modalities have not been utilized. (B) Observation is not appropriate as this patient has symptoms that warrant ruling out pancreatic cancer. (C) Percutaneous biopsy of the pancreas is sometimes used to obtain tissue for pathologic diagnosis in suspected cancer. However, a lesion to biopsy has not yet been identified in this patient. (D) This patient needs further workup. Repeating the abdominal CT scan would not be appropriate and would simply allow more time for a potential tumor to grow.

13 A 45-year-old woman presents for a routine checkup. She is in good medical condition but seems anxious. She inquires about the causes of acute pancreatitis because her husband recently was hospitalized with an episode. Which of the following may you advise her is the most common cause of acute pancreatitis in western populations?

(A) Alcohol consumption
(B) Gallstone disease
(C) Hypercalcemia
(D) Hypertriglyceridemia
(E) Trauma

The answer is B: Gallstone disease. Biliary disease is the most common cause of acute pancreatitis in western populations and is estimated to account for approximately 30% to 50% of cases. The pancreatic injury is secondary to bile stone blockage the ampulla of Vater. The blockage results in increased pressures in the pancreas, which may ultimately lead to the episode of acute pancreatitis.

(A) Alcohol consumption is a close second most common cause of acute pancreatitis in developed countries such as the United States and accounts for approximately 35% of cases. Alcohol is thought to cause pancreatic damage by several mechanisms including causing an accumulation of digestive enzymes in the pancreas, increasing permeability of the ductules which allows enzymes to reach the parenchyma, and increasing protein content of pancreatic juice which leads to formation of protein plugs that block pancreatic outflow. (C) Hypercalcemia secondary to many diseases (hyperparathyroidism, malignancy, excessive vitamin D, etc.) may result in acute pancreatitis. (D) Hypertriglyceridemia may occur when the triglyceride levels are significantly elevated (greater than 1,000 mg/dL). Triglycerides usually do not reach this level unless the patient suffers from familial hyperlipidemia syndromes. (E) Trauma to the pancreas in a variety of forms (penetrating, blunt, gunshots) may cause pancreatitis, although these are less common than alcohol and gallstones.

 A 41-year-old man presents to the emergency department with severe epigastric pain that radiates to his back. He has also been vomiting severely over the last several hours. The initial physical examination, imaging, and laboratory studies suggest a diagnosis of acute pancreatitis. The patient is started on careful intravenous support and receives nothing by mouth. Over the next hour, the patient develops hypotension, hypoxemia, and multiorgan failure. His blood pressure fails to respond after infusion of 8 L of normal saline over 8 hours. Which of the following is the most likely cause of this patient's hypoxemia?

(A) Acute lung injury from aspiration
(B) Overzealous intravenous hydration
(C) Pneumonia
(D) Sepsis
(E) Systemic cytokine release

The answer is E: Systemic cytokine release. This patient is most likely suffering from acute respiratory distress syndrome secondary to systemic cytokine release following severe pancreatitis. During severe necrotizing pancreatitis, there is often massive third-spacing of fluid due to pancreatic inflammation and systemic inflammatory response syndrome. These cytokines may affect the lung tissue through diffuse alveolar damage, microvascular injury, and an influx of inflammatory cells into the lung parenchyma. The inflammatory response also increases endothelial and epithelial permeability with resulting protein-rich leakage of exudate into the alveolar space. This exudate hinders oxygen exchange resulting in the respiratory symptoms. Physicians must be careful to distinguish adult respiratory distress syndrome (ARDS) secondary to acute pancreatitis from overhydrating as the treatment is significantly different. (A) Although the patient was vomiting, he has other systemic signs along with acute pancreatitis indicating a different etiology. (B) Overhydrating this patient is a less likely cause of hypoxemia since the patient's blood pressure is unresponsive to fluids and there are other signs of systemic failure. (C) Although pneumonia may cause respiratory distress, this patient's symptoms are coinciding with an episode of acute pancreatitis and have evolved much more rapidly than typical for pneumonia. (D) Although sepsis may cause a systemic inflammatory response and resulting respiratory distress, this patient's presentation is more suggestive of respiratory distress secondary to severe necrotizing pancreatitis.

---

 15 A 59-year-old woman with a long history of smoking presents with painless jaundice and pruritus. A workup including abdominal computed tomography imaging reveals a 2-cm mass in the head of the pancreas. Besides the new found mass, the patient is in otherwise excellent medical condition. Which of the following is a contraindication to performing a pancreaticoduodenectomy in this patient?

(A) Liver serosa involvement
(B) Lymph nodes positive for cancer
(C) Tumor abutment of the superior mesenteric artery
(D) Tumor in the head of the pancreas
(E) Tumor size of 2 cm

The answer is A: Liver serosa involvement. Pancreatic cancer generally has a poor prognosis due to the tendency of patients to show symptoms only when the disease is advanced. However, in some cases surgical removal of the tumor provides significant morbidity and mortality benefits. Good candidates for surgery include those with an absence of extrapancreatic disease, a patent superior mesenteric vein confluence, and no direct tumor extension to the celiac axis or superior mesenteric arteries. Local extension of the tumor to involve the liver serosa is a contraindication to performing a Whipple procedure since there is little mortality benefit. Other contraindications include liver metastasis, invasion of the colonic mesentery, invasion of the hepatoduodenal ligaments, metastasis to the portal vein, fixation by the tumor of the duodenum to underlying structures, and metastasis to the aorta or vena cava.

(B) Positive lymph nodes are not necessarily a contraindication to performing a Whipple procedure. (C) Abutment of the tumor to the superior mesenteric artery is not always a contraindication to surgery. (D) Involvement of the pancreatic head by the tumor is not a contraindication to performing a Whipple procedure. (E) Tumor size of 2 cm is not a contraindication to performing a Whipple procedure. However, tumor diameters greater than 3 cm are associated with a poor prognosis.

---

 16 A 65-year-old man is brought to the emergency department following a motor vehicle accident with blunt abdominal trauma. Although he complains of abdominal pain, he appears hemodynamically stable. CT imaging of the chest, abdomen and pelvis reveals a grade 4 splenic laceration with contrast extravasation and no evidence of other organ trauma. His past medical history is remarkable for coronary artery disease with several stents in place. Which of the following is the next best step in management?

(A) Embolization
(B) Focused assessment with sonography in trauma (FAST) examination
(C) Medical management
(D) Observation
(E) Splenectomy

The answer is E: **Splenectomy.** This patient has a significant splenic injury with contrast extravasation. Contrast extravasation is an indication of significant splenic trauma. Thus, the next best step in management for this patient is splenectomy with surgical exploration as he is not a good candidate for embolization and observation.

(A) Although embolization is a good option for patients with low-grade splenic injuries that are hemodynamically stable, this patient is over 55 with significant medical comorbidities and is not a good candidate for embolization. Embolization has a high failure rate in these patients. (B) FAST examination is more useful in hemodynamically unstable patients. Additionally, a negative FAST examination does not exclude splenic injury. (C) Medical management generally does not have a role in splenic trauma. (D) There are several nonoperative management options for splenic injuries that encompass both observation and embolization procedures. These options work best for lower grade splenic injuries. Contraindications to nonoperative management include high-grade splenic injuries (which may be indicated by contrast extravasation), hemodynamic instability, generalized peritonitis, or patients with additional intraabdmominal injuries that require surgical repair/exploration.

17 A 31-year-old man with a history of immune thrombocytopenic purpura is evaluated for splenectomy after corticosteroids and intravenous immunoglobulin (IVIG) have failed to maintain his platelet counts. His platelet count is currently 6,000/μL. Which of the following is the most appropriate step in preparing this patient for surgery?

(A) Lifelong amoxicillin prophylaxis
(B) Lifelong penicillin prophylaxis
(C) Pneumococcal, meningococcal, and Haemophilus influenzae Type B vaccine (HIB) vaccine 2 weeks prior to surgery
(D) Pneumococcal, meningococcal, and HIB vaccine 14 days after surgery
(E) Pneumococcal, meningococcal, and HIB vaccine immediately following surgery

The answer is C: Pneumococcal, meningococcal, and Haemophilus influenza Type B vaccine (HIB) vaccine 2 weeks prior to surgery. Loss of splenic functional tissue places individuals at high risk for infection (overwhelming postsplenectomy sepsis) with encapsulated organisms such as *Streptococcus pneumoniae, Haemophilus influenzae* type b, and *Neisseria meningitidis*. Although the timing of vaccine administration with splenectomy is a topic of long-standing debate, current guidelines recommend prophylactic vaccination with polyvalent pneumococcal, meningococcal, and haemophilus b conjugate vaccines at least 2 weeks prior to elective splenectomy to allow an adequate immune response.

(A) Prophylaxis with amoxicillin may sometimes be utilized in select asplenic patients but is not indicated in this patient. (B) Lifelong penicillin prophylaxis may sometimes be utilized in select asplenic patients but is not indicated in this patient. (D) This is not the current recommendation for patients undergoing elective splenectomy. (E) Although this may be appropriate in certain situations (patient fails to receive vaccine dose before surgery), this is not the recommended schedule for the vaccinations with elective splenectomy.

18 A 60-year-old male immigrant complains of fatigue, malaise, and abdominal pain. On physical examination, the spleen is palpable and prominent below the costal margin. A CT examination reveals a massively enlarged spleen estimated to weigh approximately 2,500 g. Which of the following is not a potential cause of massive splenomegaly?

(A) Cirrhosis
(B) Lymphoma
(C) Malaria
(D) Myelofibrosis
(E) Polycythemia vera

The answer is A: Cirrhosis. Massive splenomegaly is defined as a spleen size of greater than 1,000 g. Causes of massive splenomegaly include (among others) thalassemia, chronic myelogenous leukemia, chronic lymphocytic leukemia, lymphomas, myelofibrosis, polycythemia vera, various metabolic diseases (Gauchers disease, Niemann-Pick disease, etc.), sarcoidosis, auto-immune hemolytic anemia, and malaria. Cirrhosis is not a cause of massive splenomegaly but still may cause an enlarged spleen secondary to vascular congestion.

(B) Lymphomas may cause massive splenomegaly due to infiltration by tumor cells. (C) Malaria is a potential cause of massive splenomegaly in patients, especially with repeated episodes. The syndrome is called "tropical splenomeg-aly syndrome" and patients with this disease may have quite impressive spleen sizes. The spleen in tropical splenomegaly enlarges secondary to an exaggerated stimulation of polyclonal B lymphocytes producing vast amounts of immu-noglobulin M. (D) Myelofibrosis is a bone marrow disorder where the mar-row is replaced with collagenous connective tissue. In this disease, the spleen may become the primary site of hematopoiesis. It is possible for the spleen to become markedly enlarged weighing up to 4,000 g. (E) Polycythemia vera is a myeloproliferative disease characterized by a trilineage expansion of hemato-poiesis. A significant portion of patients with polycythemia vera present with splenomegaly, and a significant portion of these with massive splenomegaly.

---

19   A 30-year-old white man is rushed by paramedics to the emergency department after being stabbed in the abdomen by a jealous girlfriend. On arrival, the patient is hemodynamically stable and complaining of severe abdominal pain. On examination, there is a single penetrat-ing stab wound to the upper left quadrant of the abdomen. Imaging reveals a grade 5 splenic laceration with a significant amount of free blood in the abdomen. The patient is emergently brought to the oper-ating room for exploratory laparotomy, splenectomy, and hemostasis. Which of the following is not a function of this patient's spleen?

(A) Clearance of microorganisms and particulate from the bloodstream
(B) Development site for T lymphocytes
(C) Embryonic hematopoiesis
(D) Removal of abnormal RBCs
(E) Synthesis of immunoglobulin

The answer is B: Development site for T lymphocytes. Although T lym-phocytes are found within the spleen, the development site for T lymphocytes is in the thymus.

(A) One function of the spleen in mechanical filtration of particulate matter and microorganisms from the bloodstream. (C) While the bone mar-row is the primary site of hematopoiesis in adults, the spleen also continues to function and is a major site of hematopoiesis in the developing fetus and neonate. (D) The red pulp in the spleen functions to mechanically filtrate abnormal red blood cells. (E) A major function of the spleen is with the active immune response through both humoral and cell-mediated pathways. B lymphocytes located within the spleen produce a significant portion of the body's immunoglobulin.

 20 A 70-year-old homeless man with a history of chronic alcoholism presents with severe pain in his upper belly that started several hours prior. He characterizes the pain as "10/10," with a "stabbing" like quality and radiation to the back. His serum lipase and amylase are greatly elevated. Which of the following physical examination findings are associated with severe necrotizing pancreatitis?

(A) Chronic papulovesicular eruptions on the extensor surfaces
(B) Edema and bruising in the subcutaneous tissue around the umbilicus
(C) Enlarged nodule in the left supraclavicular fossa
(D) Palpable nodule bulging into the umbilicus
(E) Visible swollen venous vessels that resolve and appear around the body

The answer is B: **Edema and bruising in the subcutaneous tissue around the umbilicus.** Acute necrotizing pancreatitis is a severe form of acute pancreatitis. The natural history of acute pancreatitis is often described in the literature of consisting of two phases with an initial systemic inflammatory response resulting in release of inflammatory mediators and possible organ failure. The second phase, usually described as a sepsis picture with organ failure, usually occurs several weeks later. Several physical examination findings are associated with acute necrotizing pancreatitis including Cullen sign and Grey-Turner sign. Cullen sign is characterized by superficial bruising and edema in the subcutaneous tissues surrounding the umbilicus. Grey-Turner sign is characterized by retroperitoneal hemorrhage and flank bruising. Other signs may include subcutaneous nodules as a result of fat necrosis.

(A) This physical examination finding is a description of dermatitis herpetiformis, a skin condition associated with celiac disease. (C) This physical examination finding is a description of Virchow node, which also may represent malignant disease (often gastric cancer) in the abdomen. (D) This description is that of a Sister Mary Joseph nodule, which classically represents metastatic cancer in the pelvis or abdomen. (E) This physical examination finding is a description of Trousseau sign of malignancy, associated with pancreatic adenocarcinoma.

Skin and Soft Tissue

1 A 45-year-old man is cut on his right palm with a knife while removing a fishing knot. He immediately drives to a local urgent care for evaluation. On examination, there is a clean 2 cm in length by a 0.5-cm-deep laceration on his palm with minimal bleeding. Which of the following wound closure methods would best facilitate healing in this man's laceration?

(A) Amputation
(B) Quaternary intention
(C) Primary intention
(D) Secondary intention
(E) Tertiary intention

The answer is C: Primary intention. This patient has a clean wound with edges that may easily be approximated. In this case, the wound edges may be approximated by suture and undergo primary intention healing. Primary intention healing is the shortest and most efficient method of wound healing. Epithelialization occurs as early as 24 hours after wound closure. This method of closure minimizes scarring and heals rapidly.

(A) Amputation would not be appropriate for this patient's wound as the hand is not gangrenous or necrotic and blood supply is maintained. (B) Quaternary intention is not a type of wound healing. (D) Secondary intention describes when a wound is not approximated and instead allowed to granulate. This type requires a much longer phase of healing than primary intention. Granulation results in a wider scar formation. Wound care is typically performed to remove debris and allow granulation tissue to form. This patient's laceration is clean and small with easily approximated edges; thus secondary intention is not necessary. (E) Tertiary intention is defined as delayed primary closure. In tertiary intention, the wound is left open for cleaning and observation for several days. After a set time period, the edges are approximated so that the remainder of healing may occur. This patient's laceration is clean and small with easily approximated edges; thus tertiary intention healing is not necessary.

2 A 29-year-old woman falls down an escalator while shopping in high heals. She sustains several lacerations and bruises on her arms and torso. Her friends bring her to the emergency department for evaluation. Fortunately, only minor injuries are found during evaluation. She is discharged from the emergency department several hours later. Which of the following is not a feature of normal wound healing for this patient's minor injuries?

(A) Contraction
(B) Collagen deposition
(C) Denaturation
(D) Maturation
(E) Proliferation

The answer is C: Denaturation. Denaturation is a process of protein breakdown including loss of secondary and tertiary structures. Although it may happen in wound healing, it is not a described phase of wound healing.

(A) Contraction occurs to some degree in all healing wounds during the proliferative phase, which occurs approximately 5 to 10 days after wound occurrence. In contraction, the wound shrinks due to the action of myofibroblasts (differentiated fibroblasts). However, if contraction phase is extended too long, there may be disfigurement and loss of tissue function. However, this usually occurs to a greater degree in more serious wounds. (B) Collagen deposition occurs during the proliferative phase of healing as a function of fibroblasts. The result is increased strength of the wound and better facilitation of healing. (D) Maturation is an important part of the healing process. It occurs after the levels of collagen production (type 1 from type 3) equalize through the processes of creation from fibroblasts and destruction by collagenases. This process may take up to 2 years to complete. (E) Proliferation is the second stage of healing and occurs after the inflammatory phase. It typically begins within 48 hours of injury and involves angiogenesis, granulation, contraction, and epithelialization.

3 A 27-year-old woman with a history of severe asthma is stabbed by her boyfriend during an argument over who is the best professional baseball player. She presents to the emergency department in severe pain and clutching her stomach. On examination, there is a large laceration over her abdomen with moderate bleeding. Her wound is operatively repaired and she is discharged several days later. During a follow-up visit, her medications are reviewed. Which of the following medications will most likely prevent optimal healing in this patient?

(A) Ceftriaxone
(B) Gentamicin
(C) Methylprednisolone
(D) Retinoic acid
(E) Vitamin E

The answer is C: Methylprednisolone. Glucocorticoids including methylprednisolone are known to cause impaired wound healing by directly blunting the cellular response that naturally takes place. Impaired cellular response results in impaired fibroblast proliferation and decreased collagen deposition. Studies have also shown decreased granulation tissue, extracellular matrix, epithelialization, and wound contraction. Although this effect is often decreased with inhaled glucocorticoids for asthma, it occurs in greater frequency in patients with severe asthma that are inhaling or receiving intravenous medications frequently. Some other medications and substances that impair wound healing include anticoagulants, antihistamines, nonsteroidal anti-inflammatory drugs, immunosuppressive drugs (phenytoin, chemotherapy agents, azathioprine, etc.), penicillamines, some retinoids, and colchicine.

(A) Ceftriaxone is not associated with impaired wound healing. In some cases it may increase wound healing by clearing infection. (B) Gentamicin is not associated with impaired wound healing. In some cases it may increase wound healing by clearing infection. (D) Several studies have shown that vitamin A may even help wound healing. Particularly in patients on glucocorticoids, administration of vitamin A may help reverse some of the wound impairing effects. (E) Studies have shown that vitamin E may assist in wound healing.

 4 A 27-year-old man is burned by an iron while using this instrument to iron his pants. He is immediately brought to the emergency department for evaluation. On examination, the skin over a 5 cm area on his anterior left leg appears red and blistering. Although the involved area is tender to touch, the skin blanches with pressure. An image of the leg is shown in *Figure 13-1*.

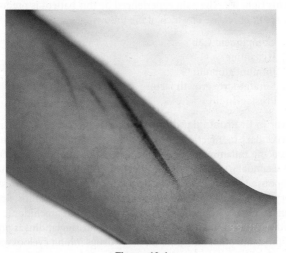

Figure 13-1

Which of the following most likely describes the attributes of this burn?

(A) It extends into the dermis
(B) It involves the entire dermis and extends into subcutaneous tissue
(C) It involves the epidermis only
(D) It will require excision and grafting
(E) The patient's mother should be reported to child protective services

The answer is A: It extends into the dermis. The description of this patient's burn is that of a second-degree burn. Second-degree burns are often red, wet, and very painful and tend to evolve over time. In second-degree burns, there may be an enormous variability in the depth ranging from the papillary to reticular dermis. They are prone to infections, scarring, and contractures, and may occasionally require excision with skin grafting.

(B) Burns that involve the entire dermis and extend into the subcutaneous tissue are defined as third- or fourth-degree burns. (C) Burns that involve the epidermis only are usually minor and defined as first-degree burns. (D) Although second-degree burns may require excision and grafting, they do not always require it. (E) This clinical vignette does not give enough information to determine whether child protective services should be involved.

5 A 19-year-old male construction worker presents with pain in his right lower leg that has occurred over the last several days and has been getting worse. He currently rates the pain as 7/10. Several days earlier, he recalls scratching his foot on a nail while at work. Examination of his leg reveals swollen, erythematous, and warm skin extending partially up his right leg. The pain experienced by this patient is predominantly the result of release of which of the following?

(A) Compliment C3b
(B) Histamine
(C) Immunoglobulin G
(D) Keratinocyte growth factors
(E) Prostaglandin

The answer is E: Prostaglandin. This patient is most likely suffering from cellulitis secondary to infection introduced by his earlier injury. With cellulitis there is an acute inflammatory response with infiltration by neutrophils and exudation secondary to the bacterial infection. Along with this acute inflammatory response is release of numerous chemical mediators that result in the warmth, erythema, swelling, and pain associated with the cellulitis. Prostaglandins are unsaturated carboxylic acids synthesized from arachidonic acid that are released with inflammation. One function of prostaglandins is production of pain. Aspirin and other anti-inflammatory drugs inhibit cyclooxygenase, an enzyme involved in the production of prostaglandins.

(A) Compliment C3b acts as an opsonin but is not known to be directly involved in pain. (B) Histamine is a vasodilator and does not directly cause the pain. (C) Immunoglobulin G (IgG) is involved in the immune response and vasodilation. It is not directly responsible for this man's pain. (D) Keratinocyte growth factors are involved in keratinocyte migration, proliferation, and differentiation. They are not directly involved in pain.

 6 A 48-year-old woman presents with new onset of seizures and behavioral changes that started approximately 6 months ago. Advanced imaging reveals multiple round metastatic lesions in her brain. Her past medical history is remarkable for a black lesion on her toe she had excised 20 years prior. A thorough workup and multiple additional imaging studies reveal no primary malignancy. A lesion on the arm is noted and shown in *Figure 13-2*.

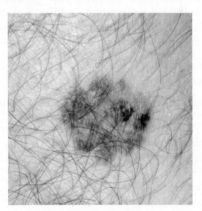

Figure 13-2

Which of the most likely characterizes this type of malignancy?

(A) Originates from cells in the stratum basalis
(B) Negative staining for HMB45
(C) Prognosis typically determined by amount of horizontal spread
(D) Signet ring cells are commonly seen on histology
(E) Tends to metastasize to the lungs, bone, and liver

The answer is A: **Originates from cells in the stratum basalis.** This patient is most likely suffering from metastatic malignant melanoma. Her description of a black lesion on her toe that was removed many years prior suggests a long latency between metastasis, which is not usually seen with other tumors. Malignant melanoma may often metastasize to areas that other tumors do not typically metastasize to. Malignant melanoma originates from melanocytes in the stratum basalis layer of the epidermis.

(B) Malignant melanoma tumors usually stain positive for HMB45 and S100, which may assist in the diagnosis. (C) Prognosis with malignant melanoma is typically determined by vertical rather than horizontal spread. (D) Although signet ring cells may be rarely seen in malignant melanoma, they are more often associated with adenocarcinomas. (E) Melanoma tends to metastasize to the dermis, lungs, liver, and brain. Although melanoma may metastasize to bone, the most common sites of prostate cancer metastasis include the lungs, bone, and liver.

7 A 29-year-old man presents to the emergency department with complaints of fever and painful swelling in his scrotum for the last 3 days. He reports that he had a minor injury of his scrotum 5 days previously for which he received no treatment other than acetaminophen. His current blood pressure is 110/75 mmHg, pulse 110 beats/min, respirations 19 breaths/min, and temperature 38.2°C. Local examination of the genitals reveals an edematous and tender scrotum with palpable crepitation and foul smelling discharge. Laboratory studies show:

> Leukocytes: 19,000/mm³
> Hemoglobin: 14 g/dL

Which of the following best explains the path of infection in this patient?

(A) Along fascial planes
(B) Hematogenous spread
(C) Localized spread
(D) Lymphatic spread
(E) Transcutaneously

The answer is A: Along fascial planes. This patient is suffering from Fournier gangrene, a necrotizing soft tissue infection that spreads along fascial planes. The most common origin is usually a genitourinary or perianal source, although other less common origins are possible. The morbidity and mortality in this infection are high; thus, prompt surgical debridement is necessary as part of the treatment.

(B) Hematogenously is an uncommon way for Fournier gangrene to initially spread. However, once patients become septic, hematogenous spread may occur. (C) Although the infection may be initially localized, Fournier gangrene tends to quickly spread along fascial planes. If left alone, patients will quickly become septic. (D) Lymphatic spread is uncommon in Fournier gangrene. (E) Although the initiating event may occur transcutaneously (such as this patient's initial injury), the infection does not typically spread along the skin.

8 A 69-year-old man with a history of diabetes mellitus presents with painful swelling of his scrotum for the last 8 days. His temperature is 38.4°C, blood pressure 100/50 mmHg, pulse 135 beats/min, and respirations 22 breaths/min. On examination, he is pale and confused. His scrotum is grossly edematous with multiple areas of gangrenous patches of skin leaking foul-smelling discharge. He is started on aggressive intravenous hydration with crystalloids, and antibiotics are ordered just prior to being rushed to the operating room for surgical debridement. To which organism(s) should initial antibiotics be targeted?

(A) Group A *Streptococcus*
(B) Polymicrobial
(C) *Pseudomonas*
(D) *Staphylococcus aureus*
(E) *Vibrio vulnificus*

The answer is B: Polymicrobial. This patient is suffering from Fournier gangrene, a necrotizing soft tissue infection of the scrotum and surrounding tissues. Wound cultures from patients with Fournier gangrene are almost always polymicrobial with a mixture of anaerobic and aerobic organisms. The most common anaerobic organism is *Escherichia coli* while *Bacteroides* is the most common anaerobe. There are multiple predisposing conditions that lead to an increased risk of Fourneir gangrene including diabetes mellitus (such as in this patient), obesity, alcoholism, elderly age, HIV infection, and other conditions characterized by immunosuppression. Broad-spectrum antibiotics should be initiated as soon as possible and provide gram-positive, gram-negative, anaerobic, and aerobic coverage.

(A) Although group A (β-hemolytic) *Streptococcus* (gram-positive coccus) is known to cause Fournier gangrene, initial antibiotics in this patient should include other organisms since the majority of the time the infection is polymicrobial. If the cultures return as predominantly group A *Streptococcus*, then the antimicrobial coverage may be targeted toward this organism. (C) Although *Pseudomonas* (gram-negative rod) is known to cause Fournier gangrene, the initial antibiotics should be directed at a polymicrobial source of infection. If the cultures return as predominantly *Pseudomonas*, then the antimicrobial coverage may be targeted toward this organism. (D) Although *Staphylococcus aureus* (gram-positive coccal bacterium) is known to cause Fournier gangrene, the initial antibiotics should be directed at a polymicrobial source of infection. If the cultures return as predominantly *S. aureus*, then the antimicrobial coverage may be targeted toward this organism. (E) *Vibrio vulnificus* is also a known but rare cause of Fournier gangrene. It is a gram-negative rod typically present in marine environments. However, this is a relatively rare cause and initial antibiotic choice should cover a polymicrobial source.

9　A 26-year-old man presents to the physician after finding a lump on his left thigh. He reports that he noticed the lump about 6 months ago and that since that time it has not increased in size or changed. He says that several of his siblings also have similar lumps under their skin in various places over their body. On examination, there is a soft, mobile mass measuring about 2 cm in the anterior left thigh felt just below the skin but above the muscle. The skin over the mass appears normal. Which of the following is the most likely diagnosis?

(A) Leiomyosarcoma
(B) Lipoma
(C) Liposarcoma
(D) Lymphoma
(E) Malignant melanoma

The answer is B: Lipoma. This patient's description of a soft tissue mass below the skin and above the muscle best fits the diagnosis of lipoma. Lipomas are the most common form of benign soft tissue tumors occurring in approximately 1% of the population. They originate in fat cells and are generally soft, mobile, and painless to palpation. They typically range from under 1 cm to greater than 6 cm. There are multiple subtypes of lipomas. They are not necessarily hereditary, but may be in some cases. Treatment is generally unnecessary unless the mass becomes painful or restricts movement.

(A) Leiomyosarcoma is an uncommon malignant soft tissue tumor (5% to 10% of soft tissue sarcomas) that most commonly occurs in areas where smooth muscle is found. (C) Liposarcomas are malignant tumors that also arise from fat cells but occur much less commonly than lipomas. They are typically large and bulky tumors and grow more aggressively than described in this scenario. (D) This patient's presentation is not typical of lymphoma. Although lymphomas may present as a soft tissue tumor, other systemic symptoms are usually present. (E) This patient's tumor is presenting subcutaneously with no overlying skin changes. This presentation is not consistent with a malignant melanoma.

10　A 56-year-old man presents with a growing subcutaneous mass in his right thigh. He reports that he does not remember how long the "lump" has been there. Although he smoked heavily as a young adult, he denies current smoking or alcohol use. His family history is unremarkable. Which of the following characteristics favor a more malignant potential for this man's tumor?

(A) Mobile
(B) Nondiagnostic pathology
(C) Painful
(D) Size greater than 7 cm
(E) Smoking history

The answer is D: Size greater than 7 cm. Soft tissue masses greater than 5 to 7 cm favor a diagnosis of a malignant soft tissue tumor. Other characteristics that suggest a malignant potential include rapid increase in size, fixation to underlying structures, increased age, associated lymphadenopathy, and others.

(A) Mobility of the mass does not suggest malignancy. Many benign soft tissue tumors such as lipomas are mobile with palpation. (B) Nondiagnostic pathology does not suggest malignancy. If the biopsy returns as nondiagnostic, the biopsy may need to be repeated. (C) Both malignant and nonmalignant soft tissue tumors may be painful. Benign tumors may cause pain through compression of local structures. (E) Smoking is not a known risk factor for the development of soft tissue sarcomas.

11 A 35-year-old man presents with acute abdominal pain. He is subsequently diagnosed with severe small bowel obstruction and is scheduled for surgery. Which of the following describes the layers of skin that the surgeon will cut through from in order of superficial to deep?

(A) Epidermis → Papillary dermis → Reticular dermis → Subcutaneous fat → Muscle

(B) Epidermis → Papillary dermis → Subcutaneous fat → Reticular dermis → Muscle

(C) Epidermis → Reticular dermis → Papillary dermis → Muscle → Subcutaneous fat

(D) Epidermis → Reticular dermis → Papillary dermis → Subcutaneous fat → Muscle

(E) Epidermis → Reticular dermis → Subcutaneous fat → Papillary dermis → Muscle

The answer is A: Epidermis → Papillary dermis → Reticular dermis → Subcutaneous fat → Muscle. The correct sequence of structures from superficial to deep includes the layers of the epidermis (stratum corneum, stratum lucidum, stratum granulosum, stratum spinosum, stratum basale), papillary dermis, reticular dermis, subcutaneous fat, and finally muscle.

(B) This is not the correct sequence of structures as the subcutaneous fat is found below the reticular dermis. (C) This is not the correct sequence of structures as the reticular dermis is found below the papillary dermis and subcutaneous fat below the reticular dermis. (D) This is not the correct sequence of structures as the reticular dermis is found below the papillary dermis. (E) This is not the correct sequence of structures as the papillary dermis is found above the reticular dermis and both are found above the subcutaneous tissue.

12 A 45-year-old man is injured while setting a beam at his construction job. He returns home and attempts to manage the wound at home with bandaging and left over narcotic pain medication from a previous hospitalization. Several days later his wife brings him to the emergency

department for evaluation. He is afebrile and his vitals are within normal limits. Examination of the wound reveals an irregular laceration on his lower calf with some debris within the cut. Which of the following is a relative contraindication to debriding the wound?

(A) Blisters around the wound
(B) Laceration involving callus
(C) Minimal foreign material within the wound
(D) Presence of healthy granulation tissue
(E) Presence of necrotic tissue

The answer is D: Presence of healthy granulation tissue. The presence of healthy granulation tissue within the wound is a relative contraindication to debridement. Other relative contraindications include presence of viable tissue, when the wound involves stable and dry heel ulcers, presence of healthy deep tissues, pyoderma gangrenosum, or dry/stable or ischemic gangrene from peripheral arterial disease.

(A) The presence of blisters around the wound is an indication for debridement. (B) Wounds involving callus are an indication for debridement. (C) Debris or foreign material within a wound is an indication for debridement. (E) Presence of necrotic tissue is an indication for debridement. Dry gangrene should not be debrided until vascular status is evaluated.

---

13 A 55-year-old farmer presents with a "mole" that has been increasing in size over the last several months. He says that the mole is not painful but has caused his wife some alarm. On examination, there is a 2×1 cm^2 dark brown area of pigmentation on the right forearm. Biopsy shows malignant cells that stain positive for S100 and invade to a depth of 2.3 mm. There are no lymph nodes identified as positive for malignancy on a sentinel lymph node biopsy. A chest x-ray is also negative. Which of the following provides the most definitive treatment for this patient?

(A) Adjuvant therapy with interferon-α 2b
(B) Dacarbazine
(C) Ipilimumab
(D) Surgical excision with 0.5 cm margins
(E) Surgical excision with 2.0 cm margins

The answer is E: Surgical excision with 2.0 cm margins. This patient has a localized malignant melanoma with a greater than 2.1 mm depth. Surgery is the definitive treatment of early melanoma with wide surgical excision. Surgical excision for tumors greater than 2.1 mm should have at least 2.0 cm margins.

(A) Adjuvant therapy with interferon-α is sometimes used with deep primary tumors (greater than 4 mm or regional lymph node involvement) after surgical excision. Studies have shown an increase in disease-free survival with interferon-α 2b. However, this drug is associated with toxicities and patients are typically closely monitored. (B) Dacarbazine is the first medication approved for treatment of metastatic melanoma. This patient's melanoma does not appear to be metastatic. (C) Ipilimumab is a humanized antibody directed against a down-regulatory receptor on activated T cells. It is currently approved for nonresectable metastatic melanoma. (D) Surgical excision with 0.5 cm margins may be appropriate for localized melanoma in situ.

 A 50-year-old woman is involved in a motor vehicle accident. She is brought to the emergency department with multiple traumatic injuries including fractures and lacerations to her right leg. She is stabilized and brought to the operating room for repair. The repair is successful. 48 hours after her initial injuries, her wounds are evaluated. Which of the following characterizes the healing of her wounds at this stage?

(A) Granulation tissue will be found in the wound beds
(B) Lymphocytes are the predominant cell type
(C) Most collagen fibers bridge the wound edges
(D) Neutrophils are the predominant cell type
(E) Wound strength is approximately 70% of normal

The answer is A: Granulation tissue will be found in the wound beds. The stages of wound healing in order are inflammation, proliferation, and maturation. The proliferative phase begins approximately 48 hours after injury and has four major elements: angiogenesis, granulation, contraction, and epithelialization. Granulation tissue is a temporary connective tissue that fills the wound bed. Fibroblasts are important in this process and are drawn to the wound by ischemia. Granulation tissue appears as a light red or pink tissue that has abundant capillary "buds." It is composed of a variety of cell types. The initial collagen type is type 3. This collagen is later replaced with type 1 collagen, a stronger collagen found in scar tissue. Since this patient's wound is only 48 hours old, granulation tissue should be found within the wound bed.

(B) Although chronic inflammatory cells are present, the predominant cell types in the proliferative phase are fibroblasts and macrophages. (C) During the proliferative phase, most collagen fibers are vertical and do not bridge the wound edges. Wound edge bridging occurs later in the healing process. (D) Although neutrophils may still be present, the predominant cell types in the proliferative phase are fibroblasts and macrophages. Neutrophils are the predominant cell type in the acute inflammatory stage. (E) Wound strength does not reach 70% of normal until much later in the healing process. Once completely remodeled, wounds typically only regain 80% of their initial strength.

15 A 21-year-old man is hit by a car while riding his bike down the highway. He sustains a large scalp laceration from falling head first into the pavement. The laceration is cleaned and sutured closed with only moderate loss of blood. He is discharged from the hospital and receives regular follow-up visits for his injuries. After complete healing of the scalp laceration, which of the following describes the potential strength of the wound as compared to the original?

(A) 100%
(B) 80%
(C) 50%
(D) 30%
(E) 20%

The answer is B: 80%. During the maturation phase of wound healing, collagen from granulation tissue is remodeled and converted to type 1 collagen from type 3. This process may take up to 2 years to complete. Alignment takes place through both external forces based on forces applied to the wound and internal forces when collagen lines up to match the wound edges. Peak tensile strength typically occurs about 60 days after injury. Unfortunately, even after complete healing, wounds typically only regain up to 80% of their tensile strength.

(A) Unfortunately, tissue rarely regains 100% of its previous strength after injury. (C) Approximately 50% of wound strength may occur when there is interference with wound healing. (D) Although this is possible in certain conditions, wounds typically regain more than 30% of their strength after complete wound healing. (E) Although this is possible in certain conditions, wounds typically regain more than 30% of their strength after complete wound healing.

16 A 30-year-old woman is brought to the emergency department by her husband due to increasing confusion, lethargy, and fever over the last day. Her husband reports that she injured her right thigh several days ago while swimming in the lake. Her temperature is 38.5°C, blood pressure 130/85 mmHg, pulse 110 beats/min, and respirations 20 breaths/min. On examination, there is erythema and soft tissue swelling extending from her thigh to her right knee that originates from a small 2-cm defect in the skin of the right anterior thigh. The skin is warm to touch over the involved area. Over the next several hours, her blood pressure becomes increasingly unstable and her fever increases to 38.7°C despite being on broad spectrum antibiotics. Blood cultures turn positive 6 hours after the initial draw and identify group A β-hemolytic *Streptococci*. Additionally, the skin over her thigh has started to turn black and necrose. Which of the following is the next best step in management?

(A) Administration of clindamycin
(B) Administration of erythromycin
(C) Administration of vancomycin
(D) Initiation of vasopressors
(E) Surgical debridement

The answer is E: **Surgical debridement.** This patient is most likely suffering from necrotizing fasciitis. She has already been given broad-spectrum antibiotics and her health continues to decline. To avoid death, this patient will need emergent surgical debridement. Continued antibiotics will be important during and after surgery.

(A) Although clindamycin might is an acceptable treatment of necrotizing fasciitis with group A *Streptococcus*, surgical debridement is the most important next step in management for this patient since failure to do so will result in death. Once surgery is complete, the antibiotics may be narrowed to adequately cover the causative organism. (B) Erythromycin is typically not used for treatment of necrotizing fasciitis. (C) Although vancomycin may adequately cover necrotizing fasciitis secondary to staphylococcal infection, the next best step in management for this patient is emergent surgery. (D) Although the patient is hemodynamically unstable, the source of the problems must be addressed. Management of her blood pressure with vasopressors is not the priority.

17 A 73-year-old man undergoes workup for a mass in his right arm. He reports that he has had difficulty moving his arm because of the increasing size of the mass. He denies pain. On examination, there is a subcutaneous 7-cm mass in the upper right arm near the shoulder joint that seems fixed to the muscle. The overlying skin is movable. An MRI of the mass shows a heterogeneous intramuscular mass with poorly defined borders. Which of the following is the next best step in management?

(A) Biopsy
(B) Chemotherapy
(C) Observation
(D) Radiation
(E) Surgical excision

The answer is A: **Biopsy.** This patient is most likely suffering from a malignant soft tissue tumor. Based on the location and features, a sarcoma is high on the differential. The next best step in management is to perform a biopsy, as the results of the biopsy will greatly influence management.

(B) Although chemotherapy may be used for treatment depending on the characteristics and stage of the tumor, biopsy to establish a diagnosis is the most important next step. (C) Observation in this case where malignancy is strongly suspected is not an appropriate. (D) Although radiation may be used for treatment depending on the characteristics and stage of the tumor, biopsy to establish a diagnosis is the most important next step. (E) Surgical excision is the mainstay of treatment for localized soft tissue malignancies. Although an excisional biopsy may be appropriate for small soft tissue tumors, biopsy to establish the diagnosis is important before surgical management in this case since the tumor is quite large.

---

18 A 5-year-old boy presents with painless mass that has been increasing in size over the last several months. On examination, there is a fixed mass on the right upper extremity that is nonmobile to palpation. Histologic examination reveals infiltrating and malignant cells consistent with a soft tissue sarcoma. Patients with which of the following conditions are at increased risk of developing soft tissue sarcomas?

(A) Neurofibromatosis type 1
(B) Fanconi anemia
(C) Neurofibromatosis type 2
(D) Diabetes mellitus
(E) Tissue trauma

The answer is A: Neurofibromatosis type 1. Although most soft tissue sarcomas are not associated with any known risk factors or identifiable etiology, several conditions and exposures are known to increase the risk in patients. For example, exposure to certain chemicals (chlorophenols, vinyl chlorides, etc.) may increase the risk. Several inherited diseases are known to have an increased tendency to develop soft tissue sarcomas. This includes neurofibromatosis type 1 (NF1). NF1, or von Recklinghausen disease, is caused by a mutation in the NF1 gene on chromosome 17. Patients characteristically have café-au-lait spots, dermal neurofibromas, and freckling in the axillary regions along with other associated conditions. Patients with NF1 are especially at an increased risk of developing malignant peripheral nerve sheath tumors, a type of malignant soft tissue tumor. Other conditions with an increased risk of developing malignant soft tissue tumors include Li-Fraumeni syndrome, tuberous sclerosis, Werner syndrome, Gorlin syndrome, familial adenomatous polyposis, Gardner syndrome, and retinoblastoma.

(B) Patients with Fanconi anemia are not known to have an increased risk of soft tissue sarcomas. (C) Patients with neurofibromatosis type 2 are not known to have an increased risk of soft tissue sarcomas. (D) Patients with diabetes mellitus are not at increased risk of developing soft tissue sarcomas. (E) Although once thought to be a risk factor, trauma is not associated with an increased risk of developing a soft tissue sarcoma.

---

19 A 55-year-old man presents with a feeling of "pressure" in his abdomen. He denies pain or gastrointestinal symptoms. On examination, there is a palpable mass in his left abdomen. CT imaging reveals a large left retroperitoneal mass. Biopsy shows malignant spindle-shaped cells consistent with a leiomyosarcoma. Which of the following characteristics of this tumor is not associated with a worse prognosis?

(A) Higher histologic grade
(B) Increased age
(C) Lymph node involvement
(D) Presence of metastasis
(E) Size greater than 2 cm

The answer is E: Size greater than 2 cm. The prognosis of soft tissue sarcomas usually depends on the stage of the tumor along with other features such as the grade and comorbid medical conditions. The staging system for retroperitoneal sarcomas takes into account the histologic grade, tumor size, depth of the tumor relative to the superficial muscular fascia, presence of lymph node involvement, and presence/absence of distal metastasis. However, 5 cm rather than 2 cm is considered the cutoff for a poorer prognosis with soft tissue sarcomas.

(A) Higher histologic grade suggests a poor prognosis for patients with soft tissue sarcoma. (B) As with many malignancies, increased age is associated with a poorer prognosis. (C) Lymph node involvement is associated with a poorer prognosis. (D) Tumor metastasis is associated with a decreased survival with soft tissue sarcomas.

 20 An 83-year-old nursing home patient with severe Alzheimer dementia is brought to the physician after a nursing aid finds an area of "skin breakdown on her back." On examination, she appears thin and frail. Her vitals are within normal limits. There is an area of skin loss with moderate tissue necrosis over her sacral area that extends into the subcutaneous tissue and fascia. The underlying muscle and bone are not involved. Which of the following is not necessarily part of the management for this patient?

(A) Repositioning the patient approximately every 2 hours
(B) Administration of antibiotics
(C) Surgical debridement
(D) Nutritional optimization
(E) Daily inspection and skin drying

The answer is B: Administration of antibiotics. Decubitus or pressure ulcers are a type of pressure sore that occurs from prolonged pressure exertion on the skin, soft tissue, muscle, or bone of the patient. In patients with normal mobility, mental capacity, and sensitivity, pressure ulcers rarely occur. Management of pressure ulcers depends on several factors including the stage, cause, and presence of infection. Although antibiotics may be used when infection is present, biopsy should be performed prior to administration of antibiotics to determine the presence of infection versus simple contamination.

(A) Repositioning the patient approximately every 2 hours is the cornerstone of pressure sore prevention. Even in the presence of specialty beds or other surfaces, the importance of repositioning should be emphasized. (C) Surgical debridement most often required for stage III or IV ulcers. Stage III ulcers are characterized by full-thickness skin loss with extension into the subcutaneous tissue but not through the underlying fascia. It usually appears as a "crater" on physical examination. Stage IV pressure ulcers are characterized by full thickness loss of skin and extension of the pressure ulcer into muscle, bone, tendon, or joint capsules. Osteomyelitis may often be present with stage IV pressure ulcers. (D) Nutritional status for patients with pressure ulcers should always be optimized if possible since this is the only way healing is sustained. This may require even parenteral feedings if nutrition cannot be corrected through less invasive methods. (E) Daily inspection with skin drying is very important for the healing and prevention of pressure ulcers.

Vascular Surgery

1. A 70-year-old man presents with right flank pain that radiates to his groin. He has a long history of heavy smoking and alcohol use and reports passing a kidney stone approximately 20 years prior to this event. His past medical history is also remarkable for diabetes mellitus, high cholesterol, and obesity. A computed tomography scan reveals a right 7-mm ureteral stone. In addition, coronal imaging was obtained, and is shown in *Figure 14-1*.

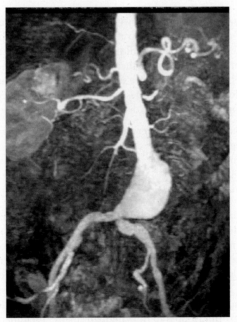

Figure 14-1

Which of the following is the greatest risk factor for the development of this patient's additional findings on the imaging study shown?

(A) Age
(B) History of smoking
(C) History of urolithiasis
(D) Metabolic syndrome
(E) Male sex

The answer is B: History of smoking. In this patient, smoking is the greatest risk factor for the development of aortic aneurysm. Studies have shown that it increases the risk approximately eight times that of nonsmoking adults. Other tobacco use also increases the risk. Other risk factors include the patient's age, atherosclerotic disease, hypertension, hypercholesterolemia, and connective tissue diseases such as Ehlers-Danlos or Marfan syndrome.

(A) Age greater than 65 is associated with an increased risk of aortic aneurysms. (C) Urolithiasis is not a risk factor for abdominal aortic aneurysms. (D) Metabolic syndrome is considered a risk factor for aortic aneurysms, although not as great as smoking. (E) Although men have a four- to five-fold increased risk of developing aortic aneurysms over that of women, smoking is a greater risk factor than gender.

 2 A 77-year-old man presents with a painful area in his groin following femoral artery catheterization after a motor vehicle crash. On examination, there is a painful pulsatile mass over the common femoral artery. The skin over the mass is erythematous. Duplex ultrasonography shows a pocket of hypoechogenicity surrounding the artery containing active blood flow that communicates with the underlying artery. Which of the following is the most likely diagnosis?

(A) Common femoral artery aneurysm
(B) Hemangioma
(C) Hematoma
(D) Inguinal hernia
(E) Pseudoaneurysm

The answer is E: Pseudoaneurysm. This patient's presentation is most consistent with that of a pseudoaneurysm. Pseudoaneurysms are hematomas that form outside the arterial wall, entrapped by surrounding tissue. The hematoma communicates with the artery and will often present as a painful pulsatile mass. The overlying skin may sometimes be edematous and erythematous. The most common causes of pseudoaneurysms are traumatic, and often a result of medical procedures. Diagnosis is often made with imaging such as duplex ultrasonography. Although many pseudoaneurysms may resolve by themselves, surgical correction may also be required.

(A) Although common femoral artery aneurysm may also present as a pulsatile groin mass, this patient's lesion has developed in the site of recent catheterization. Thus, an iatrogenic pseudoaneurysm is a more likely explanation for this patient's presentation. (B) Although a hemangioma may also form over a site of catheterization, it takes time to grow and would generally not present as acutely. (C) Hematomas commonly occur after catheterization and would also be in the differential of this patient's groin mass. However, hematomas do not typically have active blood flow since they do not communicate with the artery. (D) An inguinal hernia should be in the differential of any patient presenting with a groin mass. However, it is not the most likely diagnosis as this has developed acutely in an elderly patient after femoral catheterization.

3 A 55-year-old man presents with an acute onset of chest pain. He describes the pain as severe and of a "tearing" quality with radiation to his back. His blood pressure is 190/95 mmHg, pulse 120 beats/min, and respirations 20 breaths/min. He appears pale and diaphoretic. Which of the following findings will support a diagnosis of a thoracic aortic dissection?

(A) Difference in blood pressure between right and left arms
(B) Increased troponin levels
(C) Pain with palpation of the chest wall
(D) Systolic murmur on cardiac examination
(E) ST elevations on ECG

The answer is A: Difference in blood pressure between right and left arms. This man's clinical history along with a finding of blood pressure differences between the right and left arms would suggest a diagnosis of aortic dissection. Other features that suggest that the aortic dissection in the patient is the quality of the pain and hypertension. The diagnosis may be confirmed with transesophageal echocardiography or spiral CT imaging.

(B) Increased troponin levels would support a cardiac etiology for this man's chest pain. (C) Pain with palpation of the chest wall would suggest a musculoskeletal etiology of this man's pain. (D) Systolic murmur does not suggest a diagnosis of aortic dissection. Occasionally, the dissection may involve the aortic valve resulting in aortic insufficiency. If this occurs, a diastolic murmur best heard in the right second intercostal space may be present. (E) ST elevations do not usually occur with aortic dissection. If present, they would more support a cardiac etiology for this man's chest pain.

4 A 66-year-old man presents for a routine checkup several months following a shoulder surgery. He has a 30-pack-year smoking history but quit approximately 10 years ago. His current medications include aspirin and a multivitamin. He received a colonoscopy 7 years ago and his cholesterol was checked and within normal limits 3 years ago. He is not sexually active. His blood pressure today is 130/75 mmHg, pulse 60 beats/min, and respirations 15 breaths/min. The physician uses the visit to assist the patient in catching up with routine screening recommendations. Which of the following screenings are indicated at this time?

(A) Abdominal ultrasound
(B) Chest x-ray
(C) Colonoscopy
(D) HIV screening
(E) Lipid panel

The answer is A: **Abdominal ultrasound.** This patient is over 65 with a history of smoking. The United States Preventative Task Force (USPTF) recommends a single screening for abdominal aortic aneurysm with an abdominal ultrasound for men age 65 to 75 years who have a history of smoking.

(B) Chest x-rays have been proposed in the past for lung cancer screening. Unfortunately, they are not an effective screening tool and are not currently recommended. (C) This patient had a colonoscopy 7 years ago which is within the recommended 10-year interval. Thus, no colon cancer screening is indicated at this time. (D) HIV screening is only indicated for high-risk adults. This patient is not sexually active and thus at low risk for acquiring HIV. (E) According to the USPSF recommendations, lipid panels are indicated every 5 years. This patient's last lipid check was performed approximately 3 years ago.

 5 A 50-year-old woman complains of a "bulge in her stomach" that she can feel when she lies down. She denies pain or discomfort, but is worried about it because she has never felt it before. Her past medical history is unremarkable and she is generally in good health. On examination, there is a pulsatile mass palpable below the umbilicus just to the left of the midline. An aortic aneurysm is suspected. If confirmed, which of the following features will support an elective repair of the aortic aneurysm?

(A) Growth of 0.2 cm a year
(B) History of smoking
(C) High risk of mortality with repair
(D) Palpable aneurysm
(E) Size of 4.7 cm in diameter

The answer is E: **Size of 4.7 cm in diameter.** This patient is most likely presenting with an asymptomatic abdominal aortic aneurysm. Elective repair for good surgical candidates provide a significant mortality benefit. Indications for elective repair include a diameter greater than 5.4 cm in men and 4.5 cm in women. Patients also are candidates for elective repair when the aneurysm enlarges greater than 0.5 cm in 6 months or 1 cm in 1 year. For patients with significant comorbidities such as congestive heart failure, severe chronic obstructive pulmonary disease, symptomatic coronary artery disease, and a life expectancy less than 2 years, the risks of the operation may outweigh the benefits of repair. However, patients with significant comorbidities and aneurysms greater than 7 cm may sometimes be treated with elective repair.

(A) Growth of 0.2 cm a year does not necessarily indicate necessity for repair. Current recommendations indicate elective repair for growth greater than 0.5 cm in 6 months or 1 cm per year. (B) A history of smoking is not necessarily an indication for elective repair. Patients currently smoking should be strongly encouraged to quit smoking as this increases the chance for rupture. (C) Patients with a high risk of mortality from repair are generally not candidates for repair. (D) Aneurysms are more likely to be palpable when the patient is thin or with large size. However, it is not part of the criteria for elective repair.

 6 A 68-year-old woman presents to the surgical clinic with significant pain in her right calf after walking 30 feet. She reports that the pain goes away with rest and can be reproduced with additional walking. She has a history of smoking ½ pack per day for the last 40 years. Her other medical problems include diabetes mellitus, obesity, and a recent urinary tract infection. Her blood pressure today is 130/80 mmHg. Doppler pulses can be found in both extremities and ankle–brachial indices are 0.6 and 0.5 in the left and right extremities, respectively. Which of the following is the next best step in management?

(A) Anticoagulation with warfarin
(B) Arteriogram of her right leg
(C) Femoral-popliteal bypass surgery
(D) Observation
(E) Smoking cessation and exercise

The answer is E: Smoking cessation and exercise. This patient is presenting with symptoms of claudication. Intermittent claudication is caused by atherosclerotic blockage in the peripheral arteries. It is a separate entity than neurogenic claudication, which is often confused due to the similarity of symptoms. First-line treatment for this patient includes smoking cessation and an aggressive exercise regimen that should include walking. Walking will improve circulation and help collateral circulation form. Smoking cessation will prevent additional atherosclerotic disease. Medications such as antiplatelet agents, lipid-lowering agents, and pain relievers may also be used in management. Surgery for peripheral artery disease is always a last resort.

(A) Anticoagulation with warfarin has been shown to not prevent the heart complications of peripheral artery disease. Additionally, it greatly increases the risk of life-threatening bleeding. (B) Although an arteriogram of this patient's leg may reveal atherosclerotic disease, the test is invasive and not necessary to diagnose intermittent claudication. (C) Bypass surgery is generally performed only when the disease is severe. Surgery is never the first-line treatment for intermittent claudication. (D) Observation is not appropriate in this patient as she has risk factors (smoking, poor exercise) that can be addressed.

7 A 60-year-old man presents to the surgical clinic with pain and discomfort behind his left knee that is worse after standing for long periods of time. He also reports occasional numbness and tingling in his foot that has been occurring over the last 6 months. On physical examination, there is a palpable pulsating mass behind the patients left knee. Imaging study is obtained and is shown in *Figures 14-2A–C.*

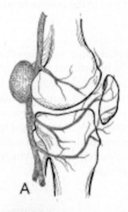

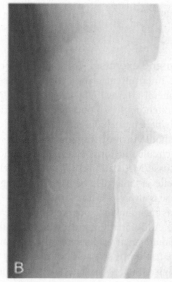

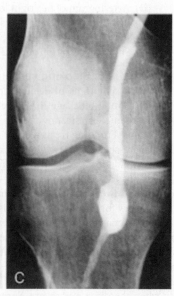

Figure 14-2

Which of the following is the most common acute complication of this patient's problem?

(A) Arteriovenous fistula formation
(B) Distal ischemia secondary to compartment syndrome
(C) Hematoma formation
(D) Rupture
(E) Thromboembolism

The answer is E: Thromboembolism. This patient is most likely suffering from a popliteal artery aneurysm. The imaging study obtained shows the popliteal aneurysm. The most common acute complication of popliteal aneurysms is thromboembolism with distal arterial occlusion. Thrombosis occurs in as many as 55% of patients with popliteal aneurysms.

(A) Arteriovenous fistula formation may rarely occur in peripheral aneurysms, but is much less common than thromboembolism. (B) If distal ischemia occurs in patients with a popliteal aneurysm, it is usually a result of thromboembolism rather than compartment syndrome. (C) Hematoma is not a common acute complication of popliteal aneurysm. (D) Rupture is a feared but uncommon complication of popliteal aneurysms. Rupture results in amputation of the limb in 50% to 70% of patients.

8 A 25-year-old woman complains of headaches, dizziness, and occasional chest pain. She reports that she was once told she had high blood pressure during a pre-employment physical. She reports that her mother also had similar symptoms and died from a stroke at age 34. Her temperature is 37.2°C, blood pressure 175/90 mmHg, pulse 65 beats/min, and respirations 18 breaths/min. Her cardiovascular examination is unremarkable. Bruits are auscultated on both sides of the umbilicus. Which of the following is the most likely diagnosis?

(A) Atherosclerosis
(B) Connective tissue disease
(C) Essential hypertension
(D) Fibrovascular dysplasia
(E) Kawasaki disease

The answer is D: Fibrovascular dysplasia. Suspect fibromuscular dysplasia in a young adult with hypertension and narrowing of the renal arteries. Fibromuscular dysplasia is an autosomal dominant disorder characterized by fibrous thickening of the arterial vessel walls. It is the most common cause of acquired renovascular hypertension in the United States. The most common artery affected by fibromuscular dysplasia is the carotid artery; however, renal arteries may also be affected. Renal artery stenosis results in activation of the renin–angiotensin system and water retention. This can further exacerbate the hypertension.

(A) Atherosclerosis is more likely in older patients but unlikely in this young woman. (B) Connective tissue diseases such as Marfan syndrome, Ehlers-Danlos syndrome, scleroderma, and others are unlikely causes of bilateral renal stenosis. (C) Essential hypertension may result in similar symptoms if severe, but would be much more common in elderly adults and unlikely to present with bilateral renal bruits. (E) Although vasculitides, such as Kawasaki disease, are important causes of renovascular hypertension in children, they are less common than fibromuscular dysplasia. Furthermore, this patient does not have other symptoms of Kawasaki disease.

 A 75 year old man is brought to the emergency department after falling off his chair while eating at the table. He is currently complaining of blurry vision. His past medical history is remarkable for hyperlipidemia and coronary artery disease. His examination in the emergency department is remarkable for limited function of his right hand. After 24 hours, his vision and strength have returned to normal. Head imaging reveals no areas of ischemic change. The patient's blood glucose is normal. Which of the following is the most likely diagnosis?

(A) Normal old age
(B) Severe dementia
(C) Stroke
(D) Temporal arteritis
(E) Transient ischemic attack

The answer is E: **Transient ischemic attack.** This patient has most likely suffered a transient ischemic attack (TIA). TIA symptoms typically last less than an hour, but may last as long as 24 hours. Patients suffering from TIAs will not have evidence of ischemic damage. The most common cause of a TIA is atherosclerotic emboli from the carotid arteries. Risk factors include family history, age 55 and older, men, African American race, hypertension, diabetes, and known atherosclerotic disease.

(A) Although elderly patients are more prone to falling, this patient's presentation is not a feature of normal aging. (B) Although severe dementia may present with neurologic manifestations, it does not present in an acute reversible manner such as this. (C) If this patient had suffered a stroke, there would most likely be evidence of permanent neurologic change or evidence of ischemia on imaging. (D) Although temporal arteritis may present with blurry vision, limited motor function is not a feature.

 A 65-year-old obese man presents with pain with walking that has recently progressed to pain at rest. He has been diagnosed with peripheral arterial disease in the past. Which of the following is not a risk factor for the development of peripheral arterial disease?

(A) Age over 50
(B) Hypertension
(C) Obesity
(D) Smoking
(E) Venous insufficiency

The answer is E: Venous insufficiency. Venous insufficiency is a condition caused by impaired venous valves resulting in pooling, dilated peripheral veins, and retrograde flow of venous blood. Common symptoms include pruritus, swelling, burning, aching, leg fatigue, and hyperpigmentation of the legs. Symptoms are often worse with walking and better with leg elevation. Risk factors include age (especially those over 50), hypertension, obesity, smoking, diabetes mellitus, hyperlipidemia, and other hypercoaguable states. However, venous insufficiency has not been shown to be a risk factor for peripheral arterial disease.

(A) Age over 50 is a known risk factor for peripheral arterial disease. (B) Hypertension is a known risk factor for peripheral arterial disease. (C) Obesity is a known risk factor for developing peripheral arterial disease. (D) Smoking is a known risk factor for developing peripheral arterial disease.

11) A 55-year-old man presents with claudication of his left calf that is reproducible with walking. He reports that this pain is very distressing because his favorite hobby is taking walks in the local park. He is subsequently diagnosed with intermittent claudication secondary to peripheral arterial disease. Which of the following medications has been shown to increase walking distance, improve HDL cholesterol, decrease triglycerides, and improve the quality of life in patients suffering from intermittent claudication?

(A) Alteplase
(B) Aspirin
(C) Cilostazol
(D) Heparin
(E) Simvastatin

The answer is C: Cilostazol. Cilostazol is a selective inhibitor of type 3 phosphodiesterase used for intermittent claudication. Studies have shown that cilostazol increases the amount of pain-free walking distance, improves HDL cholesterol by up to 13%, reduces triglycerides by up to 16%, and significantly improves the quality of life in patients suffering from intermittent claudication.

(A) Alteplase is a thrombolytic drug that may be used in acute episodes of vascular occlusion. It is not appropriate for use in intermittent claudication. (B) Aspirin is a first-line agent for intermittent claudication. However, it has not been shown to increase the amount of pain-free walking distance. (D) No benefit has been established for use of heparin for intermittent claudication. In addition, use of heparin greatly increases the risk of major bleeding events.

(E) Although Simvastatin has been shown to improve HDL and decrease triglycerides, its main effect is on LDL cholesterol and decreasing cardiovascular mortality/morbidity. Furthermore, there is not a known benefit for walking distance or quality of life improvements in patients suffering from intermittent claudication. Patients with known atherosclerotic disease should be managed with lipid-lowering agents.

 12 A 70-year-old man presents to the emergency department after his wife noticed him lose consciousness while watching television. She also reports that he has become progressively confused over the last several days. A CT examination of the patient's head shows blood in the subarachnoid space. Which of the following is the most common site for an aneurysm in the cerebral blood supply?

   (A) Anterior cerebral artery
   (B) Internal carotid artery
   (C) Middle cerebral artery
   (D) Posterior cerebral artery
   (E) Superior cerebellar artery

The answer is A: **Anterior cerebral artery.** This patient is most likely suffering from a ruptured cerebral aneurysm. The most common site for a cerebral aneurysm is the anterior cerebral artery.

   (B) The internal carotid artery is not the most common site. (C) The middle cerebral artery is not the most common site. (D) The posterior cerebral artery is not the most common site. (E) The superior cerebellar artery is not the most common site.

 13 A 60-year-old male diabetic patient with end-stage chronic kidney disease presents for preoperative evaluation for placement of an arteriovenous fistula. The patient asks the vascular surgeon what effect the fistula will have on his vascular system. Which of the following hemodynamic profiles will this patient most likely have following placement of the fistula?

	Heart Rate	Cardiac Output	Peripheral Vascular Resistance	Stroke Volume
(A)	Increased	Increased	Increased	Increased
(B)	Decreased	Decreased	Decreased	Decreased
(C)	Increased	Decreased	Decreased	Increased
(D)	Decreased	Increased	Increased	Decreased
(E)	Increased	Increased	Decreased	Increased

The answer is E: Heart Rate Increased, Cardiac Output Increased, Peripheral Vascular Resistance Decreased, Stroke Volume Increased. Arteriovenous fistulas are known to induce several hemodynamic changes. An arteriovenous fistula shunts oxygenated blood directly into venous circulation. Following fistula placement, arterial conductance increases. Consequently, cardiac output must increase. Changes include decreased total systemic vascular resistance, increased cardiac output, increased stroke volume, and increased heart rate.

(A) Although heart rate, cardiac output, and stroke volume increase with placement of a fistula, peripheral vascular resistance actually decreases when AV fistulas are present. (B) Although peripheral vascular resistance does decrease after fistula placement, heart rate, cardiac output, and stroke volume increase rather than decrease with AV fistulas. (C) Cardiac output increases rather than decreases when AV fistulas are present. (D) Heart rate and stroke volume increase while peripheral vascular resistance decreases when AV fistulas are present.

---

14 A 59-year-old man is referred to the surgery clinic after his primary care physician heard a bruit over the left carotid artery. He reports no symptoms although he admits he is currently on medication for "high cholesterol." Doppler imaging reveals 75% stenosis on the left and 30% stenosis on the right. Which of the following is the next best step in management of this patient's carotid stenosis?

(A) Anticoagulation
(B) Bilateral carotid endarterectomy
(C) Left carotid endarterectomy
(D) Observation
(E) Right carotid endarterectomy

The answer is C: Left carotid endarterectomy. This patient will require a left carotid endarterectomy. Studies show a significant benefit of surgical intervention in preventing morbidity and mortality with over 70% stenosis in asymptomatic stenosis. If patients are symptomatic, the stenosis threshold may sometimes be lowered.

(A) Although anticoagulation with medications such as aspirin may be appropriate for this patient long term to prevent complications, this patient has over 70% stenosis in the left side and will need surgery. Continued aspirin therapy after surgery will be required. (B) This patient only has 30% stenosis on the right side, which does not meet the threshold for surgical intervention on that side. (D) Observation is not appropriate for this patient as there is significant stenosis of the left carotid artery and atherosclerotic disease in the left. (E) Right carotid endarterectomy is not needed, as there is only 30% stenosis.

15 A 68-year-old man presents with pain in his legs during walking. He reports that the pain decreases with rest and will come back when he tries to walk again. He is retired from his job as a salesman and says that he sits home and watches television all day. He has smoked 2 packs of cigarettes per day for the last 40 years. His past medical history is remarkable for hypertension and obesity. His temperature is 36.9°C, blood pressure 135/85 mmHg, pulse 67 beats/min, and respirations 15 breaths/min. On examination, the pulses in his distal lower extremities are not palpable. Which of the following is the next best step in diagnosis?

(A) Angiography
(B) Ankle–brachial index
(C) Computed tomographic angiography
(D) Electrocardiogram
(E) Magnetic resonance angiography

The answer is B: Ankle–brachial index. Ankle–brachial index is an inexpensive and noninvasive test for diagnosing peripheral vascular insufficiency. The ankle–brachial index measures the systolic arterial pressure at the ankle and brachial artery using a Doppler device. A normal ankle-brachial index (ABI) is greater than 1.0. With symptoms of mild claudication, the ABI is often within 0.6 to 0.8. Severe claudication is usually characterized by an ABI of less than 0.5. Pain at rest and tissue necrosis may occur with ABIs less than 0.3.

(A) Although angiography is the gold standard for diagnosing peripheral arterial disease, it is invasive and usually reserved for patients undergoing surgical treatment for peripheral arterial disease. (C) Computed tomographic angiography might be used in certain settings for diagnosis of peripheral arterial disease but would most certainly not be the initial test for diagnosis in this patient. (D) Although patients with peripheral arterial disease often have coronary artery disease, this patient has no evidence of ischemic heart changes and would most likely have a normal EKG. (E) Magnetic resonance angiography is useful in some settings for diagnosis and imaging of peripheral arterial disease. However, it is expensive and not the initial test for workup.

16 A 59-year-old woman complains of "ugly legs." She reports that she noticed discoloration of her legs several years ago, but "doesn't like to look at them anymore." She denies ever seeing a physician before but reports that her mother died from breast cancer. Her blood pressure is 145/85 mmHg, pulse 70 beats/min, and respirations 13 breaths/min. On examination, there are several large shallow ulcers starting at the mid-calf and extending down to the lateral malleolus. The skin in her lower extremities is flaking, is thick, and has a brown discoloration. Which of the following is the most likely diagnosis?

(A) Arterial insufficiency
(B) Diabetic ulcers
(C) Gout
(D) Trauma
(E) Venous insufficiency

The answer is E: Venous insufficiency. This patient is most likely suffering from venous stasis. Symptoms that indicate chronic venous insufficiency include swelling in the lower legs, achiness, varicose veins, leathery (discolored) and thick skin, flaking/itching of the skin, and stasis ulcers. Stasis ulcers may be distinguished from other types of ulcers by their location (starting at mid-calf and extending down to the lateral/medial malleolus) and shallow ulcer bed.

(A) The ulcers of arterial insufficiency are usually located distally on the dorsum of the feet or toes. The ulcer base is covered with granulation tissue and bleeds very little with manipulation. The skin around the ulcers will show other signs of arterial insufficiency including hairlessness, pale and cold skin, and absent pulses. (B) Diabetic ulcers result from diabetic neuropathy and poor healing. They usually occur over bony prominences in the extremities. (C) Tophaceous gout often occurs in the big toe and may result in ulceration. This patient's presentation is not consistent with this diagnosis. (D) Traumatic wounds would follow a history of trauma, which this patient does not have.

17 A 66-year-old obese man presents with pain in his right leg during walking. He reports the pain will stop when he rests and returns with exercise. His past medical history is remarkable for diabetes mellitus. He smokes 2 packs per day for the last 50 years. He is retired from his job as a meat packer. He reports that his father died at age 65 from a myocardial infarction and that his sister has had several acute coronary events. His current medications include aspirin and metformin. His blood pressure today is 135/85 mmHg, pulse 70 beats/min, respirations 15 breaths/min, and temperature 37.5°C. Which of the following is the next best step in management?

(A) Cilostazol
(B) Diet change
(C) Smoking cessation
(D) Surgery
(E) Warfarin

The answer is C: Smoking cessation. The next best step in any patient with claudication is exercise and lifestyle modifications such as smoking cessation and exercise. Smoking cessation has been shown to be the most important modifiable risk factor to improve claudication symptoms. Other changes that decrease symptoms include use of lipid-lowering agents, reduction of fat intake, and management of comorbid conditions (diabetes, hypertension, etc.).

(A) Cilostazol is an antiplatelet medication that has been shown to improve walking distance in patients with intermittent claudication. Although this is an option, lifestyle modifications should always be the first-line step in management of patients with intermittent claudication. (B) Although diet change is an important lifestyle modification for patients with intermittent claudication, smoking cessation has been shown to improve symptoms more. (D) Surgery should always be the last resort for intermittent claudication. (E) Warfarin does not improve outcomes in peripheral arterial disease and increases the risk of bleeding events.

---

18 A 75-year-old man presents to the clinic with cramping in his legs. He reports that the pain has been getting progressively worse over the last year. The pain begins within 10 minutes of walking and will go away with rest. His past medical history is remarkable for coronary artery disease, excised melanoma at age 30, and diabetes mellitus. On examination, the skin on his distal extremities is dry and flaky with loss of hair. His pedal pulses are diminished. The patient's ankle–brachial index is 1.3. Which of the following is the most likely cause of this patient's symptoms?

(A) Deep vein thrombosis
(B) Neurogenic claudication
(C) Peripheral arterial disease
(D) Restless leg syndrome
(E) Venous insufficiency

The answer is C: Peripheral arterial disease. This patient's presentation is classic for arterial insufficiency. While the ankle–brachial index is usually decreased in patients with arterial insufficiency, his ankle–brachial index may be falsely elevated due to calcification and stiffening of his peripheral arteries. This is a more common occurrence in patients with diabetes mellitus.

(A) Symptoms such as pain, swelling, redness, and warmth suggesting a diagnosis of deep vein thrombosis are not present in this patient. (B) Although neurogenic claudication (caused by spinal stenosis) may be confused with intermittent claudication, neurogenic claudication will improve with hip flexion and worsen with extension. (D) Restless leg syndrome is a disorder defined by the urge or need to move the legs to stop unwanted sensation. This patient does not describe symptoms consistent with this diagnosis. (E) Venous insufficiency does not present with symptoms of intermittent cramping with exercise.

---

19 A 57-year-old man with severe arterial insufficiency is referred by his primary care physician to the vascular surgery clinic with worsening pain in the lower 1/3 of the calf. He reports that the pain is so severe that he is unable to perform his daily job duties as a security guard. He exercises and reports quitting smoking 7 months ago. His current medications include clopidogrel, hydrochlorothiazide, and simvastatin. On examination, the patient's distal pulses are not palpated. An arteriogram demonstrates occlusion of the superficial femoral and popliteal arteries. Intact flow is seen distal to the blockage. Which of the following is the most appropriate management for this patient?

(A) Amputation
(B) Anticoagulation only
(C) Aortofemoral bypass
(D) Femoropopliteal bypass
(E) Observation

The answer is D: Femoropopliteal bypass. This patient requires a femoropopliteal bypass procedure. Femoropopliteal bypass surgery has been shown to drastically improve lifestyle in patients suffering from disabling claudication. Operative mortality rate is low for those without cardiac disease. With this surgery, the anastomoses are given to the artery with the best outflow tract (often popliteal or tibial arteries). After successful reconstitution, the patient will require frequent examinations for patency of the graft and medications to reduce further atherosclerotic disease such as aspirin and lipid-lowering agents.

(A) Amputation is not appropriate for this patient as the tissue distal to the blockage is not necrotic or containing irreversible ischemia. (B) This patient is already taking anticoagulation without improvement of his symptoms. Further intervention is indicated at this time. (C) An aortofemoral bypass would not treat this patient's symptoms as the blockage is distal to the femoral artery. (E) Observation alone would not be appropriate as the patient is suffering from disabling claudication.

20   A 67-year-old man undergoes a hip replacement. His operative and immediate postoperative course is unremarkable. A week after surgery he complains of low-grade fevers and left leg pain extending from the medial thigh to the calf. On examination, the pain is worse with dorsiflexion of the foot. There is mild discoloration of the left lower extremity and pain with palpation of the calf muscle. Which of the following is the next best step in management?

(A) Compression ultrasonography
(B) D-dimer assay
(C) Helical computed axial tomography
(D) Observation
(E) Ventilation perfusion scan

The answer is A: Compression ultrasonography. This patient has a high likelihood of having deep vein thrombosis and will need venous ultrasonography for diagnosis. Venous ultrasound is the first step in diagnosis in patients with moderate to high likelihood of deep venous thrombosis (DVT).

(B) D-dimer is a degradation product of cross-linked fibrin found in blood clots. In patients with DVT, D-dimer levels are typically elevated. However, due to the many other conditions that can result in an elevation in the D-dimer levels, this test is not specific for DVT. Thus, current recommendations suggest using D-dimer assay for low probability of DVT. (C) Helical computed axial tomography is the first-line test for diagnosis of pulmonary embolism. Although deep vein thrombosis may lead to pulmonary emboli, this patient does not currently have these symptoms. (D) Observation in this patient would not be the correct choice as this patient has a high likelihood of DVT. (E) Ventilation perfusion scanning might be more appropriate in patients with symptoms of pulmonary embolism.

 A 52-year-old woman who underwent a cholecystectomy for gallbladder disease complains of left leg pain several days after her operation. Her medical history is remarkable for stage 3 lung cancer with metastasis to the colon, diabetes mellitus, and anemia secondary to mild gastrointestinal bleeding. On examination, there is a palpable cord noted on the lateral aspect of the left calf. The leg is warm and visibly swollen. Which of the following is the next best step in management?

(A) Anticoagulation with heparin
(B) Anticoagulation with heparin followed by warfarin
(C) Aspirin
(D) Low molecular weight heparin
(E) Vena cava filter

The answer is E: Vena cava filter. This patient is most likely suffering from deep vein thrombosis following surgery. Unfortunately, with her recent surgery invoking a risk of bleeding along with her comorbid conditions such as lung cancer and gastrointestinal bleeding, anticoagulation is contraindicated. Thus, the next best step in management is placement of a vena cava filter. Inferior vena cava (IVC) filters are generally placed percutaneously and accessed through the femoral or jugular vein approach.

(A) This patient recently underwent surgery and is at a high risk for bleeding; thus, anticoagulation is contraindicated. (B) Although this might be the initial step in a patient without risk for bleeding or other contraindications for anticoagulation, this patient will need an IVC filter placed. (C) Aspirin would be inappropriate for an acute treatment of deep vein thrombosis and

Which of the following is the most important next step?

(A) Chest computed tomography
(B) Obtain previous chest imaging
(C) Percutaneous biopsy of the lesion
(D) Serum carcinoembryonic antigen
(E) Transbronchial biopsy of the lesion

The answer is B: Obtain previous chest imaging. This patient is presenting with a pneumonia-like picture along with an upper lobe lesion that could potentially represent malignancy. The images shown reveal a left upper lobe lung lesion. Since he has a history of smoking, he is at greater risk for lung cancer. The next step in diagnosis is to search his medical records for a previous chest x-ray or imaging to characterize the lesion. A new lesion or one that has increased in size is more likely to represent cancer than a lesion that has not changed. This option is not only the most important first step, but is also inexpensive and less invasive compared to the other options.

(A) Although most patients with a suspicious lung lesion will eventually get a chest computed tomography, this would not be the most important initial step as looking for a previous image would be much less expensive. (C) Although a percutaneous biopsy might be appropriate if the lesion is found to be peripheral and growing in size, this would not be the initial step for an unknown lesion. (D) Carcinoembryonic antigen (CEA) is a marker for colorectal cancer and would generally not be helpful in the workup of a new lung lesion unless metastasis is suspected. (E) Although a transbronchial biopsy might be appropriate if the lesion is found to be central and growing in size, this would not be the initial step for an unknown lesion.

 A 62-year-old man with a 50-pack-year smoking history presents with worsening cough and occasional hemoptysis. He also reports he has felt more tired than usual on his morning walks in the park. His temperature is 36.5°C, blood pressure 135/75 mmHg, pulse 60 beats/min, and respirations 14 breaths/min. On examination, there are decreased breath sounds on the left lung base. Although laboratory studies are normal, a chest radiograph reveals a 3-cm mass in the left lower lobe that has a spiculated appearance. A computed tomography scan reveals a complex 3-cm mass near the left main stem bronchus and an effusion in the left lower lobe. Which of the following is the next best step in management?

(A) Bronchoscopy
(B) Magnetic resonance imaging
(C) Obtain fluid for cytology
(D) Percutaneous needle biopsy
(E) Resection of the tumor

The answer is A: Bronchoscopy. This patient has a mass that most likely represents malignancy. Prior to determining the proper treatment, tissue must be obtained for diagnosis as the type and stage of tumor significantly affect the prognosis and treatment. Along with bronchoscopy, mediastinoscopy is often performed to evaluate the lymph nodes for metastasis.

(B) This patient already has imaging revealing the nature of the mass and additional imaging is unlikely to be helpful at this time. (C) Although fluid may be obtained for cytology, the pathologist will need tissue for a definitive diagnosis. (D) Percutaneous needle biopsy is best used to obtain tissue for diagnosis from peripheral lesions. (E) Although resection of the tumor may be an option once more information about the tumor is obtained, it is not the next step in management.

 5 A 52-year-old woman with a history of smoking is referred for an incidental lung lesion seen on a chest x-ray. She denies any symptoms. Review of the chest x-ray sent with her medical records shows a lung lesion shaped like popcorn. This same lesion is seen on a previous x-ray and has the same dimensions and appearance. Which of the following is the most likely diagnosis?

(A) Chondroma
(B) Hamartoma
(C) Non–small cell carcinoma
(D) Small cell carcinoma
(E) Sarcoidosis

The answer is B: Hamartoma. Hamartomas are benign lesions classically shaped like popcorn on chest radiography. They are usually well circumscribed and do not usually grow when followed. They are the most common benign tumors of the lung and the third most common benign solitary nodule found on lung imaging. Pathologically they are composed of disorganized tissues that are normally found in the lung. The majority of hamartomas are smaller than 4 cm. Calcifications may be seen within a minority of these lesions. They almost always do not require treatment.

(A) A chondroma is a benign lesion that may be found on the chest wall and rarely in the lung. The lesions are usually peripheral and form a well-demarcated mass with central or "popcorn" calcifications. They are often multiple. This diagnosis is much less common than a hamartoma. (C) Non–small cell carcinoma of the lung may appear as an irregular mass. Mediastinal widening, atelectasis, hilar enlargement, and/or pleural effusions may also be seen. Popcorn calcifications are more common in benign lesions. (D) Small cell carcinoma, also known as "oat cell" carcinoma, is a type of tumor most common in the lung. It may be associated with paraneoplastic syndromes as the cells sometimes secrete ectopic hormones. Treatment depends on how extensive the cancer is and may include chemotherapy and radiation. Radiographically these cancers are often found centrally in the vast majority of cases and will appear as a perihilar mass or mediastinal widening. Often mediastinal lymph node enlargement may also be seen. (E) The most common appearance of sarcoidosis on chest radiography is bilateral hilar and mediastinal lymph node enlargement. Classically the "1-2-3" sign is apparent characterized by bilateral hilar and right paratracheal node enlargement. In more advanced sarcoidosis, reticulonodular opacities are not uncommon.

---

6 A 63-year-old man with a history of smoking presents with a lung mass that has doubled in size from previous imaging performed a year ago. The tumor is characterized as a large irregular mass found on the left lung near the left main bronchus. Tissue obtained from biopsy reveals sheets of small round cells with scant cytoplasm and fine granular chromatin. The patient wishes to receive treatment. Which of the following is the best treatment strategy for this patient?

(A) Chemotherapy and radiation
(B) Observation only
(C) Palliative care
(D) Radiation followed by resection
(E) Tumor resection

The answer is A: Chemotherapy and radiation. This patient is presenting with a tumor that most likely represents small cell carcinoma of the lung. Small cell carcinoma, also called oat cell carcinoma, is a highly malignant neuroendocrine tumor that most often develops centrally and has a strong association with smoking. Unfortunately, the tumors are usually nonresectable and treatment involves chemotherapy (often platinum based) and thoracic radiation.

(B) Observation only would not be appropriate for this patient as treatment may provide significant benefits. (C) Palliative care might be appropriate if the patient was older and had extensive disease. This patient requests treatment; thus palliative care is not an appropriate option. (D) Although radiation and chemotherapy may shrink the tumor, radiation only with resection is not used for treatment of small cell cancer. (E) Surgical resection has a very limited role in small cell lung cancer and is only used for early stage disease confined to the lung parenchyma.

---

7 A 65-year-old woman is referred for repeating sinopulmonary infections. She is currently complaining of occasional low-grade fevers and a persistent cough. Although previous chest radiography has been negative, a chest x-ray performed at this visit shows several new suspicious lesions. A review of her medical history reveals a diagnosis of malignancy a decade earlier, which was completely resected. Which of the following is not a common metastatic tumor to the lung?

(A) Breast cancer
(B) Choriocarcinoma
(C) Colon cancer
(D) Renal cell carcinoma
(E) Uterine cancer

The answer is B: **Choriocarcinoma.** Pulmonary metastasis most often appears on chest radiography as peripheral well-rounded nodules of variable size and scattered throughout the lungs. Although choriocarcinoma most commonly metastasizes to the lungs, it is not a common primary metastatic tumor found in patients with lung metastasis.

(A) Breast cancer is a common primary lesion found in patients with pulmonary metastasis. (C) Colorectal cancer is a relatively common primary lesion in patients with pulmonary metastasis. (D) Renal cancer is a relatively common primary lesion in patients with pulmonary metastasis. (E) Uterine cancer, including leiomyosarcoma, is one of the top five primary cancers in patients with pulmonary metastasis.

8 A 46-year-old man complains of weight loss, fatigue, and a "sweaty face." On examination of his right eye, his eyelid is drooping and his pupil does not dilate. Chest imaging reveals a tumor in the apex of the right lung. Which of the following is the most likely diagnosis?

(A) Adenocarcinoma of the lung
(B) Cluster headache
(C) Dissecting carotid aneurysm
(D) Squamous cell carcinoma
(E) Small cell carcinoma

The answer is D: **Squamous cell carcinoma.** Pancoast syndrome is caused by a tumor that arises or spreads to the superior sulcus and can represent a variety of types of lung cancer. However, squamous cell carcinoma accounts for the majority (52%) of the tumors causing Pancoast syndrome. On physical examination, these patients may present with Horner syndrome in addition to the typical symptoms suspicious for cancer. Surgical treatments for these tumors are often difficult due to the close proximity of vital structures.

(A) Squamous cell carcinoma is the most common cause of Pancoast syndrome followed by adenocarcinomas and large cell carcinomas of the lung. (B) Although cluster headaches are a cause of Horner syndrome, the patient is not complaining of the typical symptoms (i.e., headache) that should be present. Additionally, a cluster headache would not explain the radiographic findings. (C) Although a dissecting carotid aneurysm is a cause of Pancoast syndrome, it is unlikely in this scenario. (E) Small cell lung cancer is rarely in a position that causes Horner syndrome and is almost always centrally located.

9 A 23-year-old man presents with a worsening cough and fatigue during exercise. He is employed as a prison guard in Ohio and has no history of smoking. He was recently diagnosed with a sinopulmonary infection and reports getting better after antibiotics. His parents are immigrants from Eastern Europe. He denies hemoptysis. On examination, he appears well. His temperature is 36.8°C, blood pressure 118/69 mmHg, pulse 65 beats/min, and respirations 19 breaths/min. Auscultation of the lung reveals mild wheezing in the right upper lung field. A tuberculin skin test performed 2 days earlier shows 7 mm of induration. A chest radiograph shows a collapsed right upper lung lobe. Which of the following is the most likely diagnosis?

(A) Aspergilloma
(B) Bronchial adenoma
(C) Histoplasmosis
(D) Non–small cell lung cancer
(E) Tuberculosis

The answer is B: Bronchial adenoma. This is a young patient without a history of smoking, which makes lung cancer a much less likely diagnosis. His history and radiographic finding of a collapsed lung are consistent with a bronchial adenoma, which may obstruct the bronchus resulting in atelectasis and this patient's other symptoms. Bronchial adenoma is a descriptive term for several types of benign neoplasms that grow beneath the bronchial epithelium and may compress the airway. If symptomatic, the tumor may be removed surgically.

(A) Aspergilloma is a fungus ball that develops in a preexisting lung cavity. It may cause hemoptysis, but would not cause an upper lung atelectasis. (B) Although histoplasmosis does occur in Ohio and may cause pulmonary symptoms, these are usually asymptomatic or self-limiting and would result in different symptoms. This patient's presentation is more consistent with a bronchial adenoma. (C) This patient is young and does not have a history of smoking making non–small cell lung cancer less likely. (D) Since this patient does work in a prison with exposure to patients at high risk for tuberculosis, it puts him in a category where greater than 10 mm of induration would be suspicious for tuberculosis.

10 A 31-year-old woman is seen in the emergency department for right-sided pleuritic chest pain that developed suddenly while watching television. The patient also complains of dyspnea. She reports a history of this happening at least several times before with resolution after a few days in the hospital. The patient denies any additional significant medical history and does not smoke. Her temperature is 37.0°C, blood pressure 131/81 mmHg, pulse 93 beats/min, and respirations 21 breaths/min with shallow respirations. Her oxygen saturation is 99%

on 2 L of oxygen. On examination, the breath sounds are diminished on the right side and the chest is hyper-resonant to percussion. A chest x-ray shows several apical blebs and a mild right-sided pneumothorax. Which of the following is the best definitive management?

(A) Bleb excision and pleural abrasion
(B) Chest tube placement
(C) Needle decompression
(D) Observation and continued supplemental oxygen
(E) Pleurodesis

The answer is A: **Bleb excision and pleural abrasion.** This patient is presenting with recurrent spontaneous pneumothorax. Although there are a variety of treatments available for the acute episode, this patient will require surgery to prevent future occurrences. The most common method of repair is video-assisted thoracoscopic surgery to remove the blebs, and repair is occasionally performed via thoracotomy.

(B) Although a chest tube placement may help the patient get over the acute episode, this patient will need definitive surgical treatment to prevent future occurrences. (C) Although needle decompression is a good acute treatment for a tension pneumothorax, this patient will need definitive treatment to prevent reoccurrences. (D) Although continued observation and supplemental oxygen are an important part of the acute management and might be the extent of treatment in a patient suffering from a nonrecurring pneumothorax, this patient will require corrective surgery. (E) Pleurodesis is best reserved for patients with repeated pneumothoraces who are not good candidates for surgery.

11 A 46-year-old woman with a history of a heart murmur and recent diagnosis of atrial fibrillation complains of a progressive worsening shortness of breath during exercise. She does not smoke and a recent cholesterol panel was normal. On examination, there is a holosystolic murmur best heard at the apex with radiation to the back. An echocardiogram reveals mitral prolapse, a normal sized left ventricle, and an enlarged left atrium. Which of the following is the most likely diagnosis?

(A) Congenital heart disease
(B) Marfan syndrome
(C) Mitral stenosis
(D) Myxomatous degeneration of the mitral valve
(E) Valve dysfunction secondary to previous infarction

The answer is D: **Myxomatous degeneration of the mitral valve.** This patient is suffering from mitral regurgitation, which is most commonly caused by worsening mitral valve prolapse secondary to myxomatous degeneration of the valve leaflets. Mitral regurgitation in this patient most likely developed slowly over months to years. This patient may require surgical correction if there are signs of left ventricular dysfunction.

(A) Although different types of congenital heart diseases may result in mitral regurgitation, it is a less common cause of mitral regurgitation than myxomatous degeneration. (B) Although Marfan syndrome is a cause of mitral valve prolapse and possible regurgitation, this patient does not fit the description. (C) Mitral stenosis results in a diastolic murmur. (E) Acute mitral regurgitation may occur after an infarction and is often due to papillary muscle dysfunction. This patient is at low risk for infarction and does not have a history suggestive of a previous infarction.

 A 39-year-old man presents with progressive shortness of breath, coughing, and fatigue over the last several months. His medical records show that approximately 4 months ago he suffered from a respiratory infection. He denies any history of heart disease in his family and has no risk factors for heart disease. His temperature is 37.3°C, blood pressure 135/85 mmHg, pulse 100 beats/min, and respirations 20 breaths/min. A chest x-ray reveals an enlarged heart shadow. Which of the following is the next best step in management?

(A) Antiarrhythmic medications
(B) Antiviral medications
(C) Diuretics and ACE inhibitors
(D) Heart transplantation
(E) Observation and support

The answer is C: Diuretics and ACE inhibitors. This patient is most likely suffering from dilated cardiomyopathy. Physical examination findings may include tachycardia, tachypnea, hypertension, edema, signs of hypoxia, and other findings of heart dysfunction. A common cause of dilated cardiomyopathy in this age group is viral myocarditis. Patients suffering from viral myocarditis are generally middle aged and may have a history of a recent infection. The initial management of dilated cardiomyopathy includes ACE inhibitors, β-blockers, diuretics, and other agents to maximize heart function. Once medical therapy has been maximized, other treatment modalities such as left ventricular assist devices, pacing, and implantable defibrillators may assist in the management. As a last resort, heart transplant may be required.

(A) Although antiarrhythmic medications may be used in certain patients, extreme caution should be exercised as they may result in decreased heart function. (B) Antiviral medications are ineffective in treating dilated cardiomyopathy. (D) Transplant is indicated for end-stage heart failure and when medical therapy is ineffective. (E) This patient requires much more than just observation and support to prevent further damage to the heart and progression of his heart failure.

13 A 29-year-old homeless man is admitted with a history of a cough producing foul sputum, fever, and night sweats. He has a history of alcohol abuse and carries a diagnosis of schizophrenia. A chest computed tomographic scan reveals a pleural effusion and a 3-cm area with thickened walls and loculations of the right lung. Chest x-ray is obtained and shown in *Figure 15-2*.

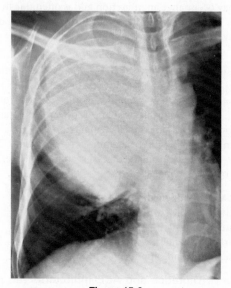

Figure 15-2

Fluid obtained from the collection reveals a pH of 6.5, glucose of 30 mg/dL, and a LDH of 1,900 IU/dL. Which of the following is the best step in management?

(A) Biopsy
(B) Intravenous antibiotics
(C) Open thoracotomy
(D) Surgical placement of a chest tube and oral antibiotics
(E) Video-assisted decortication

The answer is B: Intravenous antibiotics. This patient is presenting with imaging suggesting an empyema, possibly secondary to aspiration suggested by the patient's alcohol history and foul breath. The initial treatment for empyema is extended intravenous antibiotics and chest tube insertion. In some cases, fibrinolytics are administered intrapleurally to break up the septations. The chest x-ray reveals a mottled opacity over the right upper lung lobe.

(A) Biopsy is unnecessary in this case as the diagnosis of empyema is strongly suggested by the history, presentation, and studies. (C) Surgical debridement via the open technique may be necessary for unresponsive empyemas, although video-assisted thoracoscopic techniques are more commonly utilized. (D) Although surgical placement of a chest tube is appropriate, intravenous antibiotics, not oral, are required. (E) If more conservative measures are ineffective, surgical management may be appropriate. Video-assisted decortication is becoming more popular for surgical management of empyemas.

 14 A 59-year-old man presents with new chest pain. He has a history of high cholesterol, smokes a pack per day, and is moderately obese. The initial workup suggests possible myocardial ischemia as ST elevation is seen on the electrocardiogram. Arteriography reveals three-vessel coronary atherosclerotic disease with high-grade left main disease. His ejection fraction is found to be 35%. Which of the following is the best management for this patient?

(A) ACE inhibitor, statins, and β-blockers
(B) β-Blockers and statins
(C) Coronary artery bypass
(D) Percutaneous coronary intervention (PCI)
(E) Smoking cessation and exercise

The answer is C: Coronary artery bypass. This patient has significant three-vessel disease, which is an indication for coronary bypass surgery. Other indications include significant left main coronary artery disease and diffuse disease not amendable to treatment with PCI.

(A) Medical management alone is not recommended for this patient with active myocardial ischemia. (B) Although medical therapy with β-blockers and statins along with other agents is important in the management of those at risk for myocardial ischemia, this patient has significant three-vessel disease and evidence of ongoing ischemia. Thus, additional intervention is indicated at this time. (D) Although PCI has been shown to be more effective than medical management alone, it is not as effective for significant three-vessel disease as bypass surgery. (E) Although lifestyle changes such as smoking cessation and exercise should be part of the long-term treatment for this patient, it will not help with the acute management.

 15 A 50-year-old woman presents with dysphagia of both solids and liquids. Upper endoscopy reveals an esophageal mass near the gastroesophageal junction. Within which of the following anatomical locations is the majority of the esophagus found?

(A) Anterior mediastinum
(B) Middle mediastinum
(C) Posterior mediastinum
(D) Retroperitoneal space
(E) Superior mediastinum

The answer is C: **Posterior mediastinum.** The esophagus is found primarily in the posterior mediastinum. Other structures found in the posterior mediastinum include the thoracic aorta, azygous venous system, thoracic duct, nerves branching off the spinal cord including the splanchnic nerves, and the vagus nerve.

(A) The anterior mediastinum contains remnants of the thymus gland and mediastinal lymph nodes. It is located anterior to the pericardium. (B) The middle mediastinum is located between the anterior mediastinum and posterior mediastinum. It contains the heart and pericardium, the origins and terminations of the great vessels, phrenic nerves, and lymph nodes. It does not contain the esophagus. (D) Although the retroperitoneum does contain part of the esophagus, it is only the thoracic segment. (E) The superior mediastinum is located at the inlet of the thorax marked by the sternal angle and extends to the lower border of T4 vertebrae. It contains the brachiocephalic veins, superior vena cava, azygous vein, aortic arch and its branches, and the left and right vagus nerves.

 16 A 56-year-old man with a history of coronary artery disease is found to have significant atherosclerotic disease on angiography, including 70% stenosis of the left main coronary artery. His ejection fraction is also significantly decreased. Which of the following interventions is the best management for this patient?

(A) Bypass using internal mammary artery grafts
(B) Bypass using saphenous vein grafts
(C) Bypass using synthetic grafts
(D) Continue medical therapy alone
(E) Percutaneous angioplasty

The answer is A: **Bypass using internal mammary artery grafts.** This patient is a good candidate for coronary bypass surgery due to the presence of three-vessel disease and reduced ejection fraction. A graft utilizing the internal mammary artery has been shown to have the best patency. When performing the surgery, the internal mammary artery is left intact at its origin to the aorta and the distal end attached to the obstructed coronary vessel.

(B) Saphenous vein grafts have been shown to have lower patency rates than mammary artery grafts. (C) Although prosthetic grafts have been used for bypass in cases where more suitable grafts are not available, they are generally not recommended since function and durability are highly variable. (D) Continued medical therapy alone is not appropriate at this time since significant left main coronary stenosis is associated with a high degree of sudden death. (E) Percutaneous angioplasty, with current evidence, has been shown to be inferior to coronary artery bypass graft (CABG) for reducing death and myocardial infarction in those with significant left main coronary disease.

---

17 A 65-year-old man with a long history of smoking presents with weight loss, fatigue, and a persistent cough. A chest x-ray shows a new right lung mass. Biopsy reveals non–small cell carcinoma confined to the right middle lobe. A surgical evaluation is performed to explore the possibility of removing the right middle lobe. A ventilation perfusion scan predicts a forced expiratory velocity in 1 second (FEV1) of 400 mL in the right lung after lobectomy. The FEV1 of the left lung is 700 mL. Which of the following is the best course of action?

(A) Chemotherapy
(B) Lobectomy
(C) Palliative care
(D) Pneumonectomy
(E) Radiation and chemotherapy

The answer is B: **Lobectomy.** Preoperative evaluation of patients with lung cancer involves lung function tests that predict postoperative lung function. These may include ventilation perfusion scanning, diffusion capacity measurements, and/or spirometry. Since after surgery the patient's predicted FEV1 will be greater than 800 mL, the patient may proceed with surgery. Surgery is contraindicated when lung function is less than 800 mL since patients have a significantly higher rate of death.

(A) Chemotherapy may be an option to patients for which surgery is not indicated. (C) This patient has disease confined to one lobe and his preoperative evaluation indicates adequate postoperative lung capacity; thus, palliative care is not an appropriate course of action. (D) Since there is limited disease spread, lobectomy is a better option for this patient than complete removal of the lung. (E) Radiation and chemotherapy are both options for patients with lung cancer and contraindications to surgery.

---

18 A 55-year-old man presents with dizziness brought on with changes in position. More recently, he has also experienced dyspnea with exertion. A cardiac examination reveals a diastolic rumble that changes with movement. An electrocardiogram is normal. A transesophageal echocardiogram reveals a polypoid mass within the left atrium arising from the anterior wall with partial obstruction of the mitral valve. Which of the following is the most likely diagnosis?

(A) Lymphoma
(B) Mesothelioma
(C) Myxoma
(D) Rhabdomyosarcoma
(E) Thrombus

The answer is C: Myxoma. This patient is presenting with a left atrial mass. High on the differential diagnosis is an atrial myxoma. Myxomas account for approximately one-half of cardiac tumors and usually occur sporadically. Although often asymptomatic, patients may present with symptoms produced by mechanical interference of cardiac function or embolization. Treatment is surgical resection of the tumor.

(A) Primary cardiac lymphomas are extremely rare and unlikely account for this patient's symptoms. (B) Mesothelioma is a rare form of cancer that may arise from the mesothelium surrounding organs. It would not occur inside the atrium. (D) Cardiac rhabdomyosarcomas are less common than myxomas, accounting for approximately 1/5 of all cardiac neoplasms. (E) An atrial thrombus is also high on the differential for an atrial mass, but since this patient's mass is characterized as "polypoid," a thrombus is less likely. Ultrasonography and other advanced imaging techniques may be required to distinguish between the two. A thrombus is usually found in the posterior atrium and has a layered appearance.

19 A 55-year-old woman with a history of atrial fibrillation presents with new episodes of palpitations, shortness of breath, and dizziness. An electrocardiogram shows a recurring paroxysmal atrial fibrillation and a recent echocardiogram shows a normal left atrial volume. The arrhythmias had previously been successfully controlled with metoprolol and amiodarone, but have since started occurring again. Previous attempts at electrical cardioversion have been unsuccessful. Which of the following is the next best step in management?

(A) Cardiac catheter ablation
(B) Continue medical therapy
(C) Lifestyle changes
(D) Maze procedure
(E) Mitral valve replacement

The answer is A: Cardiac catheter ablation. This patient is presenting with paroxysmal atrial fibrillation now refractory to medical therapy. The next best step in management is to attempt cardiac ablation. Cardiac ablation is performed by passing a catheter into the heart and ablating the abnormal tissue. Catheter ablation is best used for patients with paroxysmal atrial fibrillation and structurally normal hearts.

(B) Continuing medical therapy with different agents may be an option for this patient but is less likely to result in resolution of her atrial fibrillation.

(C) Although lifestyle changes are always important, they are unlikely to resolve this patient's atrial fibrillation. (D) The Maze procedure is the most effective technique for potentially curing atrial fibrillation and involves creating a number of incisions on the left and right atrium to form scar tissue and disrupt the abnormal electrical impulse. It may be performed via open surgery or video-assisted thoracic surgery. Maze surgery is best suited for patients needing concomitant open surgery. It is rarely performed as a standalone procedure. (E) Although mitral valve dysfunction is a major cause of atrial fibrillation, there is no evidence of mitral valve dysfunction in this patient.

 A 60-year-old man presents with progressive shortness of breath, especially noticeable when attempting to walk. He says that several months ago he suffered a heart attack, but was soon "on his feet and walking about." A month afterward, he recalls a fever accompanied by fatigue that resolved on its own. On physical examination, there is hepatomegaly, increased jugular venous pressure, and ascites. A chest x-ray reveals pericardial calcifications and a thickened pericardium. Heart catheterization reveals reduced right and left ventricular end diastolic volumes and elevated diastolic pressures. Laboratory studies reveal a mildly increased brain natriuretic peptide (BNP) of 110 ng/L. Which of the following is the most likely diagnosis?

(A) Aortic stenosis
(B) Constrictive pericarditis
(C) Dilated cardiomyopathy
(D) Massive left ventricular infarction
(E) Restrictive cardiomyopathy

The answer is B: Constrictive pericarditis. This patient is most likely suffering from constrictive pericarditis, possibly secondary to Dressler syndrome, a type of pericarditis that follows a heart attack. Differentiating constrictive pericarditis from restrictive cardiomyopathy can be difficult, but is suggested in this case by the pericardial calcifications, thickened pericardium, and only mildly elevated BNP. Definitive surgical management involves pericardial stripping.

(A) Aortic stenosis may cause shortness of breath, but would cause the other findings in this patient. (C) Dilated cardiomyopathy would present with increased end diastolic volumes rather than reduced. (D) This patient's lack of acute presentations along with pericardial changes and chronic thickening of the pericardium suggests an alternative diagnosis. (E) One of the major diagnostic dilemmas in constrictive pericarditis is its easy confusion with restrictive cardiomyopathy. Some studies may assist in differentiating including brain naturetic peptide (BNP) (often much more elevated), echocardiography, advanced imaging with CT or MRI, and biopsy.

21 A 35-year-old man attends a local health screening. He fills out a questionnaire about his prior medical, surgical, and family history. His family history was positive for lung cancer in his mother who was recently diagnosed by CT scan. The patient has a 20-pack-year history of cigarette smoking. He denies fever, fatigue, night sweats, dyspnea, or hemoptysis. Which of the following is currently recommended as a screening tool for lung cancer?

(A) Computed tomography
(B) Chest x-ray
(C) No tool is recommended for screening
(D) Serum antidiuretic hormone
(E) Sputum cytology

The answer is C: **No tool is recommended for screening.** Currently, the clinical practice guidelines issued by the American College of Physicians as well as the United States Preventative Services Task Force recommend against screening asymptomatic individuals for lung cancer.

(A) Although recent studies have suggested computed tomography as an effective screening tool in high-risk individuals, it is not currently recommended for screening use in asymptomatic patients. (B) Chest x-ray has not been shown to be an effective screening tool for lung cancer. (D) Although serum antidiuretic hormone may be elevated in some small cell lung cancers, it is not a useful screening tool. (E) Sputum cytology has been shown to be an ineffective screening tool for lung cancer.

22 A 72-year-old man with a 50-pack-year history of smoking undergoes successful three-vessel coronary artery bypass surgery 3 months ago. The surgical procedure and recovery were uneventful. He rehabilitated at home for one month and now presents for a follow-up examination. He has a healed mid-sternal scar. Which of the following medications has been shown to reduce mortality and risk of ischemic complications and is routinely used after coronary bypass surgery?

(A) Aspirin
(B) Calcium channel blocker
(C) Clopidogrel + aspirin
(D) Isosorbide dinitrate
(E) Simvastatin

The answer is A: **Aspirin.** Aspirin has been shown to reduce the risk of death and ischemic complications in numerous studies. Additionally, it is considered safe and does not increase the risk of bleeding complications.

(B) Although short-term use of Ca channel blockers may be useful in patients with radial artery grafts, there is little evidence to support the routine use of Ca channel blockers after coronary artery bypass graft (CABG) to reduce patient mortality and ischemic complications. (C) The addition of clopidogrel to aspirin as dual therapy after CABG is controversial. Some research has suggested a benefit while other studies have shown no difference in mortality between patients receiving aspirin alone and combination therapy. (D) There is little evidence to support significant mortality benefits with isosorbide dinitrate after CABG surgery. (E) Although statins have been shown in some studies to reduce progression of atherosclerosis and decrease the occurrence of graft occlusion, they do not show the same mortality benefits as aspirin.

 A 6-week-old infant presents to the physician with increasing stridor, wheezing, and occasional respiratory distress. His mother reports that he has been feeding well without vomiting or choking. His birth history is unremarkable with good Apgar scores. There is a family history of asthma. On examination, there is both inspiratory and expiratory stridor and subcostal retractions. A chest x-ray reveals an anterior indentation of the trachea and an esophogram shows bilateral compression of the esophagus that is maintained during peristalsis. Which of the following is the most likely diagnosis?

- **(A)** Asthma
- **(B)** Infection
- **(C)** Pneumorthorax
- **(D)** Tracheoesophageal fistula
- **(E)** Vascular ring

The answer is E: Vascular ring. This patient is presenting with signs, symptoms, and imaging findings suggesting the presence of a vascular ring. Vascular rings are a set of rare congenital anomalies that occur during the development of the aortic arch and great vessels that may compress the trachea and/or esophagus. Symptoms of respiratory distress may occur. The barium esophogram is the most important imaging study to order and is diagnostic in the vast majority of cases. If symptomatic, patients may need surgery to correct the problem with the type depending on the specific vascular anomaly.

(A) It would be highly unusual for asthma to present this early in life. Furthermore, the imaging studies are not consistent with a diagnosis of asthma. (B) This patient does not have symptoms consistent with infection. (C) Although respiratory distress is a symptom of pneumothorax, the other findings are not consistent with this diagnosis. (D) If this patient had a tracheoesophageal fistula, they would more likely present with excessive salivation as a newborn and associated choking, vomiting, or distress associated with feeding.

 A 59-year-old man presents with an "achy" pain in his right chest aggravated by movement. He also describes the pain being worse at night. On examination, the chest wall appears normal but is tender to palpation over the anterior sixth rib. An MRI of the chest shows a 6-cm mass projecting inward from the chest wall with irregular borders and bony invasion. A biopsy is performed and sent to pathology. Histologically the tumor is composed of numerous spindle cells with moderate atypia and occasional mitotic figures. The cells do not stain with S100. Which of the following is the most likely diagnosis?

(A) Chondroma
(B) Fibrous dysplasia
(C) Malignant schwannoma
(D) Multiple myeloma
(E) Soft tissue sarcoma

The answer is E: Soft tissue sarcoma. This patient's tumor description is that of a malignant soft tissue sarcoma. These tumors are relatively uncommon and may occur in the chest wall. They often present as a painless lump but may cause symptoms if invading into the bone or compressing nerves. There are numerous subtypes of soft tissue sarcomas that appear histologically similar. The stage of the tumor depends on the size and histological grade. Surgical resection is the most common form of treatment.

(A) Chondromas are benign neoplasms of cartilage that may occasionally occur on the chest wall. They are composed of mature cartilage and would not have this histological appearance. (B) Fibrous dysplasia is a benign condition characterized by abnormal bone growth and may occasionally occur on the chest wall. Treatment options include medication to strengthen bones and pain management. Surgery does generally not have a role in treatment. (C) Although a malignant schwannoma (derived from neural tissue) may appear histologically similar to soft tissue sarcomas, they are usually S100 positive. (D) Multiple myeloma is a malignancy of plasma cells that may result in bone pain that often involves the spine or ribs. Lytic lesions may be seen on imaging. A bone marrow biopsy may show increased percentage of plasma cells. Surgery is generally not indicated.

---

25   A 19-year-old male driving a motorcycle crashes head on into a guide rail on the highway. He was ejected from the motorcycle and thrown against the concrete medial divider and sustained chest trauma. Upon arrival in the emergency department, he is unconscious. He has decreased breath sounds on the left side of the chest. Chest x-ray reveals multiple left rib fractures and evidence of a large pleural fluid collection. Chest tube placement is suggested. Which of the following describes the best location for placement of the tube?

(A) Anterior axillary line just below the fourth rib.
(B) Anterior axillary line just below the 12th rib
(C) Midaxillary line just above the fifth rib
(D) Midaxillary line just above the eighth rib
(E) Midclavicular line just below the ninth rib

The answer is C: **Mid axillary line just above the fifth rib.** Proper chest tube placement is important skill as vital structures must be avoided. Complications from improper technique may easily be avoided with an understanding of important anatomical landmarks. A chest tube should be placed in the mid- or anterior axillary line, behind the pectoralis major muscle to avoid extensive muscle dissection. Placing the tube above the fifth rib or the level of the nipple is important because the diaphragm elevates to this level during inspiration. The incision should be placed along the upper border of the rib to avoid damaging the neurovascular bundles that travel along the bottom of each rib.

(A) This chest tube placement would compromise the neurovascular bundle that runs below the fourth rib. (B) This chest tube placement would be much too low and would endanger the neurovascular bundle that runs below the rib. (D) This tube placement would be too low. (E) This chest tube would be too anterior, too low, and endanger the neurovascular bundle.

Otolaryngology

1 A 36-year-old woman presents to clinic with a complaint of trouble breathing through her nose. She denies anosmia and epistaxis, and is otherwise healthy. On nasal examination, she is found to have a large polyp coming off of the inferior turbinate and situated in the left inferior meatus. The opening to which structure is most likely obstructed by this mass?

(A) Sphenoid sinus
(B) Maxillary sinus
(C) Nasolacrimal duct
(D) Ethmoid sinus
(E) Frontal sinus

The correct answer is C: Nasolacrimal duct. The nasolacrimal duct functions to drain tears from the lacrimal sac (located in the medial canthus of the eye) into the nasal cavity. It travels from the medial canthus of the eye inferiolaterally and drains into the ipsilateral inferior meatus. It is the reason that rhinorrhea follows excessive lacrimation.

(A) The sphenoid sinus drains into the sphenoethmoidal recess. (B) The maxillary sinus drains into the middle meatus. (D) The ethmoid sinus is made up of groups of air cells with drain into the superior and middle meatuses. (E) The frontal sinus drains into the superior meatus.

2 A 17-year-old boy presents to his pediatrician with a "cold that won't quit." He has had a runny nose for a while, but lately his head and face have been hurting. He has felt feverish, which responds to Tylenol. He also has had trouble sleeping, as he wakes up several times per night coughing. On examination, he grimaces when his pediatrician presses on his maxilla. He subsequently is diagnosed with an acute sinusitis. What are the three most common pathogens in acute sinusitis?

(A) *Streptococcus pneumoniae, Haemophilus influenza*, and *Moraxella catarrhalis*

(B) *S. pneumoniae, H. influenza*, and *Staphylococcus aureus*

(C) *S. aureus, H. influenza*, and *M. catarrhalis*

(D) *Staphylococcus aureus, Streptococcus pneumoniae*, and *M. catarrhalis*

(E) *H. influenza, M. catarrhalis*, and *Escherichia coli*

The correct answer is A: **Streptococcus pneumoniae, Haemophilus influenza, and Moraxella catarrhalis.** Acute sinusitis usually occurs secondary to an upper respiratory infection, where mucosal inflammation obstructs drainage from any of the paranasal sinuses. Bacterial infection then ensues in the retained sinus secretions. Patients complain of nasal congestion, facial pain, fevers, and postnasal drip. Diagnosis is aided by endoscopic evaluation of the nasal cavity to visualize draining ostia and rule out obstructing masses. Computed tomography (CT) scanning also can be used to evaluate for mucosal thickening and the presence of air–fluid levels. The three most common pathogens of acute bacterial sinusitis are *S. pneumoniae, H. influenza*, and *M. catarrhalis*.

(B) Although *S. aureus* can cause sinusitis, it is not one of the three most common pathogens. (C) Although *Staphylococcus aureus* can cause sinusitis, it is not one of the three most common pathogens. In addition, *Streptococcus pneumoniae* is the most common pathogen. (D) Although *S. aureus* can cause sinusitis, it is not one of the three most common pathogens. (E) *E. coli* is not a common cause of bacterial sinusitis

---

3 A 12-year-old girl presents to his pediatrician with a "runny nose for a while." In addition, she has felt feverish and her head and face have been hurting. She also complains of a scratchy throat and that it feels like "something is tickling it." She is diagnosed with an acute sinusitis. What is the first-line antimicrobial treatment for acute sinusitis?

(A) Amoxicillin/clavulanic acid

(B) Amoxicillin

(C) Erythromycin

(D) Penicillin V

(E) Trimethoprim

The correct answer is B: **Amoxicillin.** Acute bacterial sinusitis is an infection of the paranasal sinuses for less than 4 weeks. It arises usually secondary to an upper respiratory infection, where mucosal inflammation obstructs drainage from any of the paranasal sinuses. It is caused most commonly by *Streptococcus pneumonia, Haemophilus influenza*, and *Moraxella catarrhalis*. The first-line agent of choice to cover these main pathogens is Amoxicillin, which is a third-generation penicillin.

(A) Amoxicillin/clavulanic acid is second line for acute bacterial sinusitis. It is also used in cases refractory to first-line therapy. (C) Erythromycin is not used to treat bacterial sinusitis. (D) Penicillin V is first line for the treatment of streptococcal pharyngitis. (E) Trimethoprim alone is not used for acute sinusitis. But when combined with sulfamethoxazole, it is a first-line treatment for acute bacterial sinusitis.

4 A 16-year-old boy presents via ambulance to the emergency department with a decreased level of consciousness (LOC). His mother relays that he recently was given antibiotics that he got from his doctor for a sinus infection. She relays he had a runny nose for a while, but did not go to the doctor until he started feeling worse. She confessed that he started feeling much better 2 days after seeing the doctor, so he stopped taking the antibiotics. He currently is febrile, and is not responding to speech. He is noncooperative with the neurologic examination, but all his reflexes are 2+. When his head is lifted, his knees also lifted off of the gurney. Which complication of sinusitis does this patient have?

(A) Orbital infection
(B) Brain abscess
(C) Meningitis
(D) Cavernous sinus thrombosis
(E) Refractory sinusitis

The correct answer is C: Meningitis. Acute bacterial sinusitis can progress to more serious and life-threatening complications involving nearby structures. Although these complications are rare, they are much more common when sinusitis goes untreated. This patient did not complete a full course of 10 to 14 days and subsequently developed a decreased LOC alongside fever. He does not have any focal neurological deficits and displayed a Brudzinski sign. All these clinical signs indicate the infection spread into the meninges. This patient requires empiric IV antibiotics and corticosteroids. Diagnosis is best made by a cerebrospinal fluid (CSF) analysis and culture.

(A) Orbital infections typically cause an edematous and erythematous orbit leading to pain with eye movement alongside normal pupil function. It does not cause a depressed LOC. (B) Brain abscesses typically cause focal neurologic deficits alongside a depressed LOC. (D) Cavernous sinus thrombosis is a clot in the cavenous sinus which drains blood into the venous system. It often leads to ptosis, ipsilateral cranial nerve palsies (III, IV, V, VI), as well as headache and sepsis. Our patient lacked focal neurological signs. (E) Refractory sinusitis does not cause a depressed LOC.

5 A 24-year-old woman presents to her gynecologist for a routine physical examination. She recently developed a sore throat as well as painful swallowing. She has had a fever as well as some "swollen glands" under her jaw. Her gynecologist decides to obtain a rapid streptococcal antigen test, which comes back positive. She is prescribed a course of penicillin for streptococcal pharyngitis. The likelihood of which possible compli-cations of bacterial pharyngitis is not decreased by treatment?

(A) Poststreptococcal glomerulonephritis
(B) Rheumatic fever
(C) Scarlet fever
(D) Endocarditis
(E) Meningitis

The correct answer is A: Poststreptococcal glomerulonephritis. Strep-tococcal pharyngitis is the most common type of bacterial pharyngitis, and is caused by Group A strep. The infection most commonly is in the palatine ton-sils, uvula, soft palate, and posterior pharyngeal wall. Patients most commonly complain of a sore throat, odynophagia, fevers/chills, malaise, and headache. A pertinent historical finding is the absence of cough. Physical examination findings include cervical adenopathy, pharyngeal edema, and erythema, gray–white tonsillar exudates, and petechiae on the soft palate. First-line treatment for strep throat is penicillin. There are several complications of strep throat which can occur after the acute infection. Poststreptococcal glomerulonephri-tis is one whose occurrence is not influenced by whether or not the patient was adequately treated for the primary pharyngeal infection.

(B) The risk of rheumatic fever is significantly decreased if the patient is adequately treated for the pharyngeal infection. (C) The risk of scarlet fever is significantly decreased if the patient is adequately treated for the pharyn-geal infection. (D) Endocarditis is not a sequela of streptococcal pharyngitis. (E) Meningitis is not a sequela of streptococcal pharyngitis.

6 A 14-year-old boy presents to the school nurse complaining of a sore throat. He recalled that it started today, and divulged that his new girl-friend shares his symptoms. He has had trouble eating due to pain-ful swallowing, as well as a low-grade fever. He also recalled that his girlfriend had some "swollen glands" under her jaw. The nurse did not appreciate swollen glands on his physical examination, but was still very suspicious of an infectious cause. For streptococcal pharyngitis, which of the following is not one of the Centor criteria?

(A) Fever
(B) Cervical adenopathy
(C) Pharyngeal erythema
(D) Tonsillar exudates
(E) Absence of cough

The correct answer is C: Pharyngeal erythema. Streptococcal pharyngi-tis is the most common type of bacterial pharyngitis, and is caused by Group A strep. The infection most commonly is in the palatine tonsils, uvula, soft pal-ate, and posterior pharyngeal wall. Patients most commonly complain of a sore throat, odynophagia, fevers/chills, malaise, and headache. A pertinent historical finding is the absence of cough. Physical examination findings include cervical adenopathy, pharyngeal edema and erythema, gray–white tonsillar exudates, and petechiae on the soft palate. The Centor criteria can be used to make the diagnosis, and consists of fever, cervical adenopathy, absence of cough, and tonsillar exudates. Pharyngeal erythema is not one of the Centor criteria.

(A) Fever is one of the Centor criteria. (B) Cervical adenopathy is one of the Centor criteria. (D) Tonsillar exudates is one of the Centor criteria. (E) Absence of cough is one of the Centor criteria.

7 A 3-year-old girl is brought by her parents into the pediatrician for an urgent evaluation. The child recently started running a high fever in addition to refusing to eat or drink anything. She appears uncomfortable on her mom's lap, leaning very far forward. She is also drooling a fair amount. A cervical radiograph is shown in *Figure 16-1*.

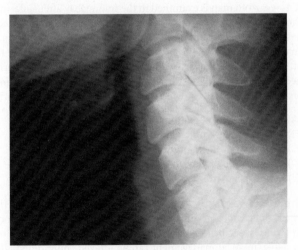

Figure 16-1

What is the most likely explanation for this finding?

(A) Thumbprint sign
(B) Batwing sign
(C) Air–fluid levels
(D) Honeycombing
(E) Steeple sign

The correct answer is A: Thumbprint sign. Epiglottitis is an infection of the epiglottis which can lead to upper airway obstruction. It is most commonly seen in ages 3 to 6 years, and is most commonly caused by *Haemophilus influenza* B (HIB). The incidence has decreased 90% since the introduction of the HIB vaccine. Children present with fever, sore throat, and severe odynophagia. They appear sitting up and leaning forward, drooling. They may have biphasic stridor, especially when presenting later. Epiglottitis can be detected radiographically with a lateral cervical plain film, which shows the characteristic "thumbprint sign." This sign is caused by the thickened epiglottis.

(B) Batwing sign is the presence of bilateral hilar shadowing, most often caused by pulmonary edema. (C) Air–fluid levels are seen in acute sinusitis or also in the abdomen in the case of small bowel obstruction. (D) Honeycombing is a collection of clustered, thick walled, cystic spaces in the lung parenchyma, and represents dilated and thick walled bronchial walls seen in bronchiectasis. (E) Steeple sign is an air shadow seen at the level of the larynx on an antero-posterior plain film caused by subglottic swelling.

---

8) A 41-year-old man is examined in the trauma bay after suffering a gunshot wound to the neck. He presented hypotensive and obtunded, and has been intubated and given bolus IV fluids. On examination, there is an entrance wound in the anterolateral right neck, 2 cm above the angle of the mandible. An exit wound is identified on the posterior right neck. Both wounds are still actively bleeding. For a penetrating injury on this part of the neck, what is the best surgical management?

(A) No surgery, observation only
(B) Angiography with embolization
(C) Open surgical exploration
(D) Angiography followed by open surgery
(E) No surgery with serial laryngoscopic examinations

The correct answer is B: Angiography with embolization. The acute management of laryngeal trauma depends on the mechanism and location of injury. In all cases, securing a stable airway is the first course of action. If the airway is stable, medical management can be utilized (humidified air, elevate head of bed, voice rest, antibiotics, steroids etc.). For unstable airways, surgical intervention is generally indicated. In the case of penetrating injuries, management depends upon the anatomical zones involved. For injuries to zone III, which is from the angle of the mandible to the skill base, angiography with embolization is typically performed.

(A) This patient is still actively bleeding, and thus surgical intervention is indicated to ensure hemodynamic stabilization. (C) Open surgery without imaging is indicated for penetrating trauma to zone II. (D) Angiography followed by open surgery is an option for penetrating trauma to zone I. (E) Serial laryngoscopic examinations are used to monitor laryngeal trauma with a stable airway.

9 A 13-year-old boy presents to an urgent care center with a painful neck mass. His father recounts a 3-day history of a "painful, red, and swollen gland on his neck." He has had difficulty swallowing as well. On examination, a 3-cm erythematous, fluctuant mass is identified on the right side of the patient's neck near the sternocleidomastoid muscle. An ultrasound shows the mass to be primarily a cystic structure. What is the most definitive treatment?

(A) Aspiration of fluid
(B) Incision and drainage
(C) Antibiotic therapy only
(D) Antibiotics and aspiration of fluid
(E) Excision

The correct answer is E: Excision. Branchial cleft cysts are caused by the failure of obliteration of the branchial clefts in the fetal period. They are nontender and fluctuant masses, which can become inflamed (as in this patient) and form into an abscess. Other symptoms that can result are dysphagia and striodor. Diagnosis can be aided by ultrasound, computed tomography, or magnetic resonance imaging (MRI) to evaluate the mass for cystic vs. solid components as well as to evaluate the location of the mass. Antibiotics are utilized if these cysts become infected, but otherwise surgical excision of the cyst is the only definitive treatment for them.

(A) Aspiration of the cyst can be helpful as it decompresses the mass, but excision is a better treatment. (B) Incision and drainage is best avoided as it makes any future attempt to excise the cyst much more difficult. (C) Antibiotics are not a definitive treatment for branchial cleft cysts. (D) Aspiration plus antibiotics is not the definitive treatment for branchial cleft cysts.

10 An 8-week-old female infant presents to her pediatrician for a well-child check. The parents immediately point out a red mass on the infant's face, stating "it appeared out of nowhere!" They recalled she did not have it when she left the newborn nursery, but then started to develop it approximately a month ago. Since then, it rapidly grew in size. On examination, the mass appears red and well circumscribed. When palpated, the child does not react negatively, and the mass is firm and rubbery. What is the best first step in the treatment of this lesion?

(A) Watchful waiting
(B) Surgical excision
(C) Laser resection
(D) Interferon
(E) Prednisone

The correct answer is A: Watchful waiting. Infantile hemangioma is the most common tumor of infancy, which is not seen in the newborn nursery and then appears during the first 6 weeks of life. It commonly shows rapid growth in the first 8 to 12 months, and then regresses slowly in the next 5 to 8 years. It is a firm, well-circumscribed, rubbery, red lesion, which usually is asymptomatic. However, these lesions can become ulcerated and bleed, become infected, cause visual defects if they grow into periorbital structures, and even cause high output heart failure. It is diagnosed clinically, and watchful waiting is the first-line treatment as most of these lesions spontaneously regress by 8 to 10 years of age.

(B) Surgical excision is reserved for cases which do not completely regress. (C) Laser resection is used for cases where the lesion causes symptoms like visual defects or heart failure. (D) Interferon is used in lesions which are refractory to corticosteroid treatment. (E) Prednisone is the first-line medical therapy for symptomatic or nonregressing lesions.

11 An 11-year-old boy presents to his pediatrician for a "checkup." On examination, the pediatrician notices a lump underneath the boy's chin. When asked about it, the boy claims "that's just how my neck is." The mass is located in the middle of the top of his neck, at the level of the hyoid bone. Neck ultrasound is obtained and is shown in *Figure 16-2*.

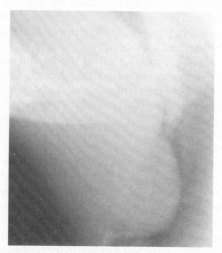

Figure 16-2

What type of tissue may be present in this congenital neck mass?

(A) Thymus
(B) Thyroid
(C) Parathyroid
(D) Lymphatic
(E) Cartilage

The correct answer is B: Thyroid. Thyroglossal duct cysts are one-third of congenital neck masses, and are usually located in the midline at the level of the hyoid bone. However, they can occur anywhere from the thyroid gland to the foramen cecum, which is the embryological origin from where the thyroid gland migrates. They are usually asymptomatic, but they can cause dysphagia, especially if they become infected. 45% of these cysts contain functional thyroid tissue. The neck ultrasound shows multiple anechoic cystic structures consistent with thyroglossal duct cyst.

(A) Thyroglossal duct cysts do not contain thymus tissue. (C) Thyroglossal duct cysts do not contain parathyroid tissue. (D) Thyroglossal duct cysts do not contain lymphatics. (E) Thyroglossal duct cysts do not contain cartilage.

 12   A 1-year-old female infant presents to her pediatrician for a well-child check. The child has been developing normally, but her mom complains of a soft swelling on the side of her neck. The patient recently had a cold which resolved, but this swelling persisted. When reviewing neck swellings, the clinician suspected his swelling is a cystic hygroma. Which chromosomal abnormality is most commonly associated with cystic hygroma?

(A) Edward syndrome
(B) Patau syndrome
(C) Turner syndrome
(D) Klinefelter syndrome
(E) Down syndrome

The correct answer is C: Turner syndrome. Cystic hygroma is a macrocytic lymphatic malformation which is usually located in the anterior or posterior triangles of the neck. These lesions are soft and compressible, but can also swell up in the case of an upper respiratory infection. Although these can be found in healthy babies, over half of them are associated with chromosomal abnormalities. The most common chromosomal abnormality associated with cystic hygroma is Turner Syndrome which is characterized by its XO genotype.

(A) Edward syndrome is caused by trisomy 18, and is not commonly associated with cystic hygroma. (B) Patau syndrome is caused by trisomy 13, and is not commonly associated with cystic hygroma. (D) Klinefelter syndrome is caused by extra copies of X chromosome leading to genotypes of 46XXY or 47XXXY, and is not commonly associated with cystic hygroma. (E) Down syndrome is caused by trisomy 21, and is not commonly associated with cystic hygroma.

 13   A 67-year-old man presents to the emergency department with worsening pain in his right ear. For the past week, he has had increasing pain and tenderness to his right ear. He stated "I can't sleep on my right

side because it hurts my ear to lean against it." He also complains of some "itchiness" of the ear, as well as occasional "stuff coming out of it." On examination, the pinna is tender to manipulation, and there is visible debris in the external auditory canal. If left untreated, this infection can spread into the skull base. Which pathogen most commonly causes this infection?

(A) Methicillin-resistant *Staphylococcus aureus* (MRSA)
(B) *Clostridium perfringens*
(C) *Pseudomonas aeruginosa*
(D) *Streptococcus pneumoniae*
(E) Methicillin-sensitive *S. aureus* (MSSA)

The correct answer is C: *Pseudomonas aeruginosa*. Otitis externa (OE) is an infection/inflammatory process of the external auditory canal. It is commonly referred to as "swimmer's ear," as swimmers are predisposed to contract this infection due to the quantity of time they spend with their ears under water. Other risk factors are heat, humidity, and trauma to the external auditory canal. It presents with otalgia, otorrhea, pruritus, and pinna tenderness. It also can cause hearing loss, due to edema of the external auditory canal. If left untreated, especially in elderly and diabetic patients, it can progress to an osteomyelitis of the skull base known as malignant otitis externa (MOE). This is most commonly caused by *P. aeruginosa* infection.

(A) *S. aureus* (both MRSA and MSSA) is the second most common cause of OE, but not commonly associated with MOE. (B) *Clostridium perfringens* is the agent that causes "gas gangrene." (D) *Streptococcus pneumoniae* is a common cause of meningitis, but not MOE. (E) *S. aureus* (both MRSA and MSSA) is the second most common cause of OE, but not commonly associated with MOE.

14 A 3-year-old girl presents to her pediatrician with fever and fussiness. Her father recounts a 3-day history of increased fussiness and fever, and yesterday he caught her pulling on her left ear. After a thorough physical examination, she is diagnosed with an uncomplicated acute otitis media. She is given a prescription for Amoxicillin and told to call the office if she does not feel relief. Two days later, the father calls the pediatrician praising the antibiotic. He claimed that all of a sudden she was pain-free today, despite some mild drainage coming out of the left ear. He said she is back to her normal self and you would not know that she was ever sick! What is the mechanism behind this patient's pain relief?

(A) The antimicrobial agent's bactericidal activity
(B) Rupture of the tympanic membrane
(C) Opening of the Eustachian tube
(D) Spontaneous regression
(E) Decreased inflammation

The correct answer is B: Rupture of the tympanic membrane. Acute otitis media is an infection of the middle ear cavity, most commonly by bacteria which are trapped up there due to dysfunction of the Eustachian tube. The most common pathogens are *Streptococcus pneumoniae*, *Haemophilus influenza*, and *Moraxella catarrhalis*. Incidence peaks at roughly 2 years of age, and patients present with fever and irritability, occasionally pulling on their ears. Diagnosis is made clinically, with pneumatic otoscopic findings of a decreased to immobile, thickened, and hyperemic tympanic membrane. In cases where patients experience rapid pain relief followed by otorrhea, the tympanic membrane has ruptured. The pain decrease is due to the release of built-up pressure. (A) Antimicrobials help decrease the pain from otitis media, but cause more gradual relief. (C) The Eustachian tube often does not open until the infection resolves further, and would not explain the otorrhea. (D) Spontaneous regression is unlikely considering the rapid relief of pain and otorrhea. (E) Inflammation certainly decreases when pockets of infection are liberated, which is secondary to the rupture of the tympanic membrane.

15 A 14-year-old boy was skateboarding home from school when he lost his balance and fell. He hit the side of his head on the sidewalk and was knocked out. The paramedics brought him to the emergency department, where he regained consciousness but was only somewhat awake. On secondary trauma survey, he was found to have some clear fluid draining from his right nostril. In addition, he had significant bruising posterior to his right ear. If he was more alert and was subjected to a hearing test using a tuning fork, what examination finding is most consistent with his injury?

(A) Weber: no lateralization; Rinne: air > bone conduction
(B) Weber: lateralization to left side; Rinne: air > bone conduction
(C) Weber: lateralization to right side; Rinne: air > bone conduction
(D) Weber: no lateralization; Rinne: air < bone conduction
(E) Weber: lateralization to right side; Rinne: air < bone conduction

The correct answer is C: Weber: lateralization to right side; Rinne: air > bone conduction. Temporal bone fractures are 20% of all skull fractures, and are most commonly due to blunt trauma from motor vehicle collisions or falls. The two most common types are longitudinal and transverse. Common physical findings are "battle sign" (postauricular ecchymosis) and "raccoon eyes" (periorbital ecchymosis), as well as a cerebrospinal fluid (CSF) leak. Fractures can cause a conductive hearing loss which is reflected with a Weber test that lateralizes toward the side of the lesion. Also, the Rinne test is typically negative. (A) With temporal bone fractures, the Weber test typically lateralizes to the side of the injury, which in this case is the right side. (B) With temporal bone fractures, the Weber test typically lateralizes to the side of the injury, which in this case is the right side. (D) With temporal bone fractures, the Weber test typically lateralizes to the side of the injury. In addition, the Rinne test is typically negative. (E) With temporal bone fractures, the Rinne test is typically negative.

16. A 53-year-old woman trips on her dog and falls forward onto her face. An ambulance brings her to the emergency department where her injuries are evaluated. She did not lose consciousness. In addition to concussive symptoms, she has marked ecchymosis of her nose and maxilla. A head computed tomography (CT) is obtained, which shows no evidence of an epidural or a subdural hematoma. However, it does reveal several minor fractures to the maxilla, in addition to a LeFort 1 fracture. In the management of a LeFort 1 fracture, what is the first step?

(A) Open reduction and internal fixation (ORIF) of the fracture immediately.
(B) Surgically place the dentition in class 1 occlusion
(C) Placement of a tracheotomy
(D) Obtain a panoramic radiograph
(E) Placement of a nasogastric tube

The correct answer is B: **Surgically place the dentition in class 1 occlusion.** There are three types of LeFort fractures in the midface, which reflect different degrees of palatal and/or midface instability. In the case of a LeFort 1 fracture, the palate is separated from the midface due to fractures involving the pterygoid plates bilaterally, allowing it mobility. This mobility can lead to airway compromise in extreme cases. After diagnosis via head CT scan, the first step is to surgically fix the dentition into class 1 occlusion. This is done via the alignment of the mesiobuccal cusp of the maxillary first molar with the mesiobuccal cusp of the mandibular first molar. The next step depends on the severity of the displacement of the fractures. For relatively nondisplaced fractures, intermaxillary fixation for 4 to 6 weeks is sufficient. For more displaced fractures, open reduction with internal fixation using titanium miniplates is indicated.

(A) ORIF is indicated for displaced LeFort 1 fractures after they are placed in class 1 occlusion. (C) Placement of a tracheotomy is only required for patients with an unstable airway. (D) A panoramic radiograph is not required for patients with LeFort 1 fractures already diagnosed by head CT. (E) A nasogastric tube may be of use in patients with facial fractures and refractory nausea. It is not the best first step for this patient.

17. A 42-year-old man is riding his bike when he inadvertently loses his balance and flips over his handle bars, slamming his face into the pavement. He is brought to the emergency department, where he is found to have substantial facial injuries. There is marked ecchymosis

of his nose and maxilla, and on examination there is mobility of his midface. In addition, some clear fluid is spotted draining out of his right nares. A head computed tomography (CT) is obtained, which shows a LeFort 3 fracture. In the management of a LeFort 3 fracture, what is the first step?

(A) Open reduction and internal fixation (ORIF) of the fracture immediately
(B) Surgically place the dentition in class 1 occlusion
(C) Placement of a tracheotomy
(D) Obtain a panoramic radiograph
(E) Placement of a nasogastric tube

The correct answer is C: Placement of a tracheotomy. There are three types of LeFort fractures in the midface, which reflect different degrees of palatal and/or midface instability. LeFort 3 fractures typically involve the pterygoid plates, the frontonasal maxillary buttress, and the frontozygomatic buttress. These fractures result from high energy trauma and lead to midface mobility. Cerebrospinal fluid (CSF) leak can also occur. After diagnosis via head CT scan, the first step is to place a tracheotomy to secure a definite airway prior to surgery to reduce the fractures. Often multiple surgical approaches are required to stabilize a LeFort 3 fracture.

(A) ORIF is indicated for LeFort 3 fractures after a tracheostomy is placed to secure a definite airway. (B) Placement into class 1 occlusion is the first step for LeFort 1 fractures. (D) A panoramic radiograph is not required for patients with LeFort 3 fractures already diagnosed by head CT. (E) A nasogastric tube may be of use in patients with facial fractures and refractory nausea. It is not the best first step for this patient.

18 A 35-year-old man presents to the emergency department demanding to immediately be seen because "my jaw is killing me!" After being calmed down by the emergency department staff, he recounts to the triage nurse that his jaw has been hurting more and more over the last 3 days on the right side. When asked about anything that may have caused it, he exclaims "Well it's probably that left hook, I suppose." He recounts getting hit in a bar fight 5 days ago. A plain facial x-ray is obtained which shows a fracture to the mandible. For mandibular fractures, what is the benefit of a Panorex radiograph series?

(A) Identify posterior displacement of a fracture
(B) Differentiate a condylar from an angle fracture
(C) Identify small fractures in the dentition
(D) Differentiate a horizontal rami fracture from an angle fracture
(E) There is no benefit from Panorex radiographs for mandibular fractures

The correct answer is B: Differentiate a condylar from an angle fracture. Mandibular fractures are often the result of trauma, and many present several days after the fracture if the injury is suffered under the influence of drugs or alcohol. Patients can complain of pain with eating, malocclusion, or even numbness of the V3 dermatome if the mandibular nerve is damaged. Diagnosis is made using plain film x-ray or computed tomography (CT) scan. Panorex radiograph series can be utilized to distinguish a condylar fracture from an angle fracture.

(A) Posterior fracture displacement can be determined using anteroposterior (AP) and lateral plain films. There is no additional benefit from a Panorex series. (C) Damage to the dentition can be determined using AP and lateral plain films. There is no additional benefit from a Panorex series. (D) Plain films or CT are sufficient to differentiate a horizontal rami fracture from an angle fracture. (E) Panorex radiograph series help to distinguish a condylar fracture from an angle fracture.

 A 38-year-old woman with a recent diagnosis of anxiety disorder presents with a slowly enlarging mass on her lower anterior neck. She also complains of heat intolerance and unintentionally losing 13 lbs of weight over the last 2 months. Her last period was approximately 6 weeks ago. Her vitals are within normal limits. On examination, her thyroid is diffusely enlarged. Which of the following is the best initial step in evaluation of this patient?

(A) Computed tomography scan
(B) Electrocardiogram (ECG)
(C) Fine-needle aspiration biopsy
(D) Thyroid ultrasound
(E) Thyroid stimulating hormone (TSH) and free T4

The answer is E: Thyroid stimulating hormone (TSH) and free T4. There are multiple causes of an enlarging neck mass. However, this patient's accompanying complaints of heat intolerance, weight loss, menstrual irregularities, and anxiety point toward a thyroid etiology as these are all symptoms of hyperthyroidism. The initial test when evaluating a patient with suspected hyperthyroidism is thyroid function testing, including TSH and free T4. In a patient with primary hyperthyroidism, thyroid function tests may show a low TSH and elevated free T4. Additional testing may be necessary, including biopsy, if the diagnosis is uncertain or secondary causes of hyperthyroidism are suspected.

(A) Although computed tomography (CT) imaging may be useful in the workup of an enlarging neck mass of alternative etiologies, it is generally not indicated or necessary in a patient presenting with signs and symptoms of hyperthyroidism. (B) Patients with hyperthyroidism may have tachycardia or present with atrial fibrillation. However, this patient does not complain of cardiac symptoms, and an ECG is not necessary. (C) Although fine-needle aspiration may eventually be required in a subset of patients with hyperthyroidism, it is not a good choice for an initial diagnostic test. (D) Thyroid ultrasound is a useful imaging modality to evaluate nodules or palpable irregularities in the thyroid and parathyroid glands. However, it is not the initial test of choice for working up a patient with hyperthyroidism.

20 A 23-year-old male college student presents with fever, chills, and a tender neck "lump" that has been increasing in size over the last day. He says this has happened multiple times, although they usually resolve and this is the first time it has been painful. He denies a history of tobacco use. His temperature is 38.3°C, blood pressure 125/75 mmHg, pulse 85 beats/min, and respirations 17 breaths/min. On examination there is a smooth, tender, and fluctuant mass on the anterior lateral neck between the sternocleidomastoid muscle and skin. A computed tomography (CT) examination of the neck reveals a cystic, well-defined, and nonenhancing water attenuation mass on the anterior border of the sternocleidomastoid. Which of the following is the most likely diagnosis?

(A) Branchial cleft cyst
(B) Papillary thyroid carcinoma
(C) Reactive lymphadenopathy
(D) Squamous cell carcinoma of the neck
(E) Thyroglossal cyst

The answer is A: Branchial cleft cyst. This patient's presentation of an intermittent neck mass along the anterior border of the sternocleidomastoid muscle and his CT findings suggest a branchial cleft cyst, most likely now infected. Branchial cleft cysts are congenital epithelial cysts that result from failure of obliteration of the second branchial cleft. Discharge may be present with these lesions if there is an associated sinus tract. Antibiotics with incision and drainage are the initial treatment for this patient. Definitive surgical removal should not be attempted while infected but may be an option for the patient after resolution.

(B) Although papillary thyroid carcinoma may present with a neck mass, the location, intermittent growth, and current fever/chills suggest an alternative diagnosis. (C) Although reactive lymphadenopathy is certainly a possibility in this patient, the CT findings and specific location of the mass suggest a branchial cleft cyst as a more likely diagnosis. (D) Squamous cell carcinoma would be exceedingly rare in a patient this age, especially without a history of tobacco use. (E) A thyroglossal cyst is also a congenital neck mass occurring from the persistence of the thyroglossal duct. This tract normally atrophies during embryogenesis. If present, the mass is located at the midline.

21 A 45-year-old man that recently visited the dentist for a cavity presents with increasing mouth pain and neck swelling. He also reports pain with swallowing and mild shortness of breath. His past medical history is remarkable for diabetes mellitus. His temperature is 38.4°C, blood pressure is 130/80 mmHg, pulse 105 beats/min, respirations 23 breaths/min, and oxygen saturation 95% on room air. On physical examination his tongue is erythematous, elevated, and slightly protruded. Which of the following is the first step in management?

(A) Blood cultures
(B) Computed tomography (CT) imaging
(C) Incision and drainage of suspected abscess
(D) Prepare airway equipment and initiate antibiotics
(E) Start penicillin

The answer is D: Prepare airway equipment and initiate antibiotics. This patient is most likely suffering from Ludwig angina, a rapidly progressive and gangrenous cellulitis of the soft tissue in the mouth. Patients often have a history of a recent dental procedure and odontogenic infections are responsible for over 90% of cases. This patient's diabetes is a predisposing condition, although most cases occur in healthy patients. The initial management of Ludwig angina should focus on airway management, as the airway may be quickly compromised by the infection. This patient's tachypnea and mild shortness of breath are worrying and preparing possible airway placement should be a top priority.

(A) Although blood cultures should be sent as part of the workup, they are not as important as securing an airway and can wait. (B) Although CT imaging may be necessary in patients who have developed suppurative complications, it would not be the initial step. (C) Incision and drainage may very well be part of the management for this patient, but the airway should be evaluated first. (E) Antibiotics should be quickly initiated in patients with suspected Ludwig angina and should be broad spectrum to cover gram positive, gram negative, and anaerobic organisms. A common combination is penicillin, clindamycin, and metronidazole. Penicillin alone would not be adequate coverage.

22 A 2-year-old boy with complaints of fever and "runny nose" is brought to the emergency department by his mother. His mother says that he has also been irritable since she got back from a trip. On examination, there is unilateral purulent, blood tinged, and foul smelling discharge. What is the most likely diagnosis?

(A) Acute sinusitis
(B) Allergies
(C) Foreign body
(D) Nasal polyp
(E) Viral upper respiratory tract infection

The answer is C: Foreign body. A child who presents with unilateral purulent, bloody, and/or foul smelling discharge should be evaluated for a foreign body. Physical examination is the primary diagnostic tool, and a proper nasal examination is extremely important. Removal in the office setting or emergency department may be attempted in most situations, but caution should be exercised and an otolaryngology specialist consulted in cases of doubt, failed removal, or damage to adjacent structures.

(A) Although acute sinusitis is certainly possible, the characteristics of the discharge and age of the child suggest a possible foreign body. (B) Allergies may be suspected in any patient presenting with rhinorrhea. However, watery discharge, sneezing, itchy eyes, and a pale boggy nasal mucosa would more suggest this diagnosis. (D) Nasal polyps are more common in elderly patients and would usually not present as unilateral purulent discharge. (E) Viral upper respiratory tract infections are usually characterized by watery to mucoid discharge accompanied by sore throat and malaise. The nasal mucosa is often erythematous on examination.

---

 23 A 60-year-old man presents with hoarseness and dysphagia that started 6 months ago. A thorough workup is performed including nasal endoscopy, and a mass is found on the larynx. A biopsy is performed and returns as nasopharyngeal carcinoma. Which of the following is the greatest risk factor for this malignancy?

(A) Asbestos exposure
(B) Cigarette smoking
(C) History of human papilloma viral infection
(D) History of tobacco use and alcoholism
(E) Poor nutrition

The answer is D: History of tobacco use and alcoholism. The risk for laryngeal cancer, usually squamous cell carcinoma, is greatest when heavy alcohol consumption is combined with tobacco use. When combined, these two risk factors have a synergistic effect. Other risk factors in addition to those listed above include age (especially greater than 65), male gender (four times more common than women), history of gastroesophageal reflux, and certain genetic syndromes.

(A) Asbestos exposure is a known risk factor for laryngeal cancer, although it has a greater association with lung cancers and mesothelioma. (B) Although the rate of laryngeal cancer has been shown to be increased 20-fold in smokers when compared to nonsmokers, alcohol consumption along with smoking has an even greater risk. (C) Human papilloma virus is a known risk factor for squamous cell carcinoma in a number of areas, including the larynx. However, this is only considered a minor risk factor. (E) Although the etiology for this risk factor is unknown, poor nutrition is considered a minor risk factor for laryngeal carcinoma.

24 A 41-year-old woman presents with a slowly enlarging painless mass on the right side of her face, located below the ear. On examination, there is a palpable smooth and well-circumscribed 3-cm mass felt in the right parotid gland. There are no facial nerve deficits and the mass does not seem to be attached to the skin. Fine-needle aspiration of the mass shows no malignant cells. Which of the following is the most likely diagnosis?

(A) Facial nerve schwannoma
(B) Mucoepidermoid carcinoma
(C) Pleomorphic adenoma
(D) Sebaceous lymphadenoma
(E) Warthin tumor

The answer is C: Pleomorphic adenoma. Pleomorphic adenomas are the most common benign salivary gland tumor, accounting for 70% to 80%. Patients are typically middle aged. Previous irradiation is a known risk factor, but they usually occur in patients without this history. Pathologically the tumor is composed of a mixture of epithelial and myoepithelial cells with varied histology, although malignant features should not be present. Treatment is excision and the prognosis is excellent.

(A) Facial nerve schwannoma is a rare tumor that often presents with facial nerve deficits such as weakness. (B) Mucoepidermoid carcinoma is a malignant salivary gland tumor, the most common type in adults. Cytomegalovirus infection has been strongly associated with this tumor. Physical examination would most likely reveal a more fixed and irregular mass and fine-needle aspiration of this tumor would most likely show cells with malignant features. (D) Sebaceous lymphadenoma is a rare and benign salivary gland tumor composed of sebaceous cells suspended in a lymphoid stroma. (E) Warthin tumors are benign salivary gland tumors often found in the parotid gland. These are the second most common parotid tumor after pleomorphic adenomas. Unlike pleomorphic adenomas, which are mostly found in middle-aged adults, Warthin tumors are most common in elderly patients.

25 A 10-year-old boy is brought to the physician by his mother for recurring nose bleeding. The mother reports that the bleeding is intermittent and usually resolves by itself after several minutes. There is no family history of bleeding disorders. On examination, there is a scab on the anterior septum. Which of the following is the most common cause of epistaxis in children?

(A) Hemophilia
(B) Nasal angiofibroma
(C) Nose picking
(D) Osler-Weber-Rendu syndrome
(E) Von Willebrand disease

The answer is C: **Nose picking.** While there are multiple causes of epistaxis, the most common cause of nose bleeding in children is nasal picking. The physical examination will often show anterior nasal mucosal ulceration, irritation, and bleeding. Many of the pathological causes of nasal bleeding can be ruled out with a careful history and proper examination.

(A) Although hemophilia may cause nosebleeds in children, it is a much less common cause of epistaxis than nasal picking. Furthermore, this patient does not have a history or family history of other abnormal bleeding. (B) Nasal angiofibromas are benign vascular tumors that can cause nasal bleeding. They are a much less common cause of nasal bleeding than nasal picking. (D) Osler-Weber-Rendu syndrome (hereditary hemorrhagic telangiectasia) is an uncommon autosomal dominant disease that may result in bleeding from a variety of places from vascular malformations. This patient's presentation is not consistent with this diagnosis. (E) Von Willebrand disease should be suspected in a patient presenting with a family history of bleeding and prolonged bleeding episodes, both of which are not present in this individual.

 26 An 18-year-old man presents to the emergency department with nasal bleeding of several hours duration. He is agitated during the interview and attributes it to a lack of sleep over the last several days. He admits to a history of alcohol and marijuana use but denies other drug use or recent trauma. He is vitally stable. A nasal examination reveals a hole in the anterior nasal septum. Which of the following diagnostic tests is the most important component of the initial workup?

(A) Activated partial thromboplastin time (aPTT)
(B) Bleeding time
(C) Complete blood count with differential
(D) Prothrombin time
(E) Urine drug screen

The answer is E: **Urine drug screen.** This patient is presenting with a perforated nasal septum, agitation, and insomnia, all symptoms of cocaine abuse and withdrawal. A urine drug screen should be performed on this patient as he is vitally stable and an extensive workup is most likely unhelpful.

(A) aPTT time is a measure of the intrinsic and common coagulation pathway. A normal aPTT time requires normal function and presence of coagulation factors I, II, V, VIII, IX, X, XI, and XII and is prolonged by heparin. This time will also be prolonged in inherited bleeding disorders such as hemophilia. As hemophilia is unlikely in this patient, a urine drug screen would be more helpful. (B) Bleeding time is a test to assess platelet function. It will be prolonged in disorders such as Von Willebrand disease, thrombocytopenia, and medications such as aspirin. This test is unlikely helpful in this situation. (C) Although a complete blood count with differential would most likely be performed on a patient presenting to the emergency department with nasal bleeding, it is unlikely to be helpful in this patient as the presentation is strongly suggestive of cocaine abuse and the patient is vitally stable. (D) Prothrombin time is a laboratory test that measures the extrinsic coagulation pathway. It is prolonged by drugs such as warfarin and coagulation factor deficits secondary to vitamin K deficiency. As this patient is most likely perforated his nasal septum from cocaine abuse, this test is unlikely to be helpful.

 27 A 55-year-old man with a history of type 1 diabetes and hypertension presents with a severe headache, vomiting, fever, blurry vision, and eyelid swelling that has become progressively worse over the last day. A complete blood count reveals neutropenia. A radiograph shows evidence of sinusitis and retronasal and retroorbital bony erosion. Which of the following is the first step in management?

(A) Immediate irrigation and debridement
(B) Obtain advanced head imaging
(C) Obtain tissue for pathological evaluation
(D) Start intravenous amphotericin B
(E) Start intravenous voriconazole and caspofungin

The answer is D: Start intravenous amphotericin B. This patient is diabetic and presenting with symptoms, radiographic evidence, and laboratory evidence of severe necrotizing fungal infection. Infection with mucormycosis (zygomycosis) should be strongly suspected. The first step is to immediately initiate empiric antifungal treatment with intravenous amphotericin B. Advanced imaging can also be obtained to evaluate the extent of the infection. Next, surgical consultation is critical to prevent the rapid spread of the infection.

(A) Although irrigation and debridement is a critical component of treating invasive mucormycosis, it would not be the initial step as empiric antibiotics and/or antifungals should be initiated and the diagnosis must be confirmed. (B) Advanced imaging with magnetic resonance imaging (MRI) or computed tomography is very helpful for suspected invasive mucormycosis, but should only be obtained once empiric treatment with antifungal medications is initiated. (C) While obtaining tissue for pathological confirmation of the fungal infection may be part of the management for this patient, empiric antifungal treatment should be initiated first. (E) Other antifungals such as voriconazole, fluconazole, and caspofungin have not been shown to have significant activity against mucormycosis fungal organisms in the initial acute phase.

 28 A 41-year-old woman presents with a slowly enlarging painless mass on the right side of her face, located below the ear. On examination, there is a palpable smooth and well-circumscribed 3-cm mass felt in the right parotid gland. There are no facial nerve deficits and the mass does not seem to be attached to the skin. Fine-needle aspiration of the mass shows no malignant cells. Which of the following is the most likely diagnosis?

(A) Facial nerve schwannoma
(B) Mucoepidermoid carcinoma
(C) Pleomorphic adenoma
(D) Sebaceous lymphadenoma
(E) Warthin tumor

The answer is C: Pleomorphic adenoma. Pleomorphic adenomas are the most common benign salivary gland tumor, accounting for 70% to 80%. Patients are typically middle aged. Previous irradiation is a known risk factor, but they usually occur in patients without this history. Pathologically the tumor is composed of a mixture of epithelial and myoepithelial cells with varied histology, although malignant features should not be present. Treatment is excision and the prognosis is excellent.

(A) Facial nerve schwannoma is a rare tumor that often presents with facial nerve deficits such as weakness. (B) Mucoepidermoid carcinoma is a malignant salivary gland tumor, the most common type in adults. Cytomegalovirus infection has been strongly associated with this tumor. Physical examination would most likely reveal a more fixed and irregular mass and fine-needle aspiration of this tumor would most likely show cells with malignant features. (D) Sebaceous lymphadenoma is a rare and benign salivary gland tumor composed of sebaceous cells suspended in a lymphoid stroma. (E) Warthin tumors are benign salivary gland tumors often found in the parotid gland. These are the second most common parotid tumor after pleomorphic adenomas. Unlike pleomorphic adenomas, which are mostly found in middle-aged adults, Warthin tumors are most common in elderly patients.

29 A 24-year-old woman presents with bilateral and slowly progressing hearing loss. She speaks quietly throughout the interview. Along with the hearing loss, she describes a recent "ringing" in her ears and says she can hear best when there is background noise. She denies a history of trauma or frequent ear infections as a child and has no other complaints. Her mother also suffered from hearing loss at a young age. On examination, she is found to have primarily conductive hearing loss that symmetrically involves both ears. Which of the following is most characteristic of this patient's likely disease process?

(A) Abnormal collagen synthesis
(B) Impingement of abnormal bone on the stapes footplate
(C) Middle ear bone remodeling and structurally disorganized bone
(D) Normal acoustic reflex
(E) Primarily high frequency hearing loss on audiometry

The answer is B: Impingement of abnormal bone on the stapes footplate. This patient is most likely suffering from otosclerosis, an inherited disease of abnormal bone growth near the middle ear. The pathophysiology involves multifocal areas of sclerosis within the endochondral temporal bone that may result in fixation of the stapes footplate to the oval window. As a result, patients typically suffer from conductive hearing loss, although sensorineural loss may also occur. Treatment options include hearing aids and surgical stapedectomy, a procedure involving removal of the sclerotic stapes footplate and replacement with an implant.

(A) Abnormal collagen synthesis is characteristic of osteogenesis imperfecta, a disease that is often associated with early hearing loss in children. (C) Middle ear bone remodeling and structurally disorganized bone are characteristic of Paget disease, a disease that is rare in individuals under the age of 25. (D) The acoustic reflex, characterized by the involuntary tensor tympani muscle contraction in response to high intensity sound, is typically abnormal in patients with otosclerosis. (E) Patients with otosclerosis almost always suffer from low frequency hearing loss on audiometry, although high frequency loss may occur later in the disease process.

---

30 A 51-year-old woman is referred to her otolaryngologist by her dentist for "dry mouth and eyes." She admits that she has recently had many cavities requiring repair. Her past medical history is remarkable for hypertension, which is controlled by a calcium channel blocker. Her review of systems is otherwise positive for dyspareunia. On examination, her conjunctiva appear injected and there is reduced tearing with Schimer test. The patient's tongue appears red, dry, and smooth, and there are fissures on her lips. Her parotid glands are bilaterally enlarged. Laboratory testing reveals an elevated erythrocyte sedimentation rate, positive rheumatoid factor, and mild anemia. Which of the following is the most likely diagnosis?

(A) Chronic sialadenitis
(B) Medication side effect
(C) Mumps viral infection
(D) Rheumatoid arthritis
(E) Sjögren syndrome

The answer is E: Sjögren syndrome. This patient is most likely suffering from primary Sjögren syndrome (SS), an autoimmune inflammatory disease that primarily affects exocrine organs. Common complaints include xerophthalmia and xerostomia, although numerous other extraglandular symptoms may develop as well. Sjögren syndrome may also occur in association with other rheumatologic diseases such as systemic lupus erythematosus, rheumatoid arthritis, and scleroderma. Sjögren syndrome is associated with numerous antibodies, although a positive anti-SSA or anti-SSB may assist in the diagnosis.

(A) Although chronic sialadenitis may cause dry mouth, it is usually unilateral and is not associated with decreased tearing. (B) Multiple medications may cause sicca-type symptoms similar to Sjögren syndrome including some antidepressants, anticholinergics, β-blockers, antihistamines, and diuretics. This patient only takes a calcium channel blocker, which is not associated with sicca symptoms. (C) Infection of the parotid glands with mumps (a paramyxovirus) may cause sicca symptoms similar to Sjögren syndrome. However, this patient's history of eye involvement and positive rheumatoid factor is more indicative of Sjögren syndrome. (D) While patients with rheumatoid arthritis may secondary develop Sjögren syndrome, this patient lacks the arthralgia normally associated with rheumatoid arthritis.

31 A 45-year-old man from Colorado presents with a painless neck mass that has slowly enlarged over the last year. Although the patient was initially asymptomatic, he has recently started complaining of hoarseness and dysphagia. His past medical history is remarkable for chronic obstructive pulmonary disease secondary to smoking. On examination, there is a palpable mass fixed to the anterior left neck. Auscultation of the mass reveals a bruit. Ultrasound shows that the mass is located on the carotid body. Which of the following studies should be part of the initial workup in this patient?

(A) Angiography of the neck
(B) Computed tomography of the neck
(C) Fine-needle aspiration of the tumor
(D) Incisional biopsy of the tumor
(E) Urinary catecholamines

The answer is E: Urinary catecholamines. This patient is presenting with signs and symptoms of a carotid body tumor (paraganglioma), a rare type of neuroendocrine tumor. Although rare, the sporadic form is the most common type especially in a middle-aged person such as this. This patient may be suffering from the hyperplastic form of the tumor, most common in chronic hypoxic patients or patient's living at higher elevations (this patient is from Colorado). Although asymptomatic in many patients, tumor growth may eventually cause cranial nerve palsy or other compressive symptoms. In patients suspected of having a carotid body tumor, urinary catecholamines should be assessed and may be elevated.

(A) Angiography of the neck may be necessary later in the workup, but is typically not a recommended first-line image modality. (B) Although computed tomography of the neck may be helpful, magnetic resonance imaging (MRI) imaging is considered the best imaging to obtain for a diagnosis, as biopsy is often difficult to obtain. The tumor has a characteristic salt and pepper appearance on a T1-weighted MRI imaging. (C) Fine-needle aspiration biopsy of the tumor is often only helpful if the tumor is not diagnosed by imaging. (D) Incisional biopsies should not be performed on patients with suspected carotid body tumors since the tumors are very vascular and may profusely bleed.

32 A 67-year-old man presents with a slow growing left parotid mass. Biopsy of the mass shows a cystic tumor lined with bilayered epithelium. There are also multiple lymphocytes with germinal centers. Which of the following risk factors is this tumor most strongly associated with?

(A) Alcohol abuse
(B) Chronic salivary gland obstruction
(C) Mumps infection
(D) Obesity
(E) Smoking

The answer is E: Smoking. The pathological description of this tumor fits that of a Warthin tumor, a benign salivary gland tumor that is most strongly associated with smoking. Other risk factors include radiation. The tumor primarily affects older individuals and will present as a slow growing painless mass. It is highly unlikely to become malignant. Treatment is surgical excision, which is highly effective.

(A) Alcohol abuse is not strongly associated with salivary gland tumors. (B) While chronic salivary gland obstruction may increase the risk for mucoepidermoid carcinoma (a type of malignant salivary tumor), it does not increase the risk for Warthin tumors. (C) Mumps infection is not strongly associated with salivary gland neoplasms. (D) Obesity is not associated with an increased risk of Warthin tumors.

33 A 60-year-old man with a history of smoking and alcohol abuse presents with several nonhealing mouth ulcers. He also reports a 15-kg weight loss over the last month, but denies dysphagia or hoarseness. On examination, there are several ulcers on the base of the tongue and soft palate. A neck examination reveals possible cervical lymphadenopathy. Biopsy of the mouth ulcers reveals squamous cell carcinoma of the neck and a radical neck dissection is planned. A radical neck dissection involves removal of which of the following?

(A) All ipsilateral lymph node levels I to V, including those around the spinal accessory nerve, internal jugular vein, and sternocleidomastoid muscle.
(B) All ipsilateral lymph node levels I to V, sparing the spinal accessory nerve, internal jugular vein, and sternocleidomastoid muscle.
(C) Lymph node levels I, II, and III.
(D) Selective removal of lymph nodes in levels II, III, and IV
(E) Selective removal of lymph nodes in levels II, III, and IV and V

The answer is A: **All ipsilateral lymph node levels I to V, including those around the spinal accessory nerve, internal jugular vein, and sterno-cleidomastoid muscle.** Cancers of the head and neck, especially squamous cell carcinoma, commonly metastasize to cervical lymph nodes. A relatively common procedure for treatment of cervical metastasis is a neck dissection. Classification of lymph nodes is described in six anatomical regions. Level I include lymph nodes in the area bounded by the mandible, stylohyoid muscle, and anterior belly of the digastric muscle. Level II include lymph nodes in the area of the upper one-third of the jugular vein, bordered by the stylohyoid muscle anteriorly and posteriorly by the sternocleidomastoid muscle. Level III includes all nodes located between the hyoid bone and the horizontal plane of the inferior border of the cricoid cartilage. Level IV includes lymph nodes in the lower 1/3 of the jugular vein, located between the inferior border of the cricoid cartilage and the clavicle. Level V describes lymph nodes found within the posterior triangle of the neck. Level VI includes all nodes in the anterior or central compartments of the neck. A radical lymph node dissection is best used for patients with advanced disease and includes complete removal of all fibrofatty tissue from the ipsilateral neck including nodes from levels I to V and those surrounding the spinal accessory nerve, internal jugular vein, and sternocleidomastoid muscle.

(B) This describes a modified radical neck dissection, in which one or more of the structures (spinal accessory nerve, internal jugular vein, and sternocleidomastoid) is preserved. This type of neck dissection is generally indicated in clinically palpable disease. (C) This describes a supraomohyoid neck dissection, a type of selective neck dissection. (D) This describes a lateral neck dissection, a type of selective neck dissection. (E) This describes a posterolateral neck dissection, a type of selective neck dissection.

Pediatric Surgery

1. A 2-week-old baby girl is brought in by her mother who says that she vomits after almost every meal and has since birth. She is now in the 10th percentile for weight although she was in the 50th percentile for weight at birth. She does not appear to be in any distress and the mother denies excessive crying. She is currently afebrile. The mother reports two to three soft, yellowish stools per day. What is the most likely problem in this patient?

   (A) Duodenal atresia
   (B) Foreign object obstruction
   (C) Gastroesophageal reflux (GER)
   (D) Pyloric stenosis
   (E) Viral gastroenteritis

The answer is C: Gastroesophageal reflux (GER). The most likely diagnosis in this patient is GER. The differential diagnosis for excessive vomiting in infants also includes infections, pyloric stenosis, duodenal atresia, and other obstructions. Severe GER can involve failure to thrive, as in this patient. Complications include recurrent aspiration pneumonias and reactive airway disease, laryngospasm and apnea, and esophagitis possibly leading to Barrett esophagus if left untreated.

(A) Duodenal atresia is characterized by the absence of a portion of the lumen of the duodenum. A child with duodenal atresia would quickly become dehydrated and would not survive for 2 weeks. Frequent vomiting after meals that has occurred since birth is most likely due to GER. (B) Ingestion of foreign objects is more likely to occur in older infants and toddlers who are able to pass such objects into their mouths. The fact that this infant's vomiting has occurred since birth also makes a foreign object much less likely than GER. (D) Pyloric stenosis presents later in life, usually between 2 and 8 weeks of age. Vomiting from pyloric stenosis is not present at birth and becomes increasingly worse from the time of onset. (E) Gastroenteritis usually causes diarrhea, not isolated vomiting. This infant has soft stools, but that is characteristic. Infant stools are normally soft and yellowish, and the absence of fever also makes infection a less likely cause of her vomiting.

2 A 5-week-old male infant is brought to the clinic by his mother who complains of the gradual onset of vomiting after meals. This has been going on for about 2 weeks and is progressively worsening. He previously had no problems during feedings. The pylorus on ultrasound examination is measured to be 18 mm × 6 mm. What is the best management for this patient's likely condition?

(A) Circumferential incision into the muscularis
(B) Excision of a wedge-shaped section of pylorus circumferentially
(C) Excision of a wedge-shaped section of pylorus longitudinally
(D) Longitudinal incision into the muscularis
(E) Removal of the pylorus followed by reanastomosis

The answer is D: Longitudinal incision into the muscularis. Pyloric stenosis is a disorder of unknown etiology but appears to have a strong genetic component. Most cases occur in male individuals, in whom pyloric stenosis is about four times as common as in female individuals. Presentation usually involves the development of vomiting after meals that was not present at birth. The vomiting is nonbilious and progresses to projectile vomiting. Jaundice occurs in about 10% of cases. Surgical treatment of this condition involves cutting into the pylorus longitudinally into the muscularis down to but not through the mucosa.

(A) A circumferential incision is not as effective as a longitudinal incision in the treatment of pyloric stenosis. The fibers of the muscularis run circumferentially so a parallel incision will not transect nearly as many fibers as a longitudinal incision. (B) Excision of a wedge-shaped section of the pylorus circumferentially is not necessary. A longitudinal incision into the muscularis is all that is necessary. (C) There is no need to excise the pylorus longitudinally, this simply requires incision of the muscle layer. (E) Reanastamosis of the pylorus and resection is not required to treat this condition.

3 A 3.2-kg male neonate born at term who is found to have a tracheoesophageal fistula is scheduled for surgical repair. The surgeon estimates how much intravenous (IV) fluid will be needed based on the infant's weight. Which of the following statements regarding fluid compartments is true?

(A) Neonates have a greater extracellular fluid (ECF) percentage of total body weight than adults

(B) Neonates have a greater intracellular fluid (ICF) percentage of total body weight than adults

(C) Neonates have a greater percentage of solid body mass than adults

(D) Neonates have the same percentage ECF of total body weight as adults

(E) Neonates have the same percentage ICF of total body weight as adults

The answer is A: **Neonates have a greater ECF percentage of total body weight than adults.** The amount of IV fluids needed by a patient can be estimated with the patient's total body weight and estimated average percentages of total body water, ECF, and ICF fluid compartments. In adults, 60% of total body weight is made up of the total body water. Of this total body water, 40% is the ICF compartment and 20% is the ECF compartment. In neonates, the percentages are different: 75% of total body weight is total body water in term infants. The ICF compartment is only 35% and the ECF is 40%.

(B) The ICF in neonates makes up about 35% of total body weight. In adults, the ICF is about 40%. (C) In neonates, solid mass makes up only about 25% of total body weight (75% is total body water). In adults, solid mass makes up 40% of total body weight. (D) The ECF in neonates makes up about 40% of total body weight. In adults, the ECF is only about 20%. (E) The ICF in neonates makes up about 35% of total body weight. In adults, the ICF is about 40%.

4 A 4-month-old male infant is found to have a bulge in his scrotum during a routine well-child examination. The mass is easily reducible. The pediatrician refers the child to a surgeon to repair the hernia. What is the most common presentation of inguinal hernias in children?

(A) Bilateral

(B) Left-sided

(C) Right-sided

(D) Right-sided and left-sided hernias occur in approximately equal incidences

(E) Congenital hernias are so rare that data are inconclusive

The answer is A: **Bilateral.** Congenital inguinal hernias are fairly common, occurring in about 1% to 3% of all children. Inguinal hernia repairs are among the most common surgical procedures in children. 60% of inguinal hernias occur on the right, 30% occur on the left, and about 10% occur bilaterally. Treatment involves reduction of the hernia and rehydration followed by herniorrhaphy as soon as possible, within 48 to 72 hours being ideal. If left untreated, hernias can become incarcerated and lead to intestinal ischemia and obstruction.

(B) 60% of inguinal hernias occur on the right, 30% occur on the left, and about 10% occur bilaterally. (C) 60% of inguinal hernias occur on the right, 30% occur on the left, and about 10% occur bilaterally. (D) 60% of inguinal hernias occur on the right, 30% occur on the left, and about 10% occur bilaterally. (E) Congenital inguinal hernias are fairly common, occurring in 1% to 3% of all children. 60% of inguinal hernias occur on the right, 30% occur on the left, and about 10% occur bilaterally.

---

5 A newborn female infant is having difficulty breathing. Chest auscultation reveals normal breath on the right but bowel sounds can be heard on the left. She is diagnosed with a congenital diaphragmatic hernia. Which of the following is true of such hernias?

(A) Bochdalek hernias are more severe
(B) Bochdalek hernias more often occur on right hemidiaphragm
(C) Morgagni hernias are more common
(D) Morgagni hernias are more posterior than Bochdalek hernias
(E) They represent an excessive amount of apoptosis during development

The answer is A: Bochdalek hernias are more severe. Congenital diaphragmatic hernias occur in approximately 1 in 4,000 live births. These hernias represent a failure of fusion of tissue during development. Presentation is often respiratory distress because the intruding bowel does not allow the lung to expand sufficiently. Bochdalek hernias are more posterior and lateral than Morgagni hernias and usually occur on the left. Bochdalek hernias are also more common and cause more severe problems than Morgagni hernias. Management includes decompression of the bowel, surgical reduction, and repair of the defect.

(B) Although they can occur on the right, Bochdalek hernias occur most often in the left hemidiaphragm. In about 10% of cases, Bochdalek hernias are bilateral. (C) Morgagni hernias are much less common than Bochdalek hernias. The defect is usually smaller as well and they cause less severe problems. (D) Morgagni hernias are caused by a defect in the anterior diaphragm. Bochdalek hernias are caused by defects in the posterolateral diaphragm. (E) The defects in congenital diaphragmatic hernias are due to failure of fusion of tissue during development. They are not caused by excessive apoptosis.

---

6 A female fetus is seen to have an abdominal wall defect on prenatal ultrasound. At birth, a large membranous sac containing loops of bowel protrudes from her abdomen at the umbilicus. Gastrointestinal decompression is started, as well as intravenous (IV) fluids and antibiotics. A representative image is shown in *Figure 17-1.*

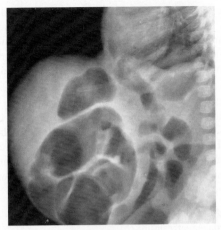

Figure 17-1

What would be the best next step in the management of this patient?

(A) Covering the viscera and sac with a sterile dressing
(B) Immediate surgical repair
(C) Protecting the viscera and sac with a plastic covering
(D) Resect the protruding bowel and repairing the defect
(E) No intervention is necessary

The answer is A: Covering the viscera and sac with a sterile dressing. Two types of abdominal wall defects exist: omphalocele and gastroschisis. Omphalocele is characterized by a membranous sac covering viscera protruding through a defect at the umbilicus. Imaging shows gas-filled loops of small bowel. Gastroschisis is characterized by a protrusion of viscera with no covering through a defect in the abdominal wall next to the umbilicus. The bowel loops in gastroschisis are generally matted together from chemical peritonitis. Management of an omphalocele involves covering the sac with a sterile dressing until surgery can be performed under the best conditions possible after decompression, IV fluids, and antibiotics have begun. Management of gastroschisis is similar except that a plastic covering is used to protect the exposed viscera and surgical closure is emergent.

(B) Emergent surgical repair is indicated in gastroschisis and ruptured omphalocele. This patient's unruptured omphalocele should be covered with a sterile dressing until surgery can be performed. (C) The membranous sac provides protection for the protruding bowels. The only covering necessary for an omphalocele is a sterile dressing. (D) The protruding bowel should not be removed unless it is necrotic. The viscera can generally be reinserted into the abdominal cavity, although this sometimes must occur in stages if the abdominal cavity cannot immediately accommodate all the protruding viscera. (E) This patient's unruptured omphalocele should be covered with a sterile dressing until surgery can be performed. The membranous sac provides some protection against moisture and heat loss, but is not as effective as skin in protecting the bowel against these and other insults such as infection.

7 The mother of a 1-week-old male infant complains that he is fussy and vomits after his feedings. The emesis is greenish in color, and the mother says "he won't eat much." Abdominal examination reveals decreased bowel sounds in the lower quadrants. An abdominal x-ray shows one pocket of air in the area of the stomach and another next to it in the upper mid-abdomen. Which of the following is the likely underlying condition?

(A) Duodenal duplication
(B) Esophageal atresia
(C) Intussusception
(D) Malrotation
(E) Omphalocele

The answer is D: Malrotation. Bilious vomiting following meals suggests gastrointestinal obstruction somewhere distal to the ampulla of Vater (where bile is secreted into the duodenum). Duodenal obstruction is most commonly caused by duodenal atresia or malrotation leading to volvulus. This type of defect is generally manifest during the first month of life. The "double-bubble" sign on x-ray corresponds to air in the dilated duodenum proximal to the obstruction and in the stomach. Emergent surgery is indicated in cases when obstruction is expected to prevent ischemia and necrosis.

(A) Duplication of any portion of the alimentary canal is rare, much less likely than malrotation. Signs and symptoms of duodenal duplication are so varied that vague that preoperative diagnosis is extremely difficult. (B) Esophageal atresia would result in vomiting after meals, but the emesis would not be bilious in nature. The "double-bubble" sign is seen in duodenal obstruction but would not be caused by esophageal atresia. (C) Intussusception is when one segment of intestine invaginates or telescopes into another and is characterized by colicky pain, bloody stool mixed with mucous, and possibly a sausage-shaped mass on physical examination. Obstruction may occur, but the "double-bubble" sign is more consistent with duodenal obstruction. (E) An omphalocele is an abdominal wall defect in which viscera covered by a membranous sac protrude through a hole at the umbilicus. This type of defect would be easily observed on abdominal examination.

8 A 38-year-old G_2P_1 woman had an abnormal quad screen at 16 weeks' gestation with an elevated human chorionic gonadotropin (hCG) level and a low alpha-fetoprotein (AFP). Amniocentesis confirms the diagnosis of trisomy 21. Which of the following defects are found in this patient type?

(A) Diaphragmatic hernia
(B) Duodenal atresia
(C) Inguinal hernia
(D) Meckel diverticulum
(E) Wilms tumor

The answer is B: Duodenal atresia. An elevated hCG level with a low AFP suggests Down syndrome, which was confirmed by amniocentesis. Trisomy 21 is associated with a number of physical defects. These include stunted growth, brachycephaly, macroglossia, umbilical hernia, and duodenal atresia. The duodenal atresia is a result of incomplete recanalization of the duodenum, which starts off patent during development, and then is occluded by epithelial overgrowth. Atresia may result in stenosis or complete obstruction.

(A) Trisomy 21 is not associated with a significant increase in the risk of developing a diaphragmatic hernia. There is, however, a strong association between trisomy 21 and duodenal atresia. (C) Trisomy 21 is not associated with a significant increase in the risk of developing an inguinal hernia. There is, however, a strong association between trisomy 21 and duodenal atresia. (D) Trisomy 21 is not associated with a significant increase in the risk of Meckel diverticulum. There is, however, a strong association between trisomy 21 and duodenal atresia. (E) Trisomy 21 is not associated with a significant increase in the risk of Wilms tumor. There is, however, a strong association between trisomy 21 and duodenal atresia.

9 An 8-hour-old newborn male infant has vomited upon every attempt at feeding. The nurse notes that he appears to salivate more than usual. The physician suspects esophageal atresia. A nasogastric tube could not be passed. This infant should also be checked closely for:

(A) Anal atresia
(B) Cleft palate
(C) Meckel diverticulum
(D) Spina bifida
(E) Esophageal atresia has no such associations

The answer is A. Anal atresia. Esophageal atresia (EA) usually occurs along with some form of tracheoesophageal fistula (TEF) because the trachea develops as an outpouching from the portion of gut tube that will become the esophagus. A number of combinations of these two abnormalities exist: in this patient, the esophagus ends in a blind pouch as demonstrated by the inability to pass a nasogastric tube. The most common combination (85% of such cases) is a distal tracheoesophageal fistula with a blind proximal esophageal pouch. These defects often occur with additional abnormalities, a phenomenon termed the vertebral, anal, cardiac, tracheal, esophageal, renal, and limb defects (VACTERL) association.

(B) Cleft palate is not known to be associated with esophageal atresia/tracheoesophageal fistula. The acronym VACTERL illustrates a known association with vertebral, anal, cardiac, tracheal, esophageal, renal, and limb defects. (C) Meckel diverticulum is not known to be associated with esophageal atresia/tracheoesophageal fistula. The acronym VACTERL illustrates a known association with vertebral, anal, cardiac, tracheal, esophageal, renal, and limb defects. (D) Spina bifida is not known to be associated with esophageal atresia/tracheoesophageal fistula. Spina bifida represents a specific spinal anomaly, distinct from the vertebral defects that make up the VACTERL association. (E) Esophageal atresia is often accompanied by a tracheoesophageal fistula and perhaps other defects as illustrated by the VACTERL acronym (vertebral, anal, cardiac, tracheal, esophageal, renal, and limb defects).

10 During the newborn examination of a 12-hour-old male infant, the physician notes the absence of an anal opening. No other abnormalities are noted on a thorough physical examination. A dark, tarry substance is noted at the urethral meatus. Imperforate anus with a fistula is suspected. Where is the most likely site of the purported fistula internally?

(A) Between the rectal pouch and bladder dome
(B) Between the rectal pouch and posterior surface of the urinary bladder
(C) Between the rectal pouch and urethra inferior to the puborectalis sling
(D) Between the rectal pouch and urethra superior to the puborectalis sling
(E) There is most likely no fistula in this patient

The answer is D: Between the rectal pouch and urethra superior to the puborectalis sling. Imperforate anus is more common in boys than girls (2:1 ratio of boys:girls) and may or may not be accompanied by a fistula. In the absence of a fistula, the rectum ends in a blind pouch. If a fistula is present, meconium may be seen at the urethral meatus in male individuals (as in this patient) or the vaginal vault in female individuals. A fistula may alternatively open anywhere along the perineum and not involve the genitourinary system at all. An easy division of fistula types involves classification in relation to the puborectalis sling: fistulae occurring superior to the sling are termed supralevator type (more common in boys) and those occurring inferior to the sling are infralevator type (more common in girls). The supralevator-type fistulae in boys form a connection between the rectal pouch and the urethra.

(A) The supralevator-type fistulae in boys form a connection between the rectal pouch and the urethra. (B) The supralevator-type fistulae in boys form a connection between the rectal pouch and the urethra. (C) A fistula inferior to the puborectalis sling would be called an infralevator type. These are more common in girls and are not likely the type present in this patient. (E) The tarry substance at the urethral meatus likely represents meconium that has passed from the rectal pouch to the urethra via a fistula.

(11)) During the newborn examination of a 12-hour-old male infant, the physician notes the absence of an anal opening. No other abnormalities are noted on a thorough physical examination. A dark, tarry substance is noted at the urethral meatus. The child is diagnosed with imperforate anus with a fistula between the rectal pouch and urinary tract. This defect often leads to which electrolyte abnormality?

(A) Hyperchloremia
(B) Hypernatremia
(C) Hypocalcemia
(D) Hypokalemia
(E) Hypophosphatemia

The answer is A: Hyperchloremia. An infant with an imperforate anus and a fistula between the rectal pouch and urinary tract is prone to developing a number of complications including urinary tract infections. The chloride excreted in the urine is also readily absorbed by colonic mucosa. Excessive chloride reabsorption leads to bicarbonate excretion to maintain charge balance and the patient may develop a hyperchloremic acidosis. Less severe cases may resolve spontaneously, but some may require urgent surgical correction even before definitive surgery can take place.

(B) Chloride excreted in the urine is readily absorbed by colonic mucosa. This may lead to a hyperchloremic acidosis as chloride is absorbed and bicarbonate excreted. Hypernatremia is not a common complication of these patients. (C) Chloride excreted in the urine is readily absorbed by colonic mucosa. This may lead to a hyperchloremic acidosis as chloride is absorbed and bicarbonate excreted. Hypocalcemia is not a common complication of these patients. (D) Chloride excreted in the urine is readily absorbed by colonic mucosa. This may lead to a hyperchloremic acidosis as chloride is absorbed and bicarbonate excreted. Hypokalemia is not a common complication of these patients. (E) Chloride excreted in the urine is readily absorbed by colonic mucosa. This may lead to a hyperchloremic acidosis as chloride is absorbed and bicarbonate excreted. Hypophosphatemia is not a common complication of these patients.

(12)) A newborn girl fails to pass meconium after 24 hours. She was born at term by spontaneous vaginal delivery and her prenatal history was benign. Her Apgar scores were 7 and 9 at 1 and 5 minutes, respectively. Abdominal x-ray reveals distended bowel but no air in the rectum.

What would a microscopic examination of tissue from the affected portion of bowel most likely show?

(A) Absence of neural ganglia
(B) Excessive proliferation of neural ganglia
(C) Hyperplastic smooth muscle fibers
(D) Hypertrophic smooth muscle fibers
(E) Muscularis replaced by fibrous tissue

The answer is A: Absence of neural ganglia. Hirschsprung disease can be suspected in any infant who has not passed meconium in the first 24 hours of life, but also in any child who has had abnormal bowel patterns since birth. Physical examination will reveal a distended abdomen and an abdominal x-ray will show air-fluid levels, distended loops of bowel, and an absence of air in the rectum. Hirschsprung disease is caused by the failure of development of parasympathetic ganglia in the colonic submucosa, without which the muscularis layers cannot relax. Diagnosis is aided by biopsy which will show the presence of Auerbach plexus but no Meissner plexus. (In normal anatomy, Auerbach plexus contains sympathetic and parasympathetic fibers, whereas Meissner contains only parasympathetic fibers. Auerbach plexus will be visible because even though the parasympathetic fibers are absent, the sympathetic fibers will pick up the stain.)

(B) Parasympathetic neural input stimulates relaxation of the smooth muscle fibers in the gastrointestinal (GI) tract. It is the absence of these relaxing stimuli that lead to Hirschsprung disease. (C) The smooth muscle fibers in Hirschsprung disease are normal; they are neither hyperplastic nor hypertrophied. The reason why they do not relax is the absence of parasympathetic input. (D) The smooth muscle fibers in Hirschsprung disease are normal; they are neither hyperplastic nor hypertrophied. The reason why they do not relax is the absence of parasympathetic input. (E) There is no replacement of muscle fibers with scar tissue in early Hirschsprung disease. The reason why the rectum is constricted is that there are no parasympathetic neurons to mediate relaxation.

---

(13) A female infant is born prematurely to an obese mother at 32 weeks of gestation. Prenatal care was poor—the mother showed up for only two visits. After birth, her Apgar scores were 2 and 5 at 1 and 5 minutes. An abdominal x-ray reveals pneumatosis intestinalis. In addition to being premature, which of the following is a known risk factor for her condition?

(A) Formula feeding
(B) Low Apgar scores
(C) Female sex
(D) Obese mother
(E) Trisomy 21

The answer is A: Formula feeding. Necrotizing enterocolitis (NEC) is a disease whose etiology has not been completely elucidated but appears to stem from a combination of ischemia and bacterial overgrowth in the setting of an immature intestine and immune system. The typical picture is a premature or low birth weight infant with feeding intolerance and abdominal distention. Abdominal x-ray will often show the pathognomonic pneumatosis intestinalis, or air within the bowel wall. Premature infants fed formula are 10× more likely to develop NEC than those fed breast milk alone.

(B) Although low Apgar scores often correlate with prematurity, they are not known risk factors for the development of NEC. (C) No correlation between sex and development of NEC has been observed. Some studies have reported a weak correlation among races with the black population being more susceptible, but this result is not consistent among all NEC studies. (D) Obesity in the pregnant mother can lead to macrosomia and birth difficulties stemming from that, but obesity is not known to be a risk factor for NEC. (E) Infants with trisomy 21 are known to be at risk for a number of defects, including endocardial cushion defects and duodenal atresia. A correlation between trisomy 21 and NEC has not been observed, however.

14 A 4-week-old male infant is brought to the clinic because of increasingly frequent vomiting after meals. He had been feeding without any problems for the first 2 weeks of life. The vomit is not bilious. His skin appears yellow. A round, movable mass can be palpated in the epigastrium. Barium study is obtained and shown in *Figure 17-2*.

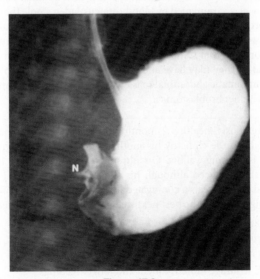

Figure 17-2

What is the most likely etiology of this patient's condition?

(A) Biliary atresia
(B) Duodenal atresia
(C) Intussusception
(D) Nephroblastoma
(E) Pyloric stenosis

The answer is E: Pyloric stenosis. Pyloric stenosis is a disorder of unknown etiology but appears to have a strong genetic component. Most cases occur in male individuals, in whom pyloric stenosis is about four times as common as in female individuals. Presentation usually involves the development of vomiting after meals that was not present at birth. The vomiting is nonbilious and progresses to projectile vomiting. Jaundice occurs in about 10% of cases. An olive-shaped mass may be palpated in the epigastric area in these patients. Such palpation is greatly aided by decompression of the stomach and practice. A barium study shows dilation of the stomach with pyloric channel narrowing. Surgical treatment of this condition involves cutting into the pylorus longitudinally into the muscularis down to but not through the mucosa.

(A) Biliary atresia is a cause of progressive jaundice that appears during the first few weeks of life. The liver may be enlarged, but biliary atresia does not lead to the formation of an epigastric mass. The child's stool will be pale. (B) Duodenal atresia leads to bilious vomiting present at birth. An abdominal x-ray will show the "double bubble" sign, or an air bubble in the stomach next to an air bubble in the early patent segment of the duodenum. (C) Intussusception generally presents as intermittent episodes of abdominal pain and sleepiness that may be accompanied by bloody, mucus-laden stool. The child is often most comfortable lying down with knees drawn up to chest. A sausage-shaped mass may be palpated on abdominal examination. (D) Nephroblastoma or Wilms tumor is a renal tumor generally discovered in children between the ages of 1 and 5. They may have abdominal pain, but more often they present with an asymptomatic abdominal mass. Vomiting and jaundice are not usually associated with nephroblastomas.

15) A previously healthy 2-month-old breastfed white male infant is brought to the clinic by his mother who is concerned that her baby's skin is turning yellow. On physical examination, the child indeed appears jaundiced although his skin tone was normal 1 month ago. Blood work reveals a conjugated hyperbilirubinemia. Which of the following would be the best next step in the care of this patient?

(A) Abdominal x-ray
(B) Blood smear
(C) Discontinue breastfeeding and start formula feeding
(D) Encourage more frequent and longer feedings
(E) Ultrasonography of the abdomen

The answer is E: Ultrasonography of the abdomen. The cause of biliary atresia is still unknown, but it is characterized by a conjugated hyperbilirubinemia caused by the degeneration of the bile ducts. It almost always occurs after birth with most cases present between 4 weeks and 4 months of age. Ultrasonography is a primary test of choice in patients with persistent jaundice because the presence or absence of the biliary tree can often be determined. Biliary atresia can be divided into two types: correctable and uncorrectable. The correctable type constitutes about 20% of all cases and involves only a small region of the biliary tree such that the atretic segment can be resected and the remaining ducts can be anastomosed. In the uncorrectable type, few or no remnants of the biliary tree can be found. The current method to drain the liver in patients with the uncorrectable type is the Kasai procedure in which a loop of duodenum is anastomosed to the liver where the common bile duct should be.

(A) An abdominal x-ray would not be useful in evaluating biliary atresia. The atretic segment is not generally calcified so it would not be visible on x-ray. The abdomen of a child with biliary atresia would look like the abdomen of a normal child on x-ray. (B) A blood smear would be useful if hereditary spherocytosis was suspected, but hereditary spherocytosis produces an unconjugated hyperbilirubinemia because of the increased turnover of red cells. (C) Breast milk jaundice usually appears during the second week of an infant's life. The cause is not completely understood, but there is no evidence that continuing breastfeeding is harmful. The child's age (2 months or about 8 weeks) makes this unlikely. (D) Breastfeeding jaundice, which is really a lack of adequate intake, occurs soon after birth within the first week of an infant's life. It is corrected by increasing the infant's oral intake. This child's age (2 months or about 8 weeks) makes this unlikely.

---

16 A 2-year-old girl is brou ght to the emergency department (ED) by her mother. The mother reports that the girl has been clutching her stomach intermittently throughout the day. She becomes very sleepy in between each attack of pain and lies on her side with her knees drawn up when the pain becomes severe. What is the most likely ailment in this infant?

(A) Appendicitis
(B) Intussusception
(C) Gastroenteritis
(D) Mesenteric adenitis
(E) Ruptured ovarian cyst

The answer is B: Intussusception. Evaluating an acute abdomen in an infant is often more difficult than in an adult because of a lack of effective communication. In spite of this, details from the parents can be pieced together to see telltale patterns that suggest specific disease processes.

The intermittent nature of this girl's pain accompanied by her sleepiness is suggestive of intussusception. It is common for patients with intussusception to present with knees drawn to chest during the episodes of pain as this patient did. Intussusception may also be accompanied by bloody stools mixed with mucus and a sausage-shaped mass may be palpated on abdominal examination.

(A) Appendicitis is rare in patients under age 4 years. The intermittent, colicky nature of this patient's pain is also suggestive of intussusception rather than appendicitis. (C) Gastroenteritis is characterized by diarrhea and possibly vomiting. The intermittent nature of this patient's pain accompanied by sleepiness is classic for intussusception. (D) Mesenteric adenitis is characterized by fluctuating levels of pain but not so much colicky bouts of pain as in intussusception. The sleepiness present in between the episodes of pain is also characteristic of intussusception. (E) Ruptured ovarian cysts occur in postmenarchal patients, which is extremely unlikely in a girl of this age. This patient's presentation of colicky pain interspersed with periods of sleepiness is characteristic of intussusception.

 17 A 16-month-old male toddler is brought to the emergency department (ED) by his parents. The mother says that he has been clutching his abdomen off and on throughout the day. The parents report that he is sleepy in between each attack of pain and lies on his side with his knees drawn up to his chest when the pain is most severe. What is the best treatment for this patient's most likely problem?

(A) Barium enema
(B) Laparoscopic partial bowel resection
(C) Nasogastric tube placement for bowel decompression
(D) Ten-day course of oral vancomycin
(E) No treatment necessary

The answer is A: Barium enema. This patient's presentation is most consistent with intussusception. The child is usually aged between 6 and 18 months and presents with intermittent abdominal pain. They often become sleepy between attacks and may pass bloody stools. A sausage-shaped mass may be palpated in the abdomen. The most common area of intussusception involves the distal ileum protruding into the lumen of the cecum (ileocolic intussusception). A barium or air contrast enema is diagnostic and usually therapeutic because the increased pressure from the contrast material in the colonic lumen functions to push the ileum back into place. Surgical reduction in the intussusception is the next step if an enema fails.

(B) Laparoscopic partial bowel resection would be the treatment of choice for a symptomatic Meckel diverticulum. While a Meckel diverticulum can act as a lead point for intussusception, the diverticulum itself often presents as a painless gastrointestinal (GI) bleed in a young child. (C) There is no need for nasogastric tube placement or other bowel decompression in the treatment of intussusception. A barium or air contrast enema is often sufficient to reduce the intussusception. (D) Antibiotics of any kind do not play a role treatment of intussusception unless surgery is required. Even then oral vancomycin would be a poor choice, but it may be useful in treating clostridium difficile colitis. But this patient's history and presentation are most consistent with intussusception. (E) Spontaneous reduction in intussusception is uncommon. Without reduction, necrosis of the bowel ensues. A barium or air contrast enema will often reduce the defect.

 A 20-month-old female infant is brought to the emergency department (ED) by her father with 4 hours of painless rectal bleeding. Abdominal examination reveals no masses, organomegaly, or tenderness. Rectal examination reveals dark blood in the rectal vault but no tenderness or evidence of trauma. The physician suspects a Meckel diverticulum. What would be the best study to confirm the suspected diagnosis?

(A) Abdominal ultrasound
(B) Abdominal x-ray
(C) Barium enema
(D) Small bowel follow-through
(E) Technetium scan

The answer is E: **Technetium scan.** As mentioned in the question stem, this patient's presentation is most suspicious for a Meckel diverticulum. The "rule of 2s" gives an overview of Meckel diverticula: they occur in about 2% of the population, are found within 2 feet of the ileocecal valve, and often present around 2 years of age. The diverticulum exists as a remnant of the vitelline duct and may contain gastric or pancreatic tissue. Ectopic gastric mucosa which secretes acid leads to the formation of ulcers and causes the painless bleeding often associated with Meckel diverticula. Technetium pertechnetate shows increased uptake in gastric tissue and is useful in evaluating suspected Meckel diverticula.

(A) This patient's age and history of painless rectal bleeding are suspicious for a Meckel diverticulum. These diverticula are not readily visualized on ultrasound. A technetium scan will show increased uptake in a Meckel diverticulum containing gastric tissue. (B) An abdominal x-ray would not be a good test to evaluate a possible Meckel diverticulum because these diverticula are poorly visualized on plain film. A technetium pertechnetate scan would be the best study to evaluate a possible Meckel diverticulum. (C) A barium enema may be useful in the evaluation (and treatment) of intussusception, but is not as sensitive as a technetium scan for evaluating a Meckel diverticulum. (D) A small bowel follow-through would not be as good a test as a technetium scan in identifying possible Meckel diverticulum. Technetium scanning provides the best visualization.

19　A 3-week-old male infant has been spitting up after meals since his birth. The rest of the history obtained from the mother includes many clues that raise suspicion for gastroesophageal reflux (GER). He has not been gaining weight as expected and is failing to thrive. What would be the best next step in the evaluation of the patient?

(A) Barium swallow
(B) Endoscopy
(C) Manometry
(D) pH study
(E) None needed—suspicion alone based on clinical clues is sufficient to justify surgical correction

The answer is A: Barium swallow. The most likely diagnosis in this patient is GER because his vomiting has been present since birth. A physical obstruction may cause similar symptoms. Severe GER can involve failure to thrive, as in this patient. Complications (in addition to failure to thrive) include recurrent aspiration pneumonias and reactive airway disease, laryngospasm and apnea, and esophagitis possibly leading to Barrett esophagus if left untreated. A patient with severe symptoms that are not sufficiently controlled medically may benefit from surgery if the symptoms can be attributed to GER. A barium swallow would be the best next step in the evaluation of this patient because it will likely show reflux if present and would elucidate other possible causes of his symptoms such as obstruction.

(B) Endoscopy would be useful to evaluate possible esophagitis in a patient known to have longstanding GER. The initial evaluation of this patient would be better served by a barium swallow. (C) Manometry is not as easy to perform as a barium swallow in children and would likely not provide additional information. A barium swallow would be the best next step in the evaluation of this patient. (D) A pH study is not as easy to perform as a barium swallow in children and would likely not provide additional information. A barium swallow would be the best next step in the evaluation of this patient. (E) Symptoms of this kind may be from GER, but may also be from other causes such as obstruction or otherwise abnormal esophageal anatomy. Before surgery for GER is performed, a diagnosis of GER should be established by barium swallow.

20　A 5-year-old male child presents with his mother who mentions a "hole" in his chest. On physical examination, a deep depression is seen in his mid-chest. A diagnosis of pectus excavatum is made. Most children with pectus excavatum suffer from which of the following difficulties?

(A) Excessive joint laxity
(B) Impaired upper body strength
(C) Obstructive pulmonary disease
(D) Severe cardiovascular impairment
(E) Most children with pectus excavatum suffer from none of these.

The answer is E: **Most children with pectus excavatum suffer from none of these.** Pectus excavatum occurs in up to 1 in 400 births and is seen in both male individuals and female individuals. There is a strong hereditary tendency from this deformity. The deformity is usually purely cosmetic, although some children may develop symptoms of restrictive pulmonary disease such as decreased endurance and easy fatigability. These symptoms usually appear later in childhood or in adolescence. Most children with pectus excavatum do not suffer from cardiovascular impairment.

(A) Joint laxity is seen in children with Marfan syndrome and Ehlers-Danlos syndrome. There is, however, no association between pectus excavatum and joint laxity. (B) Pectus excavatum alters the chest wall anatomy but does not cause significant impairment in strength. (C) Pectus excavatum may cause symptoms of restrictive lung disease, not obstructive lung disease. Causes of obstructive lung disease include smoking and α-1 antitrypsin activity. (D) Any symptoms from pectus excavatum generally arise from restrictive lung disease, not cardiovascular impairment. Most children with pectus excavatum do not suffer from cardiovascular impairment.

 A 7-year-old girl with severe pectus excavatum is brought to the clinic by her parents to be evaluated for possible surgical correction. She has a prior medical history of gastroesophageal reflux (GER) which has been managed with medical therapy. Consideration for surgical repair of the pectus excavatum is now considered by her physician. What is a benefit of the Nuss procedure for this patient as compared with traditional costal cartilage resection?

(A) The Nuss procedure avoids impairment in chest wall growth
(B) The Nuss procedure carries less chance of damage to thoracic organs
(C) The Nuss procedure carries significantly lower risk of infection
(D) The Nuss procedure carries significantly lower risk of pneumothorax
(E) The Nuss procedure carries significantly lower risk of recurrence of pectus excavatum

The answer is A: **The Nuss procedure avoids impairment in chest wall growth.** The traditional operation involves resection of the affected costal cartilage, a wedge osteotomy to enable anterior elevation of the sternum, and placement of hardware to maintain the new configuration for a few months while healing occurs. In the "Nuss" procedure, a semicircular bar is thoracoscopically inserted under the sternum and ribs to hold the sternum in a neutral position and is left in place for 2 years to allow remodeling of the chest wall. Both procedures carry similar risks of infection, recurrence, pneumothorax, and other damage to thoracic organs, but the "Nuss" procedure does not impair growth of the chest wall, whereas this is a common complication of the traditional operation.

(B) Both procedures carry similar risks of infection, recurrence, pneumothorax, and other damage to thoracic organs. Thoracic organs can be damaged during thoracoscopic insertion of the bar during a Nuss procedure. (C) Both procedures carry similar risks of infection, recurrence, pneumothorax, and other damage to thoracic organs. (D) Both procedures carry similar risks of infection, recurrence, pneumothorax, and other damage to thoracic organs. (E) Both procedures carry similar risks of infection, recurrence, pneumothorax, and other damage to thoracic organs.

 A 3-year-old female child is brought to the ambulatory care unit of the emergency department for evaluation of a neck mass. The parents noted a neck mass while bathing the child. She has a prior surgical history of a left inguinal hernia repair at age 2. Physical examination reveals a soft, compressible mass about 2 cm × 2 cm in size but with poorly defined borders. The mass is located just posterior to the middle of the body of her left sternomastoid muscle. What is the most likely diagnosis?

(A) Congenital malformation of lymphatic vessels
(B) Failure of obliteration of the thyroglossal duct
(C) Failure of resorption of the branchial clefts
(D) Hematologic malignancy with metastatic deposit
(E) Torticollis, congenital

The answer is A: Congenital malformation of lymphatic vessels.
Neck masses can be grouped according to their location: midline or lateral. Midline neck masses include thyroglossal duct cysts or ectopic thyroid gland tissue. Lateral neck masses include cystic hygromas, branchial cleft cysts, lymphadenopathy, and torticollis. This child's mass most closely fits the description of a cystic hygroma. Cystic hygromas are congenital malformation of lymphatic vessels. They have poorly defined borders and are soft and compressible.

(B) Thyroglossal duct cysts are the result of the failure of thyroglossal duct obliteration. Furthermore, a thyroglossal duct cyst is a midline lesion. (C) A branchial cleft cyst is a lateral neck lesion. It results when the branchial clefts that arise during embryogenesis on the sides of the neck fail to regress completely. They have well-defined borders and are found along the anterior border of the sternomastoid muscle or possibly near the ear. (D) Lymphoma is a hematologic malignancy than can have metastatic deposits. The typical cervical lymph node is palpable as a hard, fixed, lateral neck lesion. (E) Torticollis refers to a fibrosis and shortening of the sternomastoid muscle. The fibrotic region may present as a mass found in line with the sternomastoid muscle and accompanied by the head being twisted toward the contralateral side.

23 A 6-month-old male infant is brought to the pediatric clinic for evaluation of a red lesion on his forehead. The mother of the child is concerned because the lesion has been rapidly increasing in size and the infant's maternal grandmother died of melanoma in her 60s. On physical examination, a red, raised lesion about 1 cm × 3 cm with irregular borders can be seen about 3 cm superior to his left eyebrow. What is the best treatment option for this child?

- **(A)** Do no further treatment other than routine follow-up examinations
- **(B)** Embolization via superficial temporal artery
- **(C)** Excision with 2.5-cm-wide margins
- **(D)** Laser photocoagulation and adjuvant chemotherapy
- **(E)** Systemic corticosteroid therapy

The answer is A: Do no further treatment other than routine follow-up examinations. This presentation is most consistent with a capillary hemangioma. These vascular tumors most often appear within the first few weeks of life and rapidly increase in size for about a year after which they begin to spontaneously regress. Most of these hemangiomas, including the one in this question stem, should be left alone because they will most likely regress and pose no threat to the child's health. Indications for intervention include lesions that threaten to interfere with the eyes or airway or lesions so large they cause thrombocytopenia, congestive heart failure, or significant facial distortion. All of the responses represent possible appropriate interventions, but this patient's lesion does not currently require treatment of any kind.

(B) Embolization of the superficial temporal artery may be an appropriate option in another scenario. (C) Excision of the hemangioma may be an appropriate option in another scenario. This patient's lesion is currently not threatening the infant's health and should not be treated at this time. (D) Laser photocoagulation may be a good option in another scenario. This patient's lesion is currently not threatening the infant's health and should not be treated at this time. (E) Systemic corticosteroid therapy may be a good option in another scenario. This patient's lesion is currently not threatening the infant's health and should not be treated at this time.

24 A 2-year-old male child is found to have hypertension during a checkup. The child was brought to the clinic because of recurrent fevers. He is in the 10th percentile for weight. The child was born at term via C-section. The mother was a former smoker and intravenous (IV) drug user during pregnancy. A careful abdominal examination reveals an abdominal mass. What is the most likely diagnosis?

(A) Ewing sarcoma
(B) Nephroblastoma
(C) Neuroblastoma
(D) Rhabdomyosarcoma
(E) Teratoma

The answer is C: Neuroblastoma. Neuroblastomas are the most common extracranial solid tumors of children. These tumors arise from neural crest cells. Most are found in the abdomen, usually in the adrenal medulla. An abdominal mass can often be felt. Systemic symptoms, such as the fevers, hypertension, and failure to thrive seen in this patient, are common. Urine will have elevated levels of catecholamines and their breakdown products. Treatment may involve surgery, chemotherapy, and radiation as most children have metastases by the time of presentation.

(A) Ewing sarcoma is a tumor of the bone. It is most commonly found in the limbs, pelvis, or ribs and would not present as an abdominal mass. Furthermore, hypertension is associated with neuroblastoma but not Ewing sarcoma. (B) Nephroblastoma, or Wilms tumor, generally presents as a painless, asymptomatic abdominal mass. Nephroblastomas may cause hypertension and other symptoms, but this occurs much more commonly with neuroblastomas. Neuroblastomas are more common in general than nephroblastomas. (D) Rhabdomyosarcomas are generally asymptomatic tumors of skeletal muscle and are classified into two subgroups: embryonal (found in younger children in the head, neck, and genitourinary tract) and alveolar (found in older children in the trunk and extremities). Neuroblastomas are more common than rhabdomyosarcomas. (E) Teratomas are tumors made up of cells from more than one of the germ layers. In children, they are usually found around the sacrococcygeal area or ovaries. Neuroblastomas are more common overall and more commonly associated with systemic symptoms such as hypertension and fevers.

---

25 A 4-year-old male child is brought to the pediatric clinic by his father because the father reports feeling hard mass in the abdomen while bathing the child 2 days ago. The father denies fevers and the child has been otherwise growing normally. He is in the 60th percentile for weight. A hard, golf ball-sized lump can be palpated in his right upper quadrant. There is no evidence of guarding or rebound tenderness. Which of the following additional findings may also be identified in this patient?

(A) Aniridia
(B) Clubbed feet
(C) Cryptorchidism
(D) Imperforate anus
(E) Webbed digits

The answer is A: **Aniridia.** Wilms tumor, also known as nephroblastoma, is a type of renal tumor seen in children. It most often presents as a painless and otherwise asymptomatic abdominal mass in a child between the ages of 1 and 5 years. In 10% of patients, it presents bilaterally. Wilms tumor is often associated with other abnormalities, including aniridia, hypospadias, and hemihypertrophy. Treatment is surgical resection plus postoperative chemotherapy and possibly radiation therapy depending on the stage and grade of the tumor. Prognosis is generally good.

(B) Abnormalities known to be associated with Wilms tumor include aniridia, hypospadias, and hemihypertrophy. Clubbed feet are not known to be associated with Wilms tumor. (C) Abnormalities known to be associated with Wilms tumor include aniridia, hypospadias, and hemihypertrophy. Cryptorchidism is not known to be associated with Wilms tumor. (D) Abnormalities known to be associated with Wilms tumor include aniridia, hypospadias, and hemihypertrophy. Imperforate anus is not known to be associated with Wilms tumor. (E) Abnormalities known to be associated with Wilms tumor include aniridia, hypospadias, and hemihypertrophy. Webbed digits are not known to be associated with Wilms tumor.

1 A 19-year-old man with diabetes is undergoing evaluation for a possible pancreatic transplant. Along with other routine tests, which of the following should be done in this patient before the operation?

(A) Check serum amylase level
(B) Check serum C-peptide level
(C) Check serum carcinoembryonic antigen (CEA) level
(D) Check serum lipase level
(E) Check serum renin level

The answer is B: **Check serum C-peptide level.** All transplant recipient candidates undergo a careful evaluation to ensure that the condition leading to organ failure in the first place does not recur posttransplant. General health and related organ systems are also evaluated to ensure that the condition leading to the organ failure has not affected other organ systems to the extent that the potential recipient's life expectancy is significantly shortened. In addition to these considerations, specific issues are addressed for certain transplant recipients, including pancreas recipients. Most pancreatic transplants are performed for type 1 diabetes mellitus, so checking a C-peptide level before the operation to confirm that the potential recipient is indeed suffering from type 1 diabetes and not some other condition.

(A) The C-peptide level is checked to confirm that the potential recipient has type 1 diabetes mellitus and not some other condition. There is no need to check a serum amylase level in a patient hoping to receive a pancreas transplant. (C) The C-peptide level is checked to confirm that the potential recipient has type 1 diabetes mellitus and not some other condition. There is no need to check a serum CEA level in a patient hoping to receive a pancreas transplant. (D) The C-peptide level is checked to confirm that the potential recipient has type 1 diabetes mellitus and not some other condition. There is no need to check a serum lipase level in a patient hoping to receive a pancreas transplant. (E) The C-peptide level is checked to confirm that the potential recipient has type 1 diabetes mellitus and not some other condition. There is no need to check a serum renin level in a patient hoping to receive a pancreas transplant.

 2 A 23-year-old woman with renal failure is a candidate for a kidney transplant. Her monozygotic twin sister volunteered to donate a kidney. This exchange would qualify as which type of transplant?

   (A) Allograft
   (B) Autograft
   (C) Cadaveric
   (D) Isograft
   (E) Xenograft

The answer is D: Isograft. The relationship between the donor and recipient of an organ transplant is important because this relationship dictates whether or not immunosuppression is required following the operation. Allografts and xenografts do require immunosuppression to prevent organ rejection. An allograft is a transfer between genetically different individuals of the same species while a xenograft refers to transfer of an organ or tissue between individuals of different species (such as a porcine or bovine heart valve). Autografts and isografts do not require immunosuppression. An autograft is a transfer of tissue within a single individual (such as a skin graft), while an isograft is a transfer between two genetically identical individuals (such as the monozygotic twins in the question stem).

(A) An allograft refers to transfer of an organ or tissue between two genetically different individuals of the same species. Transfer between genetically identical twins would be classified as an isograft. (B) An autograft refers to transfer of tissue from one place to another within the same individual (as in a skin graft). Transfer between genetically identical twins would be classified as an isograft. (C) A cadaveric transfer simply means the organ or tissue came from an individual whose brain has ceased functioning. It does not refer to a specific graft type. Transfer between genetically identical twins would be classified as an isograft. (E) A xenograft refers to transfer of tissue between two members of different species. Transfer between genetically identical twins would be classified as an isograft.

 3 A 58-year-old man is the recipient of a kidney transplant. He later undergoes an abdominal CT scan for an unrelated issue and is surprised to learn that his transplanted kidney is down in his pelvis. This is most likely an example of what?

(A) Heterotopic transplantation
(B) Medical malpractice
(C) Organ prolapse
(D) Orthotopic transplantation
(E) Syngeneic graft

The answer is A: Heterotopic transplantation. An orthotopic transplantation means that the old organ is removed and the new organ is implanted into the same location. A heterotopic transplantation means that the new organ is implanted in a location different from the native location. Many kidneys are heterotopically transplanted into the pelvis, which makes for a much simpler operation and less difficulties reconnecting the ureter. This man's kidney represents a heterotopic transplantation.

(B) Kidneys are commonly transplanted heterotopically. The fact that this man's new kidney is located in his pelvis does not suggest malpractice. (C) "Prolapse" is a general term used to describe an organ that has fallen out of place. More likely is that this man received a kidney that was transplanted heterotopically and the organ is in the same position that the surgeons placed it in. (D) An orthotopic transplantation would mean an old kidney was removed and the new kidney was placed in the same location near the costovertebral angle. This man has undergone a heterotopic kidney transplantation. (E) A syngeneic graft is another name for an isograft. "Syngeneic" and "isograft" refer to the relationship between the donor and recipient (namely that the transfer is between two genetically identical individuals) and has no bearing on the location of the transplanted organ.

 4 A healthy 38-year-old man who has previously expressed and documented his desire to be an organ donor is severely injured during a motor vehicle accident. Which of the following would make him ineligible to donate?

(A) A normal body temperature
(B) Absence of respiratory effort
(C) Decreased cerebral blood flow
(D) No pupillary reaction to bright light
(E) Presence of deep tendon reflexes

The answer is B: Absence of respiratory effort. An organ can only be harvested from a donor body once brain death has been ascertained and certain additional criteria (such as normal body temperature) are met. Criteria for brain death vary from state to state in the United States, but sets of criteria require the absence of brainstem reflexes such as the gag reflex, corneal reflex, and pupillary reaction to light. An "apnea test" must also be negative, which refers to the absence of respiratory effort despite a high pCO_2.

(A) A normal body temperature is actually required to harvest organs from a donor. Having a normal body temperature makes this patient eligible to donate. (C) Electroencephalogram (EEG) and cerebral blood flow studies are generally optional. In any case, decreased cerebral blood flow would not preclude organ donation as this is also a sign of brain death. (D) The absence of the pupillary reaction to light is generally one of the prerequisites for organ donation. Lack of this reaction would certainly not make him ineligible. (E) Deep tendon reflexes may be seen in a brain-dead patient because these reflexes are mediated by peripheral nerves and connections in the spinal cord only. The presence of these reflexes would not make this patient ineligible to donate.

5 A harvested organ is rapidly flushed with 4°C saline as soon as it is removed from the body. Which organ is routinely treated in this manner before its transplantation?

   (A) Heart
   (B) Kidney
   (C) Liver
   (D) Lungs
   (E) These organs are all generally treated in this manner

The answer is E: These organs are all generally treated in this manner. Any time an organ is removed from its native location for transplant, it risks ischemic damage and may experience irreversible impairments in function. This risk is decreased by minimizing ischemic time. All organs are more tolerant of cold ischemia than they are of warm ischemia because of the reduction in metabolism and oxygen demand. For this reason, donor organs are flushed with cold (4°C) saline to cool them down as soon as they are harvested.

(A) Donor hearts are routinely flushed with cold saline to minimize potential ischemic damage. All organs are more tolerant of cold ischemia than they are of warm ischemia. (B) Donor kidneys are routinely flushed with cold saline to minimize potential ischemic damage. All organs are more tolerant of cold ischemia than they are of warm ischemia. (C) Donor livers are routinely flushed with cold saline to minimize potential ischemic damage. All organs are more tolerant of cold ischemia than they are of warm ischemia. (D) Donor lungs are routinely flushed with cold saline to minimize potential ischemic damage. All organs are more tolerant of cold ischemia than they are of warm ischemia.

6 An organ donor patient at a small community hospital is declared brain dead and a surgical transplant team arrives to harvest needed organs. A patient in a neighboring state is awaiting the availability of one of the organs harvested from the donor but lives 2 hours away by helicopter.

Which of the following organs can tolerate the greatest amount of cold ischemia?

(A) Heart
(B) Kidney
(C) Liver
(D) Lung
(E) Pancreas

The answer is B: Kidney. All organs are more tolerant of cold ischemia than they are of warm ischemia. There is, of course, no specific time an organ can remain ischemic after which it immediately dies. The shorter the duration of time an organ is ischemic, the better the chance it has of functioning properly for the remainder of the recipient's life once the transplant is performed and the organ's blood supply is reestablished. However, practical limits to cold ischemia time have been established after which the risks for impaired function or death of the organ increase dramatically. This period of time is around 4 hours for a heart, 6 hours for a lung, 12 hours for a liver, 36 hours for a pancreas, and 40 to 48 hours for a kidney.

(A) The practical limit of cold ischemia for a heart is around 4 hours. Kidneys can tolerate the largest amount of cold ischemia time at over 40 hours. (C) The practical limit of cold ischemia for a liver is around 12 hours. Kidneys can tolerate the largest amount of cold ischemia time at over 40 hours. (D) The practical limit of cold ischemia for a lung is around 6 hours. Kidneys can tolerate the largest amount of cold ischemia time at over 40 hours. (E) The practical limit of cold ischemia for a pancreas is around 36 hours. Kidneys can tolerate the largest amount of cold ischemia time at over 40 hours.

 7 A 55-year-old female candidate for a heart transplant has type O blood. A donor heart is available from a patient with type B blood. She is eager to undergo the transplant. What should she be told?

(A) Blood type is not a factor in this type of organ transfer
(B) Her ability to receive this organ depends on the results of a cross-match between her blood and the donor patient's blood
(C) She can receive this organ if it is thoroughly rinsed from all donor blood
(D) She can receive this organ if she is placed on immunosuppressants afterward
(E) She cannot receive this organ

The answer is E: She cannot receive this organ. Immunologic compatibility is an important topic regardless of the type of organ or tissue transplantation. Incompatibility will lead to organ rejection and ultimately organ failure. Under some circumstances, incompatibility can be overcome by recipient immunosuppression. ABO incompatibility cannot be overcome by immunosuppression because incompatible recipients have preformed anti-bodies against antigens on the donor tissue. A transplant in this case would result in rapid rejection.

(A) The ABO antigens are found on all human tissues so organ transplants follow the same rules as blood transfusions with regard to blood type. This patient with type O blood would not be eligible to receive tissue from a person with type B blood because she carries preformed anti-B antibodies. (B) A further cross-match between the blood of these two patients would not be necessary. A patient with type O blood has anti-A and anti-B antibodies and could not receive blood or tissues from a type A or a type B patient. (C) The ABO antigens are found on all human tissues so rinsing all blood from the donor heart would have no effect on its ABO compatibility. A patient with type O blood has anti-A and anti-B antibodies and could not receive blood or tissues from a type A or a type B patient. (D) ABO incompatibility cannot be overcome by immunosuppression because incompatible recipients have preformed antibodies against antigens on the donor tissue. The donor organ would be rapidly rejected even if she were immunosuppressed.

8   A 61-year-old man with end-stage renal disease (ESRD) hopes to be the recipient of a kidney transplant. A donor has the same blood type and they share closely matching human leukocyte antigen (HLA) types. The recipient has a low panel reactive antibody (PRA) reactivity. Which of the following should also be performed before the transplant can take place?

(A) Cross-match of recipient serum and donor lymphocytes
(B) No further immunologic testing need to be performed in this case
(C) The HLA match must be identical; this patient cannot receive the donor organ
(D) The donor organ should be processed to render it acellular
(E) The recipient should undergo plasmapheresis

The answer is A: Cross-match of recipient serum and donor lympho-cytes. General guidelines direct the pre- and postsurgical management of all organ transplants, but certain organs also have more specific guidelines. For example, patients involved in a kidney transplant should have closely matching HLA types, whereas HLA typing is not important for heart or liver transplants. Kidney transplant patients should also have a negative cross-match before surgery to avoid hyperacute rejections. This is performed by mixing recipient serum with donor lymphocytes and monitoring for lymphocyte death (due to cytotoxic antibodies present in the donor serum). Low PRA reactivity is not necessary for a kidney transplant, but high PRA reactivity puts the recipient at increased risk for delayed graft function and graft failure.

(B) Cross-matching is not considered mandatory in cases of liver or heart transplants, but it is mandatory in kidney transplants. This patient must demonstrate a negative cross-match before receiving a donor kidney. (C) The closer the HLA type, the less likely the graft rejection following transplant. However, HLA types are rarely identical and are not necessary for successful transplantation. (D) An acellular graft would certainly be at decreased risk for rejection following transplant, but an acellular kidney would be worthless as the function of a kidney rests on the combined activity of millions of cells that make up nephrons. (E) Plasmapheresis would remove antibodies currently present in the recipient's serum but would not prevent the possible continued production of antibodies by plasma cells. The best way to check for the presence of these antibodies is a cross-match.

9 A 34-year-old woman is being evaluated for a possible kidney transplant. She has a brother with the same human leukocyte antigen (HLA)-A type as her and is willing to be a living donor for his sister. Which additional HLA gene would be most useful in assessing the compatibility of the transplant?

(A) HLA-B
(B) HLA-C
(C) HLA-DP
(D) HLA-DQ
(E) HLA-F

The answer is A: HLA-B. There are six important HLA genes, HLA-A, -B, -C, -DR, -DP, and -DQ. Each person has two copies (alleles) of each of the six genes and hundreds of alleles exist in the population. Identical matching of HLA types is rare because of the large number of possible combinations, even among family members. In spite of this, many successful organ and tissue grafts can occur because exact matching is not necessary. HLA-C, -DP, and -DQ do not appear to play a significant role in transplantation. The closer the other three match, the less likely graft rejection is to occur. This recipient and donor already have a match of the HLA-A gene. An additional match of the HLA-B gene would make a successful transplant more likely.

(B) The HLA-C gene does not appear to play an important role in transplantation. A match at this gene is not as important as match at the HLA-A, -B, or -DR genes in assessing compatibility. (C) The HLA-DP gene does not appear to play an important role in transplantation. A match at this gene is not as important as match at the HLA-A, -B, or -DR genes in assessing compatibility. (D) The HLA-DQ gene does not appear to play an important role in transplantation. A match at this gene is not as important as match at the HLA-A, -B, or -DR genes in assessing compatibility. (E) The HLA-F gene is a minor gene and does not appear to play an important role in transplantation. A match at this gene is not as important as match at the HLA-A, -B, or -DR genes in assessing compatibility.

10. A 57-year-old gentleman undergoes a kidney transplant. Six hours after the operation he is noted to be oliguric. The oliguria worsens over the next 6 hours. The team fears that his body is rejecting the graft organ. What is the best treatment at this time?

(A) Azathioprine
(B) Cyclosporine
(C) High-dose steroids
(D) Azathioprine, cyclosporine, and high-dose steroids in combination
(E) There is no treatment available at this point; the graft will be lost

The answer is E: There is no treatment available at this point; the graft will be lost. A hyperacute rejection is one that occurs in the first 24 hours following surgery. It is due to the presence of preformed, cytotoxic antibodies against the graft tissue. This type of reaction can be predicted by a positive cross-match, which is the reason cross-matching is performed before kidney transplantations. There is no way to treat a hyperacute rejection because immunosuppressive drugs do not modify the action of preformed antibodies. They can, however, be avoided by careful selection of recipients and donors based on cross-matching.

(A) Azathioprine is a purine antimetabolite. Antimetabolites are usually reserved as third addition to a regimen of a steroid and a calcineurin inhibitor such as cyclosporine or tacrolimus is maintenance therapy. Azathioprine would have no effect on a hyperacute rejection. (B) Cyclosporine is a calcineurin inhibitor that blocks helper T-cell activation. It is used as maintenance therapy. It would have no effect on a hyperacute rejection. (C) Some steroids are used for maintenance therapy, while others are used for induction or antirejection therapy. No steroid would be useful in a hyperacute reaction. (D) A hyperacute reaction is the result of preformed antidonor antibodies. There is no treatment for a hyperacute reaction once it has started.

11. A 24-year-old man receives a liver transplant following fulminant hepatic failure from a hepatitis C infection and is placed on tacrolimus and prednisone. One month later, his aspartate aminotransferase (AST), alanine aminotransferase (ALT), and bilirubin levels are elevated. A biopsy confirms graft rejection. What is the best next step in this patient's management?

(A) Azathioprine
(B) Methotrexate
(C) Methylprednisolone (high-dose)
(D) No intervention necessary—this flair will likely resolve spontaneously on his current drug regimen
(E) This condition is untreatable

The answer is C: Methylprednisolone (high-dose). A liver transplant recipient may have elevated aminotransferases and bilirubin for a variety of reasons including cytomegalovirus (CMV) infection, graft rejection, or a more routine cause such as viral or alcoholic hepatitis. In other words, elevated liver enzymes are not specific for graft rejection. Although a number of biomarkers are being investigated for monitoring graft rejection, the current gold standard is liver biopsy. This patient is found on biopsy to be rejecting his organ graft 1 month after his operation. Based on the timing, this is most likely an instance of acute rejection. Cases of acute rejection usually occur between 6 days and 3 months posttransplant. Acute rejections can be treated with a short course (less than 3 weeks) of high-dose immunosuppressants such as methylprednisolone, antilymphocyte serum, or monoclonal antibodies.

(A) Azathioprine is an antimetabolite that impairs purine handling by cells. Antimetabolites are not as efficacious as calcineurin inhibitors or even steroids and are not used for treating acute rejection. Antimetabolites may be added as a third agent to a drug maintenance regimen. (B) Methotrexate is an antimetabolite used in treating certain cancers and autoimmune disorders but is not used in treating acute organ rejections. Antimetabolites such as azathioprine or mycophenolate may be added as a third agent to a drug maintenance regimen. (D) This scenario likely represents an episode of acute rejection. If so, it will not resolve spontaneously. Treatment with methylprednisolone, antilymphocyte serum, or monoclonal antibodies is often sufficient to halt and reverse the rejection. (E) This scenario likely represents an episode of acute rejection. Treatment with methylprednisolone, antilymphocyte serum, or monoclonal antibodies is often sufficient to halt and reverse the rejection.

 A 58-year-old woman receives a kidney transplant. As part of her antirejection regimen, she is prescribed the IL-2 receptor blocker basiliximab. How often does she need to take this medication?

(A) Daily for 6 months
(B) One dose before surgery and one dose after
(C) Only once, 2 hours before surgery
(D) Only for a few weeks at a time in response to episodes of acute rejection
(E) She will need to take this medication daily for the rest of her life

The answer is B: One dose before surgery and one dose after. There are currently two interleukin-2 receptor blockers used in antirejection regimens: basiliximab and daclizumab. When used in conjunction with a steroid and a calcineurin inhibitor, IL-2 receptor blockers have been shown to decrease the frequency of episodes of acute rejection in kidney transplant recipients. Basiliximab is dosed once within 2 hours before the operation, then again 4 days later. Daclizumab is dosed within 24 hours of the transplant then again at 14-day intervals for four more doses.

(A) Basiliximab requires only two doses for efficacy—once at the time of surgery then once 4 days later. (C) Basiliximab is given within 2 hours before surgery, then again 4 days post-op. A single dose is not as efficacious. (D) Basiliximab is dosed once within 2 hours before the operation, then again 4 days later. It is not indicated for treatment of acute rejection episodes. (E) Basiliximab is dosed once within 2 hours before the operation, then again 4 days later. The patient is not required to take any more doses.

13 48-year-old male receives a liver transplant and is started on an immunosuppressive drug regimen. Four months later, his liver enzymes are elevated and he appears jaundiced. A biopsy suggests cytomegalovirus (CMV) infection. Which would be the best way to manage this episode?

(A) Acyclovir
(B) Corticosteroids in high dose
(C) Ganciclovir
(D) Hold immunosuppressants until the infection is cleared
(E) No treatment is necessary; this flair will resolve spontaneously

The answer is C: Ganciclovir. CMV is an extremely common virus, infecting between 50% to 80% of all US adults (determined by the presence of anti-CMV antibodies). In a healthy adult host, these infections are generally mild and unnoticed. The virus can remain latent for many years in a host's body. Congenital infections can cause birth defects. CMV infections in adults are much more serious in patients immunocompromised from HIV infection or organ transplant drug regimens. Ganciclovir (or valganciclovir, which has higher oral bioavailability) is the treatment of choice for CMV infections.

(A) Acyclovir is an antiviral agent effective against herpes simplex infections. It is a prodrug and requires a viral thymidine kinase to be activated. CMV lacks this kinase and so is unaffected by acyclovir. (B) High-dose corticosteroids are the mainstay of treatment for acute rejection but would not suppress CMV replication. Ganciclovir (and valganciclovir) do impair viral replication and are useful against CMV infections. (D) Holding immunosuppressants alone at this point would not likely be sufficient to allow the patient's immune system to clear this infection. Ganciclovir would be the drug of choice in this case. (E) CMV infections can be lethal in immunocompromised individuals. This patient should be given ganciclovir or an equivalent.

14 A 28-year-old woman received a lung transplant about a year ago. She has been compliant with her antirejection regimen and is hoping to get pregnant. Which of the following describes her situation as a transplant recipient?

(A) Her baby would likely suffer from a birth defect
(B) Her risk of spontaneous abortion would be much higher than average
(C) She has a high likelihood of conceiving twins
(D) She will likely be infertile
(E) She would likely have no major complications

The answer is E: She would likely have no major complications. Many patients requiring transplant are infertile before surgery due to endocrine abnormalities from the failing organ. These patients often become fertile after the transplantation. Infertility is not a common complication of the antirejection therapy itself, nor are most of the drugs used for this purpose known to cause birth defects, increase the incidence of twinning, or cause any other obstetric complications. Female patients on antirejection regimens often give birth prematurely, but this appears to be related to graft problems or other comorbidities. This patient, who is otherwise healthy and has had no issues with her graft, will likely have no major complications.

(A) Women who are transplant recipients and on antirejection regimens do not have an incidence of birth defects above population baseline. This woman would likely have no major complications were she to get pregnant. (B) Women who are transplant recipients and on antirejection regimens do not have an incidence of spontaneous abortions above population baseline. This woman would likely have no major complications were she to get pregnant. (C) Women who are transplant recipients and on antirejection regimens do not have an incidence of twinning above population baseline. This woman would likely have no major complications were she to get pregnant. (D) Many patients requiring transplant are infertile before the operation because of endocrine abnormalities secondary to the failing organ. Many of these patients become fertile after their operation.

 15 A 6-month-old male infant is experiencing heart failure of unknown etiology. He is a candidate for a heart transplant and is on the waiting list. Which of the following are the most common indications for heart transplant?

(A) Coronary artery disease (CAD) and cardiomyopathy
(B) Congenital heart disease and cardiomyopathy
(C) Congenital heart disease and neoplasms
(D) Neoplasms and CAD
(E) Valvular disease and cardiomyopathy

The answer is A: Coronary artery disease (CAD) and cardiomyopathy. Heart transplants are considered for patients with end-stage heart disease (New York Heart Association class III or IV) and are likely to die from their heart disease within 2 years without a transplant. Heart transplants are performed for a variety of reasons in patients from neonatal age to adults in their mid-60s. Common indications include valvular disease, congenital heart disease, CAD, and cardiomyopathy. Of these, CAD and cardiomyopathy make up about 40% each of all cases requiring transplant. The remaining diagnoses make up the other 20% of cases requiring a heart transplant.

(B) Congenital heart disease makes up less than 20% of all cases requiring heart transplant. Cardiomyopathy and CAD each make up about 40% of all cases. (C) Neoplasms of the heart are rare and do not contribute significantly to cases of heart failure requiring heart transplant. Congenital heart disease makes up less than 20% of cases. Cardiomyopathy and CAD each make up about 40% of all cases. (D) Neoplasms of the heart are rare and do not contribute significantly to cases of heart failure requiring heart transplant. Cardiomyopathy and CAD each make up about 40% of all cases. (E) Valvular heart disease makes up less than 20% of all cases requiring heart transplant. Cardiomyopathy and CAD each make up about 40% of all cases.

 16 A 55-year-old man with significant coronary artery disease (CAD) and a history of multiple heart attacks has end-stage heart disease and undergoes a heart transplant. Periodically checking which of the following would best allow for monitoring of organ rejection?

(A) Biopsies are not performed in heart transplant cases
(B) Echocardiogram to evaluate ejection fraction
(C) Percutaneous endomyocardial biopsy
(D) Routine physical examination
(E) Transthoracic myocardial biopsy

The answer is C: Percutaneous endomyocardial biopsy. Acute rejection of heart transplant is difficult to accurately assess clinically. Standard measures of cardiac function and routine clinical examination findings do not adequately distinguish acute organ rejection from other cardiac pathologies. For this reason, patients with heart transplants undergo routine surveillance testing to check for evidence of organ rejection. This involves a percutaneous (usually via the internal jugular vein into the right ventricle) endomyocardial biopsy.

(A) Percutaneous endomyocardial biopsies are routinely performed on transplanted hearts. This is currently the best method to check for graft rejection. (B) Measuring ejection fraction with an echocardiogram does not adequately distinguish organ rejection from other cardiac pathologies. The current best method for monitoring graft rejection is an endomyocardial biopsy. (D) A routine physical examination does not adequately identify organ rejection as there are no physical findings specific for rejection. The current best method for monitoring graft rejection is an endomyocardial biopsy. (E) A transthoracic myocardial biopsy would be much more dangerous and prone to complications than a percutaneous endomyocardial biopsy. The current best method for monitoring graft rejection is an endomyocardial biopsy.

A 58-year-old woman with end-stage heart disease is on the waiting list for a heart transplant. A potential cadaver donor is identified. Which of the following are routinely matched for heart transplant donor–recipient pairs?

(A) Blood type and body size
(B) Blood type and human leukocyte antigen (HLA) type
(C) Blood type, HLA type, and body size
(D) Blood type only
(E) HLA type only

The answer is A: Blood type and body size. Donor hearts, as with any donor organ or tissue, must match the recipient's ABO blood type. A mismatch of the ABO blood groups will lead to hyperacute rejection which occurs within 24 hours of graft placement and cannot be treated. Many transplants require matching of HLA type as well, but matching the HLA types does not appear to be as important in heart transplants. The organ should be matched for body size, however—both the donor and the recipient should be of similar height and weight.

(B) HLA typing does not appear to be an important factor in heart transplants. Donors and recipients are matched based on ABO blood type and body size. (C) HLA typing does not appear to be an important factor in heart transplants. Donors and recipients are matched based on ABO blood type and body size. (D) Blood typing is essential for any transplant procedure as an incompatible match will lead to a hyperacute rejection. For heart transplants, donors and recipients are also matched by body size. (E) HLA typing does not appear to be an important factor in heart transplants. Donors and recipients are matched based on ABO blood type and body size.

 A 56-year-old man presents with 4 weeks of night sweats, fevers, and weight loss accompanied by a progressively worsening cough. He denies any recent travel and finished a full course of azithromycin last week prescribed by another provider. Chest x-ray is shown in *Figure 18-1*.

Which of the following is the most common reason for lung transplant?

(A) Bronchiolitis obliterans organizing pneumonia (BOOP)
(B) Chronic obstructive pulmonary disease (COPD)
(C) Cystic fibrosis
(D) Interstitial lung disease
(E) Primary pulmonary hypertension

The answer is B: Chronic obstructive pulmonary disease (COPD). This patient's symptoms are nonspecific but potentially concerning for BOOP, which clinically presents like a pneumonia but does not respond to

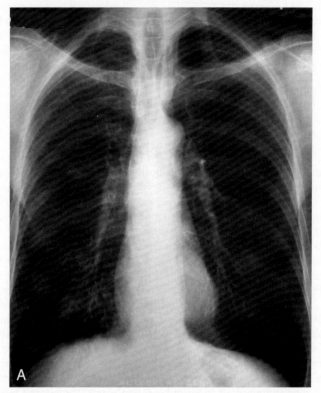

Figure 18-1

antibiotic therapy. The question asked for the most common indication for lung transplant, however. The treatment BOOP is a simple course of steroids, not a lung transplant. The most common indication for lung transplant is COPD which constitutes about 45% of lung transplant cases. The x-ray shown reveals evidence of lung hyperinflation with flattening of the diaphragm. Primary pulmonary hypertension makes up around 12% of cases and cystic fibrosis about 10%.

(A) The presentation of this patient raises concern for BOOP, but BOOP is not generally treated by lung transplantation. The most common reason for transplantation is COPD. (C) Cystic fibrosis cases make up about 10% of lung transplant cases. COPD cases on the other hand make up about 45% of cases. (D) Interstitial lung disease is not a common reason for lung transplantation. The most common indication for lung transplantation is COPD. (E) Primary pulmonary hypertension cases make up about 12% of lung transplant cases. COPD cases on the other hand make up about 45% of cases.

19 A 59-year-old woman with end-stage pulmonary disease secondary to longstanding chronic obstructive pulmonary disease (COPD) is scheduled for a lung transplant. Which of the following will most likely be a feature of her procedure?

(A) Bilateral lung transplantation
(B) Cardiopulmonary bypass during the operation
(C) Combination heart–lung transplantation
(D) Early extubation postoperatively
(E) High-dose steroids for the first week postoperatively

The answer is D: **Early extubation postoperatively.** Most lung transplants are single regardless of the indication. The exception to this rule is cases of bilateral infections because replacing only one allows the infection to easily spread to the new lung. Most cases do not require the use of cardiopulmonary bypass during the operation. Combination heart–lung transplants are only for special cases such as when cardiac function is very poor or surgically uncorrectable congenital defects are present. Multiple studies have demonstrated improved outcomes or fewer complications with early extubation following lung transplantation, and this is now the standard procedure. High-dose steroids are avoided in lung transplants because steroids severely impair healing of the bronchial anastomoses.

(A) Most lung transplants are single regardless of the indication. The exception to this rule is cases of bilateral infections because replacing only one allows the infection to easily spread to the new lung. This patient would likely receive a single lung. (B) Most lung transplants do not require cardiopulmonary bypass during the operation. An exception would be deterioration of blood gases when the pulmonary artery is clamped. (C) Combination heart–lung transplants are only for special cases such as when cardiac function is very poor or surgically uncorrectable congenital defects are present. This patient would likely receive a single lung. (E) High-dose steroids are avoided in lung transplants because steroids severely impair healing of the bronchial anastomoses. Induction therapy often involves antilymphocyte serum.

20 A 43-year-old man is scheduled for a liver transplant. He has been on the transplant waiting list for 5 years and has developed worsening hepatic encephalopathy over the past 2 weeks. Which of the following is the most common chronic diseases leading to liver transplant in the United States?

(A) Alcoholic cirrhosis
(B) Chronic hepatitis B
(C) Chronic hepatitis C
(D) Primary biliary cirrhosis
(E) Primary sclerosing cholangitis

The answer is C: Chronic hepatitis C. There are three major complications of chronic liver disease that signify end-stage disease and warrant transplantation: ascites that has become too complicated to effectively manage (e.g., refractory to treatment, ascites with hydrothorax, ascites with spontaneous bacterial peritonitis), hepatic encephalopathy, and recurrent esophageal varices. This man's encephalopathy signifies a pressing need for transplant. The most common chronic disease leading to transplant in the United States is chronic hepatitis C, comprising about 40% of all cases of liver disease leading to transplant.

(A) Alcoholic cirrhosis comprises about 15% of liver disease leading to liver transplant. The most common chronic disease leading to transplant is chronic hepatitis C. (B) Chronic hepatitis B comprises less than 10% of liver disease leading to liver transplant. The most common chronic disease leading to transplant is chronic hepatitis C. (D) Primary biliary cirrhosis comprises less than 10% of liver disease leading to liver transplant. The most common chronic disease leading to transplant is chronic hepatitis C. (E) Primary sclerosing cholangitis comprises less than 10% of liver disease leading to liver transplant. The most common chronic disease leading to transplant is chronic hepatitis C.

---

 21 A 39-year-old woman with chronic hepatitis C has been on the waiting list for transplantation for 6 years. Her Model for End-Stage Liver Disease (MELD) score recently increased to 38 and she undergoes a liver transplant. What is the best way to prevent recurrence of hepatitis C infection in the graft organ?

(A) Lamivudine
(B) Liver transplantation cures chronic hepatitis C
(C) Plasmapheresis
(D) Recurrence is unavoidable
(E) Vaccination against hepatitis C

The answer is D: Recurrence is unavoidable. Liver transplants priority is based on the MELD score rather than time on the waiting list. The MELD score is a value calculated from a patient's bilirubin, creatinine, and international normalized ratio (INR) and predicts survival without transplant. A score between 30 and 40 corresponds to a 3-month mortality over 50%. A score of 40 or more carries a 3-month mortality over 70%. A liver transplanted into a patient with hepatitis C will become infected with the virus and, as before, may progress to cirrhosis and possibly require retransplantation. There is currently no method to vaccinate against or otherwise avoid this recurrence.

(A) Lamivudine is a nucleoside analog reverse transcriptase inhibitor. It is used to treat HIV and hepatitis B infections but is not effective against the hepatitis C virus, which does not have a reverse transcriptase enzyme. (B) Liver transplantation does not cure hepatitis C. Hepatitis C virions are still present in the recipient's blood and rapidly lead to infection of the transplanted liver. (C) Plasmapheresis removes proteins such as antibodies from the plasma and is used in the management of certain autoimmune disorders but would not remove all the virions from the recipient's blood. Plasmapheresis is not an effective treatment for viral infections. (E) There is currently no vaccine effective against hepatitis C infection. Recurrence of hepatitis C after liver transplantation is unavoidable.

 A 62-year-old man with end-stage kidney disease has been on hemodialysis for 6 years is preparing for a kidney transplant. Which of the following is the most common indication for renal transplantation in the United States?

(A) Diabetic nephropathy
(B) Glomerulonephritis
(C) Hypertensive nephropathy
(D) Polycystic kidney disease
(E) Pyelonephritis

The answer is B: Glomerulonephritis. Kidney transplants in the United States are generally elective procedures because all patients have access to dialysis. Kidney transplantation is often a preferred alternative to the hassles and cost of long-term dialysis. Unstable patients can be dialyzed to allow for the best possible surgical outcome. Glomerulonephritis is the most common cause for renal transplantation in the United States at over 40% of cases. Diabetic nephropathy constitutes about 16%, polycystic kidney disease about 13%, and hypertensive nephropathy about 12%. Pyelonephritis makes up less than 10% of cases leading to kidney transplantation.

(A) Diabetic nephropathy constitutes about 16% of cases of kidney disease leading to transplantation. Glomerulonephritis is the most common cause, making up over 40% of cases. (C) Hypertensive nephropathy constitutes about 12% of cases of kidney disease leading to transplantation. Glomerulonephritis is the most common cause, making up over 40% of cases. (D) Polycystic kidney disease constitutes about 13% of cases of kidney disease leading to transplantation. Glomerulonephritis is the most common cause, making up over 40% of cases. (E) Pyelonephritis constitutes less than 10% of cases of kidney disease leading to transplantation. Glomerulonephritis is the most common cause, making up over 40% of cases.

 A 36-year-old woman with autosomal dominant polycystic kidney disease (ADPKD) is considering a kidney transplant. A sibling unaffected by ADPKD is willing to be a living donor. What is the chance that her sibling (from the same set of parents) will be a perfect human leukocyte antigen (HLA)-type match?

(A) 10%
(B) 25%
(C) 50%
(D) 75%
(E) 90%

The answer is B: 25%. Although many HLA types exist (HLA-A, -B, -C, -DP, -DQ, and -DR) and for each type dozens of alleles are possible, the HLA types important in transplantation (HLA-A, -B, and -DR) are located close to each other on the same chromosome and are usually inherited together. This is referred to an HLA haplotype. Each parent has two haplotypes, of which one is passed on to each child, so HLA inheritance follows the rules of a simple 2 × 2 Punnett square. Each child will inherit one (of a possible two) haplotype from each parent, so there is a 25% chance a sibling donor and recipient will have the same HLA haplotypes (known as a perfect match). There is a 50% chance the siblings will share one haplotype (a half match) and a 25% chance siblings will share no haplotypes (a zero match).

(A) The three HLA types important in transplants (HLA-A, -B, and -DR) are inherited together as a haplotype. There is a 25% chance two siblings share both haplotypes, a 50% chance they will share only one, and a 25% chance they will share neither. (C) The three HLA types important in transplants (HLA-A, -B, and -DR) are inherited together as a haplotype. There is a 25% chance two siblings share both haplotypes, a 50% chance they will share only one, and a 25% chance they will share neither. (D) The three HLA types important in transplants (HLA-A, -B, and -DR) are inherited together as a haplotype. There is a 25% chance two siblings share both haplotypes, a 50% chance they will share only one, and a 25% chance they will share neither. (E) The three HLA types important in transplants (HLA-A, -B, and -DR) are inherited together as a haplotype. There is a 25% chance two siblings share both haplotypes, a 50% chance they will share only one, and a 25% chance they will share neither.

24 A 45-year-old man with significant diabetic nephropathy, retinopathy, and neuropathy secondary to longstanding type 2 diabetes mellitus is considering a pancreas transplant in hopes of curing his diabetes. Which of the following pancreatic transplantation procedures would be the best option for this patient?

(A) Kidney transplant followed by pancreas after kidney (PAK) transplantation
(B) Pancreas transplantation alone (PTA)
(C) Simultaneous pancreas–kidney (SPK) transplant
(D) Simultaneous pancreas–small bowel transplant
(E) This man is not a candidate for pancreatic transplant

The answer is E: **This man is not a candidate for pancreatic transplant.** Pancreas transplants are indicated for patients with complications secondary to type 1 diabetes mellitus. Type 2 diabetes is a contraindication for pancreas transplant. Generally, the entire pancreas is transplanted, but pancreatic islet transplants have shown success in the short term. A pancreas transplantation provides long-term euglycemia which allows for stabilization or reversal of the complications of hyperglycemia.

(A) A PAK transplantation is performed in patients with renal failure who have found matching kidney donor (e.g., a living donor) but not a matching pancreas donor. Regardless, the patient in the question stem has complication secondary to type 2 diabetes mellitus which is a contraindication to pancreas transplantation. (B) A pancreas transplant would be helpful if this man had type 1 diabetes mellitus. Type 2 diabetes mellitus is characterized by insulin resistance rather than lack of insulin production. Type 2 diabetes is a contraindication to pancreas transplantation. (C) A SPK transplant is performed in patients with type 1 diabetes mellitus and end-stage renal disease (ESRD). Type 2 diabetes is a contraindication to pancreas transplantation. (D) Small bowel transplants are not commonly performed with pancreas transplants. Regardless, the patient in the question stem has complication secondary to type 2 diabetes mellitus which is a contraindication to pancreas transplantation.

 25 A 37-year-old woman with diabetic retinopathy secondary to poorly controlled type 1 diabetes mellitus is a candidate for a pancreas transplant. Which of the following is transplanted along with the pancreas in a standard pancreatic transplant?

(A) A kidney
(B) A segment of duodenum alone
(C) A segment of duodenum and part of the common iliac artery
(D) The spleen and part of the splenic artery
(E) The pancreas alone is transplanted in most pancreatic transplant cases

The answer is C: **A segment of duodenum and part of the common iliac artery.** In a routine pancreas transplant, the donor pancreas along with a segment of duodenum containing the ampulla of Vater is transplanted into the recipient. The pancreas is placed in the recipient's right iliac fossa. A segment of donor iliac artery including the bifurcation of the common iliac artery and the initial segments of the internal and external iliac arteries is also transplanted to supply blood to the graft.

(A) A simultaneous pancreas-kidney (SPK) transplant is performed in patients with complications from type 1 diabetes and end-stage kidney disease. Routine pancreas transplants do not include a kidney. (B) A segment of duodenum containing the ampulla of Vater is transplanted along with a section of iliac artery to supply blood to the graft. (D) There is no need to transplant a spleen with a pancreas transplant. The new blood supply to the graft is provided by transplanted iliac artery. (E) A segment of duodenum containing the ampulla of Vater is transplanted with the pancreas along with a section of iliac artery to supply blood to the graft.

Orthopedic Surgery

1 A 65-year-old woman falls on an extended and outstretched hand while walking her grandchild to school. She presents to the emergency department in severe pain and holding her left wrist. On examination, there is swelling, tenderness, and deformity of the wrist in a "dinner-fork" pattern. A picture of the injury is shown in *Figure 19-1*.

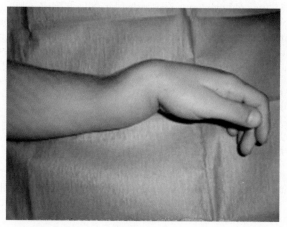

Figure 19-1

An x-ray of the injury reveals displacement and angulation of the distal radius. There is no carpal displacement. Which of the following is the most likely diagnosis?

(A) Barton fracture
(B) Chauffer fracture
(C) Colles fracture
(D) Shepherd fracture
(E) Smith fracture

The answer is C: Colles fracture. This patient has suffered from a Colles fracture. Colles fractures classically occur from falling on to a hard surface with the arms outstretched. The insult occurs to the distal radius, which results in dorsal angulation, impaction, and radial drift. The fracture is often referred to as a "dinner fork" or "bayonet" deformity due to the shape of the arm. It is most common in postmenopausal women with osteoporosis.

(A) Barton fracture is an intraarticular fracture of the distal radius. It results in dislocation of the radiocarpal joint. It usually occurs from falling on an extended and pronated wrist. Unlike Colles fractures, there is carpal displacement in a Barton fracture. (B) A Chauffer fracture (also called backfire fracture) is a fracture of the radial styloid process. It too may occur from falling on an outstretched hand. Treatment involves open reduction and internal fixation. (D) Shepherd fracture is a talar fracture and does not occur in the wrist. (E) While Smith fractures may also occur while falling on an outstretched hand, they are characterized by a distal radius fracture with volar displacement since the wrists must be flexed (rather than extended in a Colles fracture). For this reason they are known as a "reverse" Colles fracture.

---

2 A 35-year-old woman is rear-ended by a diesel truck while driving to work. She presents to the emergency department with neck pain. Computed tomography (CT) imaging reveals a nondisplaced fracture of the occipital condyles on C3. Which of the following is the best treatment for this patient?

(A) C-collar
(B) Corpectomy
(C) Halo vest
(D) Surgical decompression
(E) Vertebroplasty

The answer is A: C-collar. This patient is presenting with a nondisplaced (type 1) upper cervical spine fracture of the occipital condyles. These fractures are stable due to intact contralateral alar ligaments and the tectorial membrane. If dislocation is absent, then treatment is usually with a c-collar. Operative treatment is most often not necessary.

(B) Corpectomy is sometimes required for unstable cervical spine fractures but would not be necessary in this type of fracture. (C) Placement of a halo vest would be more appropriate in more severe occipital fractures (type 2 or 3) but is usually unnecessary for type 1 fractures. (D) Surgical decompression may be necessary in spinal fractures with significant spinal canal compromise, but not in a type 1 occipital condyle fracture. (E) Vertebroplasty is a procedure used to stabilize compression fractures in the spine. This procedure is not necessary for our patient.

3 An 18-year-old boy presents to the emergency department after a rollover motor vehicle accident. He is complaining of right upper leg pain. He is stable on arrival. On examination, there is tenderness to palpation of the upper thigh but the distal limb appears vascularly and neurologically intact. Plain radiographs reveal a femoral neck fracture, Garden grade II. Which of the following is the best treatment for this type of fracture?

(A) Closed reduction and internal fixation
(B) Hemiarthroplasty
(C) Medical management only
(D) Open reduction
(E) Traction

The answer is A: Closed reduction and internal fixation. This patient has suffered a femoral neck fracture, which are uncommon but may occur after high-energy trauma. In younger patients, femoral neck fractures are associated with a higher incidence of osteonecrosis and nonunion healing. In addition, younger individuals have a high activity level. Thus, prompt surgical treatment is important for management of these fractures. This patient will require closed reduction and internal fixation.

(B) A hemiarthroplasty is usually the best option for older and less active patients with femoral neck fractures. (C) Medical management only would not be appropriate as the patient is young and a good surgical candidate. (D) Open reduction is sometimes used if closed reduction is unsuccessful. However, closed reduction is usually attempted first. (E) Traction is contraindicated in femoral neck fractures and should not be attempted with this patient.

4 A 35-year-old man comes to the physician because of increasing right foot pain over the last 2 months. He reports that he regularly runs marathons and recently finished a 25-km marathon in Moab, Utah. He reports the pain is worse during his runs and will go away with rest. More recently, the pain has started coming sooner with exercise and becoming more intense. He reports that he tried resting for several days, but the pain started again immediately after starting his practice run. On examination, there is point tenderness over his right fourth metatarsal. There is no swelling, warmth, or bruising. An x-ray of the right foot is unremarkable. Which of the following is the most likely diagnosis?

(A) Acute metatarsal fracture
(B) Calcaneal stress fracture
(C) Metatarsal stress fracture
(D) Motor neuroma
(E) Plantar fasciitis

The answer is C: Metatarsal stress fracture. This patient is most likely suffering from a metatarsal stress fracture. This is a common injury in repetitive running athletes. Risk factors include high arched feet, osteoporosis, and poor footwear with inadequate shock absorption. Unfortunately, plain radiography is often negative, especially when performed early on. Positive radiographic findings are most often found 3 months after the fracture starts. Treatment involves rest for 3 to 12 weeks.

(A) The onset of pain would be much more acute along with swelling, bruising, and warmth over the fracture site if the patient was suffering from an acute metatarsal fracture. (B) A calcanial stress fracture would present with heal pain rather than metatarsal pain. (D) Motor neuromas usually occur between the third and fourth digits on the plantar surface. They are not tumors but rather swelling of the nerve. The most common complaints include pain, tingling, and numbness in the toes. Pain is intermittent and aggravated by exercise, thus differentiating it from a stress fracture may be difficult. On examination, there may be a "clicking" sensation when palpating the space between the digits and when squeezing the metatarsal joints. (E) Plantar fasciitis occurs when there is inflammation of the connective tissue on the bottom of the foot. Pain is usually felt on the underside of the heel and worse with weight bearing exercise. On radiography, heel spurs may be found. Treatment includes rest, stretching, anti-inflammatory medications, and physical therapy.

---

5 A 56-year-old man presents to the emergency department complaining of right ankle pain after an injury during a pick-up basketball game with some friends. He describes "rolling" his ankle when coming down after a jump shot. Immediately after the injury, he was unable to bear weight on his foot. On examination, his right ankle appears swollen with prominent ecchymosis over the lateral ankle. There is no bony tenderness on palpation of the foot, but mild pain with palpation of the lateral malleoli. In addition, there is marked laxity of the ankle joint with the talar tilt test. Which of the following is the next best step in management?

(A) Ankle support, nonsteroidal anti-inflammatory medications (NSAIDs), and physical therapy
(B) Computed tomography (CT) examination of the ankle joint
(C) Observation, rest, and pain control
(D) Plain radiographs of the foot and ankle
(E) Surgical reattachment of the ankle ligaments

The answer is D: Plain radiographs of the foot and ankle. This patient has suffered an ankle injury that could be explained by either a sprain (suggested by marked laxity of ankle joint and mechanism of injury) or fracture (inability to bear weight and point tenderness over lateral malleoli). The Ottawa ankle rules are helpful when working up an ankle injury. These rules state that radiographs should be obtained if there is pain in the malleolar zone and either one of the following:

- Bone tenderness along the distal 6 cm of the posterior edge of the tibia or tip of the medial or lateral malleolus.
- Inability to bear weight immediately after the injury and walk more four steps when being evaluated.

Since a fracture is possible, the next best step is an x-ray of the foot and ankle to assist in the diagnosis.

(A) Ankle support, anti-inflammatory medications, and physical therapy would be appropriate if this were a mild to moderate sprain. (B) While CT imaging may clearly show a fracture, it is expensive and unnecessary when plain radiography is available. (C) Reassurance, rest, and pain control might be appropriate with mild to moderate sprains. (E) In general, surgery does not improve outcome in ankle sprains.

 6 A 50-year-old woman presents to the emergency department following a motor vehicle accident in which she injured her left leg. She arrives in the emergency department in severe pain. She describes a constant deep pain distal to the site of injury with a sensation of "pins and needles" in her foot. On examination, her left leg distal to the injury is edematous and cool to touch. An x-ray reveals soft tissue swelling and a fracture of the proximal tibia diaphysis. Which of the following is the next best step in management?

(A) Arterial blood gas from the distal left leg
(B) Arteriography of the leg
(C) Computed tomography (CT) scan of the leg
(D) Emergent fasciotomy
(E) Intravenous pain control

The answer is D: Emergent fasciotomy. This patient is most likely suffering from compartment syndrome secondary to soft tissue swelling after the fracture. This diagnosis is suggested by the paresthesias, pain, and pallor distal to the fracture site. The next best step in management for this patient is an emergent fasciotomy to release the pressure and restore blood flow to the leg. Risk factors for compartment syndrome of the lower leg include tibial diaphysis fractures, soft tissue injuries, and crush injuries.

(A) Although a blood gas (if attainable) from the left leg distal to the site of injury could possibly show evidence of ischemia, it is unnecessary and would just serve to delay proper treatment. (B) Although an arteriogram of the leg would likely show decreased blood flow distal to the site of injury, it would only delay treatment and is not necessary in this patient. (C) CT imaging would only delay proper treatment and is not necessary when clinical suspicion is high and/or compartment pressures are elevated. (E) Intravenous pain control is not the most pressing intervention here as failure to release the pressure in his leg may result in limb loss.

7 A 40-year-old woman complains of weakness, burning, and numbness of her left hand, most prominent in his first three fingers. She reports the symptoms have come on slowly over the last 7 months and are worse at night. More recently, she has had trouble gripping her silverware. Her medical problems include obesity and diabetes mellitus. On examination, there is atrophy of her thenar eminence. A picture of her hand is shown in *Figure 19-2*.

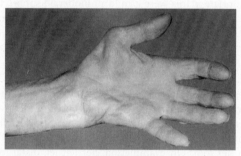

Figure 19-2

Surgery to correct the problem is scheduled. Which of the following factors may decrease the probability of successful long-term surgical outcomes?

(A) Alcohol abuse
(B) Being in good general health
(C) Decreased age
(D) Slow nerve conduction studies with retained muscle strength
(E) Symptoms that are significantly worse at night

The answer is A: Alcohol abuse. This patient is suffering from carpal tunnel syndrome most likely secondary to her diabetes mellitus. The picture shows atrophy of the thenar eminence from longstanding median nerve compression. Studies have shown that patients with poor mental status parameters or alcohol abuse problems have decreased surgical treatment outcomes for carpel tunnel syndrome than other patients.

(B) Being in good general health increases the success rate of carpel tunnel surgery. (C) Decreased age is associated with an increased surgical prognosis. (D) Having some muscle strength, even with very slow nerve conduction results, increases the chance for a successful surgery. Having very poor nerve conduction results without retained strength is associated with a decreased surgical success rate. (E) Symptoms that are significantly worse at night increase the probability that surgery will provide long-term relief.

8 A 54-year-old man with ankylosing spondylitis falls while walking on ice. He presents to the emergency department complaining of neck pain. Although a neurologic examination is normal, computed tomography (CT) imaging shows a nondisplaced fracture of C6. The patient is admitted, an orthosis is placed, and pain management is initiated. Approximately 10 hours later, he complains of increasing weakness and paresthesias of his bilateral upper and lower extremities. An emergent magnetic resonance imaging (MRI) is ordered which shows a dorsally situated epidural hematoma with mild cord compression. Which of the following is the next best step in management?

(A) Cervical laminectomy
(B) Cervical laminectomy with fusion
(C) Intravenous (IV) methylprednisolone
(D) Methylprednisolone and observation with serial advanced imaging
(E) Observation with serial advanced imaging

The answer is B: Cervical laminectomy with fusion. Patients with ankylosing spondylitis are prone to distal cervical fractures. Unfortunately, serious fractures may be difficult to diagnose since they may initially appear nondisplaced. Additionally, the bony deformities found in patients with ankylosing spondylitis make them prone to vessel damage and complications such as epidural hematomas. Since this patient has a progressing neurologic deficit along with radiologic evidence of a fracture and an expanding hematoma, treatment should involve decompression with a cervical laminectomy. Fusion is often utilized in these patients since the fracture patterns are unstable.

(A) Although a cervical laminectomy should be performed, fusion should be done along with the surgery to prevent future problems. (C) Methylprednisolone administration is often used for acute spinal fractures, best if within 3 hours of injury. A loading dose of 30 mg/kg is given over an hour followed by 5.4 mg/kg/h for the next 23 hours. This patient is presenting with spinal cord compression greater than 8 hours after the injury, for which it has not been shown to be beneficial after this amount of time. (D) Although methylprednisolone might be appropriate if given earlier in the trauma setting, it is greater than 8 hours after the injury and this patient needs surgical care. Observation with serial imaging would also not be appropriate at this time. (E) Observation with serial imaging would not be appropriate as surgery is necessary to prevent progression of this patient's condition.

9 A 15-year-old boy presents with a painful hard "bump" just above his knee. He also reports low-grade fevers, mostly occurring at night for the last several months. On examination, there is a palpable hard nodule adhered to the underlying bone of his distal femur. Biopsy of the lesion reveals a high density of eosinophilic and pleomorphic cells with enlarged nuclei and numerous mitotic figures. The malignant cells are surrounded by an osteoid matrix. Which of the following is required as part of the workup for this patient?

(A) Audiography
(B) Bone marrow biopsy
(C) Flow cytometry
(D) Genetic testing
(E) Plain films of the chest

The answer is E: Plain films of the chest. This patient's presentation and pathologic description is most likely that of osteosarcoma. Osteosarcoma is the most common type of malignant bone tumor in children and adolescents. The most common location is from the metaphysis of the distal femur or proximal tibia. The malignant cells are thought to originate from the primitive mesenchymal bone-forming cells. The primary treatment is removal of the tumor and chemotherapy. The workup for osteosarcoma includes lactate dehydrogenase (LDH) and alkaline phosphatase (ALP) (both have prognostic significance), complete blood count (CBC) with differential, platelet count, liver function tests, electrolytes levels, renal function tests, and urinalysis. In addition, an x-ray should always be performed as part of the workup to look for pulmonary metastasis.

(A) Audiography is unnecessary in the workup of osteosarcoma. (B) While bone marrow biopsies may be used for other childhood malignancies such as leukemias and lymphomas, they are not necessary with osteosarcomas. (C) Flow cytometry is not useful in the workup of osteosarcoma. (D) While some genetic abnormalities predispose patients to developing malignant tumors such as osteosarcoma, it is not a necessary part of the workup in most patients.

 A 28-year-old man is involved in an all-terrain vehicle (AVT) crash in rural West Virginia. During the accident, he sustains a neck injury. He presents to the emergency department complaining of neck pain. A computed tomography (CT) scan reveals a traumatic dislocation of his C5–C6 vertebrae with damage to one half of the spinal cord. The patient is diagnosed with Brown-Séquard spinal injury. Which of the following could represent the motor and sensory examination findings in this patient?

(A) Bilateral loss of pain and temperature sensation in upper extremities
(B) Contralateral loss of pain and temperature sensation and ipsilateral loss of motor function
(C) Contralateral loss of motor function, ipsilateral loss of pain, and temperature sensation
(D) Ipsilateral loss of motor function and pain/temperature sensation
(E) Loss of motor function and vibration sensation in the bilateral upper extremities

The answer is B: **Contralateral loss of pain and temperature sensation and ipsilateral loss of motor function.** Brown-Séquard syndrome occurs with a unilateral and usually penetrating spinal cord injuries. Motor fibers that control the muscles are found in the spinal cord on the ipsilateral side of the injury while pain and temperature fibers enter the spinal cord and cross to the contralateral side before ascending. The loss of pain and temperature sensation usually occurs at two levels below the level of spinal damage. Fortunately, the prognosis with Brown-Séquard syndrome is excellent when compared to other types of cord injuries.

(A) Since pain fibers cross to the contralateral side, there would not be bilateral loss with a unilateral spinal cord injury. (C) Motor innervation is ipsilateral while pain and temperature sensation ascends contralaterally; thus, this answer is incorrect. (D) While the motor function is ipsilateral, pain and temperature loss would be contralateral. (E) With a unilateral injury, the loss of motor function and vibration would be ipsilateral and in both upper and lower extremities.

 11 A 7-year-old boy presents with pain in his left leg. He says the pain is not always there, but rather comes and goes with varying intensities. On examination, there is a palpable nodule on the proximal left femur. Laboratory testing reveals an increased erythrocyte sedimentation rate, alkaline phosphatase, and lactate dehydrogenase. Blood cultures are negative. Plain radiography shows a lytic lesion in the proximal diaphysis of the patient's left femur with a prominent soft tissue mass extending from the bone. Biopsy of the lesion shows numerous small round blue cells that stain positive for CD99 and negative for lymphoid markers and CD45. Which of the following is a characteristic of this disease?

(A) Germline TP53 inactivation
(B) Occurs most commonly in patients less than 5 years of age
(C) Reciprocal translocation t(11;22)
(D) Tumor cells originate from myeloid precursors
(E) Tumor cells are derived from cells that produce cartilage

The answer is C: **Reciprocal translocation t(11;22).** This patient is suffering from Ewing sarcoma, a small round blue cell tumor of both mesodermal and ectodermal origins. Over 90% of these tumors result from a reciprocal translocation between chromosomes 11 and 22. They most commonly occur in the diaphysis of the femur, but the pelvis is another common area.

(A) A germline TP53 inactivation describes Li-Fraumeni syndrome. (B) Patients suffering from Ewing sarcoma are usually between the ages of 5 to 25 years of age. (D) Tumor cells for acute myeloid leukemia originate from myeloid precursors. (E) Tumor cells that originate from cartilage-producing cells form chondrosarcomas.

12 A 70-year-old man presents to the chiropractor with back pain. He says that it started several weeks earlier and seems to be getting worse lately. The pain is present at night. He is referred to the physician after several manipulation exercises resulted in increased pain. On examination, the involved lower lumbar area is mildly tender to touch. Plain radiographs reveal several well-circumscribed osteoblastic and sclerotic lesions in the lower lumbar vertebrae and ileum. Which of the following is the most likely diagnosis?

(A) Lumbar disc herniation
(B) Lumbar spondylosis
(C) Metastatic lung cancer
(D) Muscle strain
(E) Prostate cancer

The answer is E: Prostate cancer. This patient is most likely suffering from spinal injury secondary to advanced metastatic prostate cancer. The most common places for prostate cancer to spread are lymphatics and bone. Symptoms from bone metastasis are usually secondary to nerve compression or, less often, bony fractures. These metastatic lesions may be visible on x-ray, although a bone scan is the standard method for detecting bony metastasis.

(A) The radiographic description is not that of lumbar disc herniation. (B) Lumbar spondylosis is defined as bony overgrowths on the vertebrae. Spondylosis usually produces no symptoms. (C) While lung cancer may spread to the bone, it occurs less commonly than prostate cancer. Prostate cancer is responsible for 60% of all bone metastasis in men. (D) While muscle strains are a common cause of back pain, this patient has signs and radiographic evidence of something much more serious.

13 A 13-year-old girl comes to the office for a regular health checkup as part of clearance for participation in sports at school. Her vitals are within normal limits and she overall appears healthy. She denies any symptoms and reports excellent health hygiene. On examination, you note mild convexity of the spine and mild forward rotation of the right shoulder. There is approximately 10 degrees of curvature noted when the patient bends forward at the waist at 90 degrees. There is no hamstring muscle tightness and a Romberg test is negative. Which of the following is the most appropriate management?

(A) Back bracing
(B) Observation and radiographs
(C) Physical therapy
(D) Refrain from competitive sports
(E) Surgical correction

The answer is B: Observation and radiographs. This patient is presenting with mild idiopathic scoliosis of her spine. This is a common type of spinal deformity. Unfortunately, not much is known about the etiology of this condition. However, effective treatment options have been developed. For curvature less than 25 degrees, observation with interval radiographs to ensure the curvature is not progressing is an appropriate management approach.

(A) Bracing is utilized for curves between 25 and 40 degrees or rapidly progressing curves to the 20 to 25 degree range. (C) Physical therapy has not been shown to be beneficial for idiopathic scoliosis. (D) There is no reason for this patient to refrain from competitive sports. (E) Surgery is often appropriate for inflexible curves greater than 40 degrees or any curves greater than 50 degrees.

 A 56-year-old woman presents with back pain of several months duration. She reports she must bend over to relieve the pain. She also reports increased difficulty walking. She is subsequently diagnosed with severe spondylolisthesis of her lumbar spine and scheduled for surgery. During surgical decompression, there is an incidental tear of the dura matter, which is immediately repaired. The remainder of the surgery is uneventful and completed successfully. One month later, the patient returns with severe headaches. She reports the headaches are worse with standing. She also complains of nausea and rare vomiting. She says her back pain is improved and she has been able to walk much better. Her temperature is 37.2°C, blood pressure 130/85 mmHg, pulse 60 beats/min, and respirations 15 breaths/min. On examination, the incision is well healed without erythema or induration. Laboratory studies show a normal white blood cell count and an erythrocyte sedimentation rate (ESR) within normal limits. Which of the following is the most likely diagnosis?

(A) Bacterial meningitis
(B) Decreased circulating cerebral spinal fluid
(C) Lumbar epidural abscess
(D) Migraine headache
(E) Postoperative nausea

The answer is B: Decreased circulating cerebral spinal fluid. This patient's surgery was complicated by a dural tear. Although the defect was closed immediately after occurrence, there may still be leakage of the cerebral spinal fluid. The incidence of dural tears in spinal surgery is most common with repeated or revision type surgeries but may complicate up to 11% of surgeries to correct spondylolisthesis. Older patients are more susceptible to incidental dural tears. Symptoms are due to decreased circulating cerebral spinal fluid and resulting meningeal irritation.

(A) This patient is afebrile and has a normal ESR; thus, bacterial meningitis is unlikely. (C) This patient is afebrile and had a surgery complicated by a dural tear, which more likely explains this patient's symptoms. (D) This patient's presentation is not consistent with a migraine headache. (E) Although nausea may occur immediately postoperative secondary to anesthesia, this patient's nausea is likely caused by meningeal irritation secondary to decreased cerebral spinal fluid.

---

15 A 30-year-old woman with a history of resected breast cancer and leukemia is referred to her physician with painful swelling over the lateral aspect of the left ankle for the last 7 months. She denies a history of trauma or fever. The patient has already tried analgesics and nonsteroidal anti-inflammatory medications (NSAIDs), which have not relieved her symptoms. Her family history is remarkable for an early death of her mother from an unknown cancer. On examination, there is a firm 7 cm × 5 cm swelling present over her lateral malleolus. A magnetic resonance imaging (MRI) shows a large mass with soft tissue components invading the cortical bone. Biopsy of the lesion reveals spindle-shaped pleomorphic cells surrounded by an osteoid matrix. There are numerous mitotic figures noted in the pathology report. If genetic studies are performed, a mutation in which of the following genes is expected?

(A) FGFR3
(B) LMNA
(C) RB1
(D) TP53
(E) WT1

The answer is D: TP53. This patient's history of breast cancer and leukemia along with a new osteosarcoma tumor is concerning for Li-Fraumeni syndrome. Li-Fraumeni syndrome is an autosomal dominant disorder (note family history of cancer in this patient) caused by a mutation in the tumor suppressing gene p53. TP53's role is to assist in repair and destruction of mutated DNA before the cells enter the cell cycle. When mutated, cells with damaged DNA are allowed to divide resulting in increased rates of cancers in these patients. The most common cancers include sarcomas, breast cancer, brain cancers, and adrenal glands. Approximately 2% to 3% of patients with osteosarcomas have Li-Fraumeni syndrome.

(A) Mutations in the FGFR3 gene are associated with the development of achondroplasia. (B) Mutations in LMNA are associated with the development of Hutchinson-Gilford Progeria syndrome, a rare genetic disease where aspects of aging are manifested in early age. (C) Mutations in the RB1 gene are associated with retinoblastoma. (E) Mutations in the WT1 gene are associated with Wilms tumors.

16 A 16-year-old boy presents with increasing pain in the right upper arm that has been progressively getting worse over the last 4 months. He describes the pain as persistent at night. He also reports subjective fevers. On examination, there is some localized tenderness and soft tissue swelling over the proximal humerus. A plain radiograph demonstrates a large and poorly defined intramedullary diaphyseal mass permeating through the bone. The physician suspects an Ewing sarcoma. Which of the following histologic descriptions best characterize Ewing sarcoma?

(A) Malignant spindle cells forming bundles with prominent cellular atypia and mitotic figures
(B) Small round blue cells and larger eosinophilic polygonal cells with cross-striations
(C) Small round blue cells that stain positive for CD19, CD20, and CD22
(D) Small round blue cell tumor staining positive for CD99
(E) Small round blue cell tumor staining positive for S100 with Homer-Wright pseudorosettes

The answer is D: Small round blue cell tumor staining positive for CD99. Ewing sarcoma is a small round blue cell tumor, of which 80% occur in patients younger than 20. The most common sites of development are the diaphysis of the femur, tibia, humerus, ribs, and pelvis. It usually presents as a soft tissue mass. The etiology of Ewing sarcoma is a 11;22 translocation that produces the EWS/FLI1 fusion gene. Histologically, Ewing sarcomas are composed of small round blue cells with scant cytoplasm. Necrosis may be present. Cells are usually strongly positive for CD99/013 and negative for neural markers (such as S100), which may help differentiate it from primitive neuroectodermal (PNET) and neuroblastoma tumors.

(A) This is the histologic description of a soft tissue sarcoma such as leiomyosarcoma. (B) This is the histologic description of an embryonal rhabdomyosarcoma. (C) This is the histologic description of a B-cell lymphoma. (E) This is the histologic description of a neuroblastoma.

17 A 53-year-old man with a history of severe rheumatoid arthritis is referred to orthopedics by his rheumatologist for a 2-month history of right groin pain. He reports that the pain has been becoming progressively worse. He reports that at first it was present after exercise, but now hurts at rest. On examination, he walks with a limp and favors his left leg. Both active and passive ranges of motion result in the patient experiencing pain. Radiography of his right hip shows sclerosis, bone deformity, and subchondral radiolucent lines of the femoral head. Which of the following is the most likely cause of this man's condition?

(A) Factor V Leiden
(B) Iatrogenic
(C) Protein C deficiency
(D) Traumatic
(E) Vascular atherosclerotic occlusion

The answer is B: Iatrogenic. This man is most likely suffering from avascular necrosis of the femoral head secondary to long-term corticosteroid therapy for his rheumatoid arthritis. This is a well-established side effect of long-term corticosteroid use. It does not seem to occur with short-term corticosteroid use. Unfortunately, the mechanism of action is unclear. Some studies suggest it may be due to fat emboli released from hepatocytes. Another possible mechanism may be steroid-induced hypophosphatemia.

(A) Factor V Leiden is a thrombotic disorder that increases the risk of avascular necrosis of the hip. This patient's use of steroids is a more likely explanation for his condition. (C) While protein C deficiency could potentially cause avascular necrosis, it is not a likely explanation for this man's condition. (D) This patient does not have a history of trauma to explain his pain. Additionally, he is most likely being treated with long-term steroids for his rheumatoid arthritis, which is a better explanation for his symptoms. (E) While atherosclerosis may cause avascular necrosis of the femoral head, long-term steroid use is a better explanation in this patient.

18 A 33-year-old weight lifter that is training for a competition complains of numbness and tingling in his right thumb, index finger, middle finger, and thenar eminence for the last 3 months. He reports that the symptoms are worse during and after exercise, but also remain at night. On examination, there is no weakness or pain and a normal range of motion. Radiographic and neurologic studies are unremarkable. Which of the following is the most appropriate management?

(A) Rest, ice, elevation, and physical therapy
(B) Injection of corticosteroids
(C) Surgical decompression of the median nerve
(D) Oral steroids
(E) Immobilizing brace

The answer is A: Rest, ice, elevation, and physical therapy. This patient is most likely suffering from pronator teres syndrome, a compression of the median nerve secondary to increased muscle mass. Pronator teres syndrome is a compressive neuropathy that occurs in body builders. With extensive workout, muscle hypertrophy of the two heads of the pronator teres muscle may compresses the median nerve and result in the symptoms described above. Unlike carpel tunnel syndrome, the conduction velocity of the median nerve at the wrist is normal. The standard treatment for pronator teres syndrome is

"RITE," which stands for rest, ice, therapy (physical), and elevation. Patients should also discontinue exercise that would exacerbate the symptoms.

(B) Although patients may have relief of symptoms with corticosteroid injection, a strong response would more likely occur in patients with carpel tunnel syndrome. (C) Surgical decompression may be used in select cases that do not respond to rest, ice, elevation, and physical therapy. (D) Oral steroids are not effective in treating pronator teres syndrome and have numerous long-term side effects. (E) While an immobile brace is sometimes useful for treating carpel tunnel syndrome, it is not the treatment for pronator teres syndrome.

19 A 7-year-old boy is brought to the physician by his mother after several weeks of left knee pain. She reports that the pain persists and often worsens at night. The boy localizes the pain to just above the left knee. He describes it as dull and persistent without radiation. He denies fever or chills. The boy's mother says that her son has also been experiencing weight loss despite a normal appetite. On examination, there is a focal area of tenderness located over the distal femur. Plain radiography of his knee joint reveals a 1 cm in diameter lesion located in the distal femur. The lesion appears as a well-circumscribed radiolucent nidus surrounded by a border of sclerotic bone. Which of the following is the best management?

(A) Chemotherapy
(B) Nonsteroidal anti-inflammatory drugs
(C) Percutaneous radiofrequency ablation
(D) Radiation
(E) Surgical removal

The answer is B: Nonsteroidal anti-inflammatory drugs. This patient is most likely suffering from an osteoid osteoma, a relatively common and benign osteoblastic tumor. They are usually small tumors (less than 1.5 cm) and characterized by a rich and well-demarcated osteoid nidus surrounded by sclerotic bone. These tumors occur in the cortex of long bones in the vast majority of cases. Approximately 90% of osteoid osteomas occur in patients younger than 25 years of age. Initial treatment for these tumors includes non-steroidal anti-inflammatory medications (NSAIDs) or aspirin. Many tumors may resolve without operative intervention. If persistent, there are several options for additional treatment including a traditional open approach, radio-nuclide-guided excision, computed tomography (CT)-guided percutaneous excision, percutaneous laser photocoagulation, radiofrequency ablation, and others.

(A) Chemotherapy is never appropriate for osteoid osteomas. (C) Percu-taneous radiofrequency ablation has a success rate of up to 90%, with some studies supporting decreased morbidity over other approaches. However, it is best used after a trial of NSAIDs. (D) Radiation is never appropriate for osteoid osteomas. (E) Surgical removal is the gold standard for treatment of osteoid osteomas, but should be reserved for those tumors refractory to medical therapy.

20 A 14-year-old girl presents with a several-week history of low back pain. She first noticed the pain after starting her ballet class at school. She describes the pain as dull, worse with activity (especially with spine hyperextension), and relieved with rest. She denies trauma to the area, fevers, weight loss, or other symptoms. On examination, she is mildly tender to palpation of the lumbar and sacral vertebrae. There is mildly restricted lumbar range of motion and her hamstring muscles are tight on palpation. An oblique radiograph of her back shows a "Scotty Dog" sign with an interruption in the pars intraarticularis at L4. Which of the following describes the best initial treatment for this patient?

(A) Relative rest from sports activity and spinal bracing
(B) Increased extension exercises
(C) Spinal bracing only
(D) Acupuncture
(E) Surgery

The answer is A: **Relative rest from sports activity and spinal bracing.** This patient is suffering from lumbar spondylolysis, which may result in a fracture to the pars interarticularis. It most likely occurred in this patient from repetitive back hyperextension. When seen on a posterior oblique x-ray, it appears as a "collared Scotty dog" deformity. While it is asymptomatic in most patients, adolescents participating in sports may have symptoms more commonly than others. Treatment for this condition is relative rest from sports activity and spinal bracing if there is no improvement after several weeks of rest.

(B) Increased extension exercises may exacerbate the symptoms. (C) Spinal bracing may be used after 2 to 4 weeks with no improvement of symptoms. (D) Acupuncture has not been shown to be effective in managing this condition. (E) Surgical intervention may be used after more conservative treatments have been tried.

20

Neurology

(1) During morning rounds in the intensive care unit, you enter the room of a 35-year-old male patient who is intubated status post trauma. While examining him, you attempt to arouse him. He opens his eyes to sternal rub. He does not respond to your question with words or sounds. Finally, he withdraws individual extremities only when you squeeze distal digits. You are asked by your attending, at rounds, to provide this patient's Glasgow Coma Scale (GCS) score. Which of the following would be the most accurate GCS score for this patient given your prerounds examination?

(A) Seven
(B) Eight
(C) Nine
(D) Ten
(E) Eleven

The answer is B: **Eight.** Knowledge of the GCS is essential for neurosurgery as well as general surgery, particularly trauma. The score focuses on three categories (eye opening, verbal response, and motor response). The greatest possible score is 15 (individual maximums of 4, 5, and 6, respectively). This patient is described as opening his eyes in response to painful stimuli (sternal rub, i.e., score of 2), making no verbal response (i.e., score of 1), and moving in response to painful stimuli (squeezing of his digits, i.e., score of 5). The GCS score is most useful to determine a patient's immediate prognosis and long-term recovery, with scores below 8 strongly correlated with a poor outcome. The *Table 20-1* below describes GCS scoring.

(A) Seven undercalculates this patient's GCS score. (C) Nine overcalculates this patient's GCS score. (D) Ten is too great a score for this patient's condition. (E) Eleven would be considered a near-normal score, and not to be expected in a patient who is sedated for ventilatory purposes.

Table 20-1

Response	Score
Eye opening	
Opens eyes spontaneously	4
Opens eyes in response to speech	3
Opens eyes in response to painful stimulation (e.g., endotracheal suctioning)	2
Does not open eyes in response to any stimulation	1
Motor response	
Follows commands	6
Makes localized movement in response to painful stimulation	5
Makes nonpurposeful movement in response to noxious stimulation	4
Flexes upper extremities/extends lower extremities in response to pain	3
Extends all extremities in response to pain	2
Makes no response to noxious stimuli	1
Verbal response	
Is oriented to person, place, and time	5
Converses, may be confused	4
Replies with inappropriate words	3
Makes incomprehensible sounds	2
Makes no response	1

2 A 17-year-old female trauma patient status post motor vehicle accident is taken to the emergency department. She was found unresponsive at the scene. The paramedic team denies hypotensive or tachycardic episodes. They do report, however, that she has had apneic spells followed by restoration of normal breathing. She was not intubated. As her airway, breathing, and circulation are examined, you note normal respirations that become more rapid and eventually cease, with the process repeating. She has good central and distal pulses. Her pulse rate is palpated at 47. An initial blood pressure test reveals a value of 187/105 mmHg. The findings in this patient can best be described as which of the following classic triads?

(A) Beck triad
(B) Cushing triad
(C) Charcot triad
(D) Virchow triad
(E) Whipple triad

The answer is B: Cushing triad. Dr. Harvey Cushing was an American surgeon often credited as the father of modern-day neurosurgery. Cushing triad indicates neurologic trauma with increased intracranial pressure (ICP) and includes the following: hypertension, bradycardia, and irregular respirations (typically in the form of Cheyne-Stokes breathing). While trauma assessments are typically concerned with acute hemorrhage with hypovolemia, hypotension, and reflex tachycardia, the opposite (as in Cushing triad) should alert you to additional pathology. Similarly, Cushing reflex occurs when the same triad follows neurologic ischemia.

(A) Beck triad is a popularly tested triad that may occur status posttrauma, indicating cardiac tamponade due to blunt or penetrating cardiac injury. Beck triad comprises muffled heart sounds, jugular venous distention (JVD), and hypotension. All are attributed to compression of the ventricles secondary to the pericardial hematoma. (C) Charcot triad is another popular triad, but uncommon in trauma as it refers to underlying cholangitis. Charcot triad consists of fever, right upper quadrant pain, and jaundice. (D) Virchow triad differs from the remainder in that it describes pathophysiology and not physical signs. This triad embodies stasis, injury, and hypercoagulability and refers to risk factors for thrombus formation. (E) Whipple triad is a rarely tested triad. It signifies the presence of an insulinoma, and consists of hypoglycemia, vagal signs and symptoms, and relief of those signs and symptoms following glucose administration and/or meals.

3 A 32-year-old man is brought to the emergency department following a motorcycle accident in which he was unhelmeted. He was found unconscious at the scene, 30 feet away from his motorcycle. He is unresponsive, breathing simultaneously, with intact central and peripheral pulses. Vitals include a blood pressure of 135/92 mmHg and a heart rate of 94 beats/min. Focused assessment with sonography in trauma (FAST) examination is negative. Computed tomography (CT) of the brain is obtained and is shown in *Figure 20-1*.

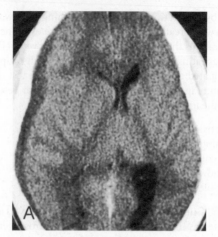

Figure 20-1

Which of the following is the most likely diagnosis?

(A) Cerebral contusion
(B) Epidural hematoma
(C) Intracerebral hemorrhage
(D) Subarachnoid hematoma
(E) Subdural hematoma

The answer is E: **Subdural hematoma.** This is a classic description of a subdural hematoma. Trauma is the most common cause of acute subdural hematoma, during which damage to the bridging veins of the brain is sheared. Coma is a common presentation of those with subdural hematoma; alternatively, signs and symptoms of increased intracranial pressure are present if the patient is conscious. Midline distortion can be associated. CT scan shows contralateral midline shift and ipsilateral contraction of the ventricles.

(A) Cerebral contusions are commonly noted in trauma and classically appear in frontal areas of the brain (a susceptible area). They are associated with hemorrhage and surrounding edema, but without defined borders like those seen in subdural and epidural hematomas. (B) Epidural hematomas are also commonly due to trauma, but these appear as convex or "lens-shaped" bleeds beneath the skull as their boundaries are made by dural attachments. This may seem subtle, but differentiating these classically tested images is very high yield. (C) Intracerebral hemorrhage generally describes a hemorrhagic cerebrovascular accident (CVA). In addition to presenting differently, it would also appear differently on computed tomography (CT), specifically, as a hyperdense wedge-shaped infarct, and in a different area than what is described in this patient's CT. (D) Subarachnoid hematomas appear as blood below the arachnoid layer, where it accumulates commonly in fissures and sulci (e.g., basal cisterns, intrahemispheric fissures, and other fissures).

 4 A 76-year-old woman is brought to the emergency department due to sudden loss of right-sided motor function in her face, arm, and leg. She has a past medical history of hypertension, hypercholesterolemia, and previous transient ischemic attack, and was recently placed on Coumadin for new-onset atrial fibrillation. A computed tomography (CT) scan is performed and is shown in *Figures 20-2A and B*.

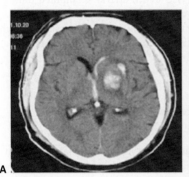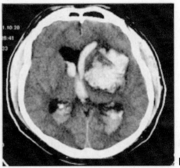

A B

Figure 20-2

Which of the following neurologic structures is most commonly involved in this patient's injury?

(A) Corpus callosum
(B) Internal capsule
(C) Putamen
(D) Thalamus

The answer is C: Putamen. This patient has a risk factor for both ischemic and hemorrhagic cerebrovascular accident (CVA); however, her recent onset of Coumadin for atrial fibrillation and imaging is suggestive of hemorrhage. Intracerebral or intraparenchymal bleeds can occur due to hypertension in the thalamus, pons, cerebellum, basal ganglia and internal capsule, and the caudate nucleus. The putamen (a basal ganglia structure) is documented as the most common area for intracerebral hemorrhage, and commonly tested in this regard.

(A) The corpus callosum is not the most common structure affected by intracerebral hemorrhage, and deficits in this region appear much differently clinically. (B) Though it may produce similar clinical signs, hemorrhage of the internal capsule is still not the most likely area for intracerebral hemorrhage. (D) Strokes that occur in the thalamus produce a wide variety of symptoms, including those of thalamic syndrome. The thalamus is not the most common area affected by intercerebral hemorrhage, but it is often affected, similar to the putamen.

 5 A 49-year-old woman is life-flighted to your trauma center after suffering a head injury in a jet ski accident. According to the flight crew, she was launched off the rolled jet ski before her head struck a rock on the water's surface. She immediately lost consciousness, during which time she was retrieved by nearby boaters. She awoke suddenly and refused emergency medical transfer. She subsequently became unresponsive prior to emergency medical service (EMS) arrival. Computed tomography (CT) of the brain in the emergency department reveals a lens-shaped hyperechoic density over the temporal region of the skull. Which of the following structures is damaged during this patient's injury?

(A) Arachnoid granulations
(B) Bridging veins of the brain
(C) Middle meningeal artery
(D) Penetrating arteries of the cerebral cortex
(E) Preexisting aneurysm within the circle of Willis

The answer is C: Middle meningeal artery. This is a fairly straight-forward question stem in which the diagnosis of epidural head bleed is suggested. Clues include the "lens-shaped" collection of blood over the temporal skull region and the lucid interval experienced by the patient. The question asks, however, to recall pathophysiology involved with epidural hemorrhage, specifically that the middle meningeal artery is the source of bleeding.

(A) Arachnoid granulations involve the flow of cerebrospinal fluid (CSF) through layers of the brain and are not commonly involved in traumatic pathology. (B) Tearing of the bridging veins in the brain is the classic buzz-phrase for subdural hemorrhage. While the history can be similar, a lucid interval is more associated with an epidural hemorrhage, and a subdural hemorrhage tends to appear more crescent shaped. (D) Hemorrhage of arteries feeding cerebral parenchyma causes intraparenchymal or intracerebral bleeds. These appear differently on CT and do not necessarily involve trauma, though they can. (E) Vascular aneurysms within the cerebral vasculature similarly do not require trauma (such as those due to uncontrolled hypertension). Additionally, bleeding in this space causes blood to pool in the subarachnoid space, not the epidural space.

 6 A 43-year-old woman with a previously diagnosed cerebral aneurysm presents to the emergency department following the rapid onset of the "worst headache of her life." Since arriving, she has noted the onset of dizziness and nausea as well. Physical examination is largely normal except for photophobia. Noncontrast computed tomography (CT) of her brain reveals blood within the circle of Willis. She was taken to the operating room by the neurosurgery service for aneurysm locating and clipping. On her eighth postoperative day, she deteriorates and becomes comatose. The pathophysiology underlying this patient's deterioration can be most likely explained by which of the following?

(A) Bleeding of another unrecognized aneurysm
(B) Postoperative cerebral edema secondary to intravenous hypertonic fluid
(C) Rebleeding of the original cerebral aneurysm
(D) Secondary vasospasm of the damaged vessel

The answer is D: **Secondary vasospasm of the damaged vessel.** One of the most common causes of mortality in subarachnoid hemorrhages is secondary vasospasm of the involved vessel. While the phenomenon is poorly understood with many possible mechanisms, a prominent theory involves calcium-dependent and calcium-independent vessel vasoconstriction. It is an often-tested phenomenon. Treatment options include calcium channel blockers, magnesium citrate, nitrous oxide donors, and endothelin-1 antagonists.

(A) While it is possible that a patient with risk factor for aneurysmal bleeding has another unrecognized aneurysm, this is not the most likely cause. (B) Hypertonic fluids are often considered cerebro-protective against cerebral edema, and would not cause cerebral edema per se as is suggested in this answer. (C) While rebleeding is a possibility, the very real and common complication of vasospasm makes this answer choice less likely.

  A 19-year-old man is involved in an all-terrain vehicle (ATV) accident with multiple rollovers as an unhelmeted driver. His friends report that he was consuming alcoholic beverages the majority of the day. Upon arrival to the emergency department, he has a Glasgow Coma Scale (GCS) score of 7. His right pupil measures 4 mm and is responsive to light. His left pupil is 7 mm and appears unresponsive and unreactive. He is hemodynamically stable, though you suspect an intracranial hemorrhage. Which of the following next steps would not be suitable in attaining your suspected diagnosis?

(A) Emergent operative exploration based on this clinical diagnosis
(B) Imaging with a noncontrast computed tomography (CT)
(C) Imaging with an increased resolution study (i.e., magnetic resonance imaging [MRI])
(D) Lumbar puncture for demonstration of xanthochromia

The answer is D: **Lumbar puncture for demonstration of xanthochromia.** The condition described in this question (dilated pupil unreactive to light and accommodation) indicates that this patient has a "blown pupil," indicating ipsilateral trauma/hematoma with contralateral uncal herniation and compression of the optic nerve. In the presence of a blown pupil, which indicates considerably increased intracranial pressure, lumbar puncture is contraindicated. This is a commonly tested and misunderstood neurosurgical concept.

(A) With a deteriorating mental status indicated by this patient's GCS score, the diagnosis is fairly certain. This patient could proceed to decompressive craniectomy. (B) CT without contrast would be the imaging study of choice, and a very acceptable, in fact, ideal, diagnostic measure. (C) Imaging with increased resolution imaging, as with an MRI study, would be acceptable, however not ideal given the time constraints imposed. This is a less desirable management plan, but much more acceptable than lumbar puncture.

 A 45-year-old otherwise healthy patient was a victim in a polytrauma event. He was found in vomitus and was intubated at the scene for what appeared to be irregular respirations. He has been hemodynamically stable. Examination in the emergency department reveals good peripheral pulses at a rate of 47 beats/minute, unresponsiveness with minimal sedation, and a fixed dilated and unresponsive right pupil. Which of the following is the best first-step option in decreasing increased intracranial pressure (ICP)?

(A) Cranial decompression surgery
(B) Diamox administered intravenously
(C) Elevation of the head of the bed
(D) Hyperventilation
(E) Peripheral rotating tourniquets

The answer is C: Elevation of the head of the bed. While there are known pharmacologic and invasive mechanisms to decrease ICP, several noninvasive maneuvers exist to provide immediate and long-lasting decreases in ICP. Elevation of the head of the bed is regularly practiced in the ICU setting, and can be performed in an emergent scenario while operative correction is currently on hold.

(A) Cranial decompressive surgery may very well be sought later in the management of this patient, but this question asks for a first-step option. (B) Diamox (acetazolamide), a carbonic anhydrase inhibitor, is known to lower ICP, but is not as simple as elevating the head of the bed. Remember to think cheaply and simply for testing purposes. (D) While hyperventilation does in fact decrease ICP in acute settings, its effects are transient at best. Additionally, the decreases seen in cerebral perfusion last longer than its effects on decreasing ICP, making it a less desirable choice clinically. (E) Peripheral rotating tourniquets (applied in trauma scenarios to patients with injuries of the limbs) have actually been shown to increase ICP. The mechanism is poorly understood, but likely involves additional blood volume from a blood-drained limb.

 A 14-year-old boy is ejected from the bed of a pick-up truck during a motor vehicle collision with rollover. He is determined to have an epidural hematoma via computed tomography (CT) and is taken immediately to the operating room (OR) for evacuation. Postoperatively, he is transferred to the pediatric intensive care unit. He has been hemodynamically stable since arrival. Current vitals read: temperature 37.5°C, heart rate 82 beats/min, respiration rate 16 breaths/min (ventilated), blood pressure 100/67 mmHg, O_2 saturation 99%. Indwelling intracranial pressure (ICP) monitor reveals an ICP of 10 mmHg. Which value best represents his calculated cerebral perfusion pressure (CPP)?

(A) 48 mmHg
(B) 58 mmHg
(C) 68 mmHg
(D) 78 mmHg
(E) 88 mmHg

The answer is C: **68 mmHg.** Calculating CPP can be done by subtracting ICP from mean arterial pressure (MAP). While ICP can be calculated with a surgically placed pressure catheter (as with this patient), MAP is typically reported by indwelling arterial lines in an ICU setting such as this one. This question, however, requires you to calculate it as well using systolic pressure (SP) and diastolic pressure (DP).

$$MAP = DP + 1/3(SP - DP) \text{ or } 67 + 1/3 (100 - 67)$$
$$MAP = 78$$
$$CPP = MAP - ICP \text{ or } 78 - 10$$
$$CPP = 68$$

(A) This number is not the correct answer based on the equations provided above. (B) This number is not the correct answer based on the equations provided above. (D) This number is not the correct answer based on the equations provided above. (E) This number is not the correct answer based on the equations provided above.

⟨10⟩ An 87-year-old woman presents with immediate-onset right-sided hemiplegia in both extremities. Her daughter noted the sudden onset of confusion and inability to speak as well. She has a past medical history of hypertension, pulmonary embolus, hyperlipidemia, diabetes mellitus, and Factor V Leiden. Her renal function is normal. Her past surgical history includes total hysterectomy status post rupture 50 years prior, and cholecystectomy 15 years prior. She is hemodynamically stable. On examination, she appears acutely distressed. Right-sided strength is 2/5 compared to 4/5 on the left. She is responsive to yes or no question, but unable to speak. Which imaging modality is most appropriate as you begin workup on this patient?

(A) Computed tomography (CT) with contrast
(B) CT without contrast
(C) Magnetic resonance imaging (MRI) with contrast
(D) MRI without contrast
(E) Cerebral angiogram

The answer is B: CT without contrast. This patient has risk factors as well as the classic presentation of cerebrovascular accident, or stroke. The standard imaging for a stroke patient remains CT of the brain without contrast.

(A) CT with contrast is contraindicated is the presence of a hemorrhagic stroke. Given that this possibility has not been ruled out, this is not a valid management option. (C) This answer is incorrect for multiple reasons, including the use of contrast as well as the imaging modality itself. (D) MRI studies have greater sensitivity and specificity for older infarcts and hemorrhages, but given the time-sensitive pathology of a cerebrovascular accident (CVA), CT is the best initial study. (E) A cerebral angiogram is the ideal imaging study for a suspected cerebral aneurysm. This would not the first step is diagnosis in stroke, which this patient is clearly presenting with. Additionally, angiograms utilize contrast dye, which should not be used.

 11 You are making morning rounds for the trauma service in the surgical ICU. You review the labs of a 23-year-old man who suffered closed head injury with subdural and subarachnoid hematomas. He has been followed by neurosurgery, who is administering hypertonic fluids and has placed an intracranial pressure monitor. This patient's sodium reads critical this morning at 119 mmol/L. Which of the following conditions best explains this patient's laboratory findings?

(A) Acute renal failure secondary to trauma
(B) Central diabetes insipidus
(C) Diuresis secondary to administration of hypertonic IV fluids
(D) Natriuresis secondary to administration of hypertonic IV fluids
(E) Syndrome of inappropriate antidiuretic hormone secretion (SIADH)

The answer is E: Syndrome of inappropriate antidiuretic hormone secretion (SIADH). Of the possible ways to test SIADH on United States Medical Licensing Examination (USMLE)-style examinations, trauma remains one of the most popular. Considered a post–head injury endocrine complication, the pathophysiology involves rupture of the pituitary stalk and with it the blood supply to the adenohypophysis (the anterior pituitary gland). Remember that SIADH leads to sodium wasting via the urine.

(A) A low serum sodium is not ideal for diagnosing acute renal failure. While it can occur secondary to trauma, more information would be needed (e.g., blood urea nitrogen to creatinine ratio, fractional excretion of sodium, etc.).

(B) Remember diabetes insipidus as the opposing pathology of SIADH, that is, water wasting via the urine. It would, therefore, proceed to hypernatremia, not hyponatremia as is suggested by this patient's serum sodium. (C) If diuresis was to occur following administration of a hypertonic solution, note that this would lead to hypernatremia, not hyponatremia. (D) Administering hypertonic fluids (cerebro-protective) is more likely to increase the serum sodium content, rather than decrease it. While natriuresis will occur with the increased sodium load on the body, it is unlikely to proceed to hyponatremia.

12 A 19-year-old woman is involved in an all-terrain vehicle (ATV) accident. She was not wearing a helmet, and the vehicle underwent multiple rollovers. She was able to walk away from the scene to her home, over one mile away. She is complaining of an intense headache and chest pain. She is neurologically intact other than being in pain. Cranial examination reveals bilateral periorbital ecchymoses. She has right hemotympanum, and was noted to have ecchymoses posterior to her ears bilaterally. Nasal examination is normal. Chest and pelvic x-rays from the trauma bay indicate multiple rib fractures. Which of the following is the most likely diagnosis?

(A) Basilar skull fracture
(B) Eustachian tube rupture bilaterally
(C) Subarachnoid hemorrhage
(D) Bilateral ethmoidal fracture

The answer is A: Basilar skull fracture. The two signs that are described in this trauma patient, raccoon eyes and battle sign, are pathognomonic for a basilar skull fracture. Either of these findings should alert you to this diagnosis. Fractures of the base of the skull are serious, as they are associated with dural tears and leaks of cerebrospinal fluid (CSF).

(B) While Eustachian tube rupture is possible in this scenario, it is more likely to occur secondary to barotrauma or penetrating trauma through the ear canal. It can occur with blunt force, such as a slap over the ear; however, bilateral Eustachian tube rupture is unlikely to be present in this patient. (C) No physical examination findings accurately indicate subdural hematoma other than late complications or deterioration. This diagnosis is made upon imaging. Note that it is possible to maintain consciousness with smaller subdural hemorrhages. (D) The buzz word for ethmoidal fractures on United States Medical Licensing Examination (USMLE)-style examinations is rhinorrhea suspicious for a CSF leak, which is not present here. Periorbital edema and ecchymoses may represent an underlying fracture, as well as physical examination findings including bony step-offs or crepitus.

13 A 19-year-old woman is brought to the emergency department after suffering a fall from a height of 30 feet. She was reportedly "free climbing" a rock-face without rope, harness, or helmet. Witnesses are unable to describe her mechanism of impact. She is given pressors en route to the hospital, with the lowest blood pressure of 90/50 mmHg and fastest heart rate of 52 beats/min. She has had no respiratory difficulty. She is responsive with improved vitals in the trauma bay and unable to move her lower extremities. She has positive spinal tenderness. Her focused assessment with sonography in trauma (FAST) examination is negative. Which of the following is the most likely level of her injury?

(A) C3
(B) T4
(C) T12
(D) L3
(E) S2

The answer is B: **T4.** Neurogenic shock occurs in traumatic injuries when spinal cord damage disrupts sympathetic outflow (predominantly from the thoracolumbar regions of the spine), allowing parasympathetic dominance to dramatically decrease blood pressure. In contrast to hypovolemic hypotension, bradycardia is more common than tachycardia (as another vagal response). As discussed in the chapter, lesions or trauma above T5 cause hypotension.

(A) While this level would certainly produce neurogenic shock, spinal cord damage to C3 would produce irregularities in respiration (as diaphragmatic innervation is found at levels C3–C5). This is not the case in this clinical presentation. (C) T12 would be too inferior a level to produce neurogenic shock. Anatomically, this would eliminate more parasympathetic tone rather than sympathetic tone. (D) L3 would be too low to result in neurogenic shock. Lower extremity reflexes would be expected to be compromised on physical examination. (E) S2 is too inferior to result in neurogenic shock. Sacral reflexes including anal wink and ankle reflex would be compromised. The patients may also complain of incontinence.

---

14. A 53-year-old man was working on his farm this evening when he experienced a sudden onset of pain and tingling in his right leg. He immediately rested and tried over-the-counter anti-inflammatory medications without alleviation. He has a past medical history of rheumatoid arthritis. He indicates the pain ceases in a diagonal pattern across his right anterior shin below his knee. Physical examination reveals paresthesia above this line as well as weakened quadriceps muscles on the affected side. The disease process described in this patient can be best localized to what vertebral level?

(A) L1–L2
(B) L2–L3
(C) L3–L4
(D) L4–L5
(E) L5–S1

The answer is C: L3–L4. This is a fairly classic description of a lumbar disk herniation. Remember that the most commonly affected areas are L4–L5 and L5–S1. However, we are given the description of an affected dermatome in the history and physical, and we can localize the injury accordingly. The presence of weak quadriceps helps localize the herniation to between L2 and L4. However, the description of paresthesia below the knee better localizes the injury to the disk L3–L4.

(A) L1–L2 disk herniations have no motor deficits and produce pain in the inguinal region as well as the medial thigh. (B) L2–L3 disk disease, despite also exhibiting quadriceps weakness, has localized pain at the region above the knee, specifically anteriorly and laterally. (D) L4–L5 herniation causes weakness in extension of the foot and great toe. The dorsal surface of the foot is affected with neurogenic pain. L4–L5 is one of the two most common levels affected by disk disease. (E) Patients who suffer herniation at the level of L5–S1 exhibit a diminished Achilles reflex and experience pain in the lateral foot. L5–S1 is one of the two most common levels affected by disk disease.

 15

A 53-year-old woman presents to the emergency department with gradual onset of worsening urinary incontinence. Her past medical history includes a history of fibromyalgia, hypertension, and cervical cancer status post-surgery and radiotherapy. Review of systems reveals minimal fecal incontinence as well. Physical examination reveals saddle anesthesia, absence of the anal wink reflex, and areflexic lower extremities. Which of the following is the most likely diagnosis?

(A) Anterior cord syndrome
(B) Brown-Séquard syndrome
(C) Cauda equina syndrome
(D) Central cord syndrome
(E) Posterior cord syndrome

The answer is C: Cauda equina syndrome. Cauda equina syndrome involves compression or inflammation surrounding the terminal nerve roots at the caudal terminus of the spinal cord. Symptoms and signs described in the question are classic (saddle anesthesia, areflexia in the lower limbs, absence of lower-root spinal reflexes, incontinence, etc.). Given her history of cervical cancer, this should raise a concern for malignant invasion of the spinal canal.

(A) Anterior cord syndrome affects the anterior spinal cord, therefore impinging on the corticospinal and lateral spinothalamic tracts. Deficits include loss of pain and temperature sensation and paraplegia. (B) Brown-Séquard syndrome, or "hemicord syndrome," causes weakness below the level of the lesion with hyperreflexia, as well as loss of pain and temperature sensation below the injury level but contralaterally (because these fibers traversing traverse the cord at a level below the injury). (D) Central cord syndrome causes upper extremity weakness as well as a cape-like distribution of loss of pain and temperature sensation. Lower extremity motor and sensory function are preserved. (E) Posterior cord syndrome, affecting the dorsal column tracts, leads to corresponding loss of proprioception and vibratory sense distally, the classic syndrome being tabes dorsalis.

 A 37-year-old woman with a history of blunt spinal trauma 1 year prior presents to clinic complaining of "numbness" from her hips to her toes, bilaterally. Besides her trauma history, she is otherwise healthy, takes no medications, and has never been hospitalized. She has no neurologic family history. Physical examination reveals a cape-like absence of pain and temperature sensation below the level of posterior superior iliac crest. Which of the following is the most likely diagnosis?

(A) Brown-Séquard syndrome
(B) Cauda equina syndrome
(C) Spinal gliosis
(D) Syringomyelia

The answer is D: Syringomyelia. Syringomyelia is the classic example used for a central cord lesion and occurs when the potential fluid space in the center of the spinal cord expands over several weeks. The classic description is a "cape-like" loss of pain and temperature sensation along with lower motor neuron signs in the same area (upper chest and back as well as arms). Dorsal column function is preserved.

(A) Brown-Séquard syndrome, or "hemicord syndrome," causes weakness below the level of the lesion and hyperreflexia as well as loss of pain and temperature sensation below the injury level but found contralaterally (because of lower-level spinal cord traversing of these fibers). (B) Cauda equina syndrome involves compression or inflammation surrounding the terminal nerve roots at the caudal terminus of the spinal cord. Symptoms and signs include saddle anesthesia, areflexia in the lower limbs, absence of lower-root spinal reflexes, etc. (C) Spinal gliosis refers to the deposition of scar tissue within the spinal cord, such as that that may occur following traumatic injury. While this phenomenon is documented, it is fairly rare.

 A 28-year-old man who suffered multiple gunshot wounds to his back and flank presents to your trauma clinic 2 weeks following his hospital discharge. He underwent extensive neurosurgical workup during his admission for spinal involvement and his neurosurgical follow-up is upcoming. His main complaints today involve inability to move his right leg, and left leg numbness. Physical examination reveals a flaccid right leg and a left leg with sensation only to vibration. Which of the following syndromes most accurately describes the findings seen in this patient?

(A) Anterior cord syndrome
(B) Brown-Séquard syndrome
(C) Cauda equina syndrome
(D) Posterior cord syndrome
(E) Syringomyelia

The answer is B: Brown-Séquard syndrome. Brown-Séquard syndrome, or "hemicord syndrome," causes weakness below the level of the lesion and hyperreflexia as well as loss of pain and temperature sensation below the injury level but found contralaterally (because of lower-level spinal cord traversing of these fibers).

(A) Anterior cord syndrome affects the anterior spinal cord, therefore impinging on the corticospinal and lateral spinothalamic tracts. Deficits include loss of pain and temperature sensation and paraplegia. (C) Cauda equina syndrome involves compression or inflammation surrounding the terminal nerve roots at the caudal terminus of the spinal cord. Symptoms and signs include saddle anesthesia, areflexia in the lower limbs, absence of lower-root spinal reflexes, etc. (D) Posterior cord syndrome, affecting the dorsal column tracts, leads to corresponding loss of proprioception and vibratory sense distally. (E) Syringomyelia is a central cord lesion that occurs when the potential fluid space in the center of the spinal cord expands over several weeks. The classic description is a "cape-like" loss of pain and temperature sensation.

18 A 47-year-old man is brought to the emergency department following the onset of reported seizures in the workplace. Antiepileptic medications were given at the scene, and the gentleman arrives conscious but slightly confused. He is able to deny previous history of seizures but does report recent worsening of his chronic headache, first noted 1 year prior. He has no significant medical history. Examination reveals a postictal man in no acute distress. An imaging study is obtained and is shown in *Figure 20-3*.
Which of the following is the most likely diagnosis?

(A) Benign astrocytoma
(B) Glioblastoma multiforme (GBM)
(C) Medulloblastoma
(D) Oligodendroglioma
(E) Pituitary adenoma

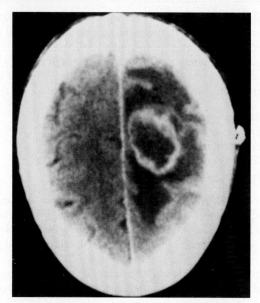

Figure 20-3

The answer is B: Glioblastoma multiforme (GBM). Of all the adult brain tumors tested on United States Medical Licensing Examination (USMLE)-style examinations, GBM is the most common for examination purposes. It is the most common and lethal glial tumor. Presentations vary and may include headaches, gait disturbances, neurologic deficits, or seizures as in this patient. Treatment of GBM consists of maximal surgical resection combined with radiation and chemotherapy. Magnetic resonance imaging (MRI) shows hemispheric lesions with enhancement. A "butterfly" appearance is classically described for GBM.

(A) Benign astrocytomas can present similar to this patient or with a host of different neurologic deficits. Their appearance, in contrast to this one, does not indicate enhancement, appear more clearly defined, and without calcification. (C) Medulloblastoma occurs for the most part in the pediatric population (75%), which is typically tested. They are typically located below the tentorium cerebelli, usually around the cerebellum with or without extension into the fourth ventricle. (D) Oligodendrogliomas are similar to GBM in that they are derived from astrocytomas. Imaging of oligodendroglioma, also via MRI, shows well-demarcated lesions that are dense with calcification. There is no butterfly description assigned. (E) Pituitary adenomas present classically with bitemporal hemianopsia, the most of which is the benign prolactin-secreting adenoma. The pituitary is not the area involved on this MRI.

---

19 A 31-year-old elite male athlete visits you in your outpatient clinic for recent onset of "tunnel vision." While he first noticed the phenomenon 2 years ago while completing a 9-hour endurance race, it ceased after the end of the event. One month ago, he noted blurry peripheral vision which progressed to bilateral peripheral blind spots currently. Visual field testing reveals diminished lateral visual acuity bilaterally. Which of the following is the most likely diagnosis?

(A) Cranial tuberous sclerosis
(B) Craniopharyngioma
(C) Physiologic devascularization due to prolonged aerobic activity
(D) Prolactinoma
(E) Empty sella syndrome

The answer is D: Prolactinoma. This patient describes classic bitemporal hemianopsia. For United States Medical Licensing Examination (USMLE)-style testing purposes, tunnel vision is a pituitary tumor until proven otherwise. Of all pituitary tumors, benign growths are much more common. Of the benign growths, prolactin-secreting adenomas ("prolactinomas") are the most common pathology involved, which this question is asking.

(A) Tuberous sclerosis involves the growth of benign hamartomas ("tubers") in the brain which are found in many anatomic locations as part of a multisystem disease. The cerebral lesions are typically found as subependymal nodules or white matter lesions. (B) Craniopharyngiomas are rare tumors that are typically diagnosed in pediatric patients and patients near their eighth decade (bimodally). While bitemporal hemianopsia does occur, prolactinomas far outweigh the incidence of these tumors. (C) While prolonged strenuous exercise as in endurance races can cause temporary visual disturbances (classically tunnel vision), these episodes are short lived and do not impose chronic visual loss. (E) Sella turcica syndrome is a tempting distracter here because its pathology is involved with structures in the same area. However, as the name implies, it is a lack of structures normally present in the area of the pituitary and commonly presents as hypopituitarism.

---

20 A 65-year-old man complains of unexplained tinnitus, vertigo, and hearing loss in his right ear. This has been progressive during the last year. Review of systems indicates worsening ringing in his left ear over 12 months, accompanied by difficulty hearing "higher notes on the radio," in his left ear, which he attributes to work exposure. Given this triad of symptoms, which of the following is the most likely diagnosis?

(A) Acoustic neuroma
(B) Acute otitis interna
(C) Acute otitis media
(D) Cranial nerve VII tumor
(E) Meniere disease

The answer is A: Acoustic neuroma. Acoustic neuroma (or vestibular schwannoma) is a Schwann cell–derived tumor that arises on the eighth cranial nerve. The triad of symptoms involved tinnitus, hearing loss, and balance disturbances, all of which are suggested in the clinical history of this patient. The next diagnostic step would be computed tomography (CT) or magnetic resonance imaging (MRI) followed by surgical resection.

(B) Acute otitis interna, or labyrinthitis, typically presents acutely with sudden onset vertigo with or without other related symptoms. The patient's presentation and chronicity suggest otherwise. (C) Acute otitis media, or the common ear infection, is unlikely here given the chronicity of his symptoms onset (6 months) as well as the symptoms themselves. (D) This is a distracting answer that tests your immediate knowledge of the cranial nerves. Neuromas of cranial nerve VII, or the facial nerve, are uncommon but do occur. A facial nerve neuroma would produce a much different picture. (E) Meniere disease is another very likely possibility given this triad of symptoms; however, episodic vertigo (two or more episodes) is required to make this diagnosis.

 An 8-year-old boy is brought to the physician with longstanding worsening headache over 1 year, dizziness, and a recent onset of frequent falling episodes. A computed tomography (CT) obtained reveals an enhancing mass located immediately adjacent to the fourth ventricle. Which of the following is the most appropriate first treatment option for this patient?

(A) Multiagent chemotherapy
(B) Palliative chemoradiation
(C) Radiotherapy
(D) Surgical resection

The answer is D: Surgical resection. Medulloblastoma occurs for the most part in the pediatric population (75%), which is typically tested. They are typically located below the tentorium cerebelli, usually around the cerebellum with or without extension into the fourth ventricle. Because of their involvement with the cerebellum, gait imbalances can occur, as with this patient. Ideal treat for medulloblastoma begins with maximal surgical resection with which staging and diagnosis can be confirmed.

(A) Despite being a mainstay in the treatment for medulloblastoma, the benefits of chemotherapy for medulloblastoma remain largely unknown. Chemotherapy typically begins after an ideal surgical resection and diagnostic confirmation. (B) There is no reason to suggest that palliative therapy should be indicated. Furthermore, proper staging and adequate resection both begin with surgical intervention, which this answer does not include. (C) Radiation therapy is also used for medulloblastoma; however, it typically begins following surgical resection and histologic confirmation and staging.

 22 A 2-hour-old female neonate is examined in the nursery following delivery. She and her mother had been followed with serial ultrasounds for a maternal history of neural tube defects. Physical examination of this infant reveals an abnormal tuft of skin at the sacral area overlying herniated meninges and neural tissue. What is the most likely diagnosis?

(A) Anencephaly
(B) Arnold-Chiari deformity
(C) Myelomeningocele
(D) Spina bifida occulta

The answer is C: **Myelomeningocele.** Myelomeningocele is a neural tube defect in which the meninges and neural tissue herniate through a vertebral defect in the lumbosacral region. The commonly tested associated anomaly is the Chiari II malformation. The defect may be open, may blend into the skin, or may be covered by a thin cutaneous membrane.

(A) Anencephaly is the most common congenital malformation and is typically detected prenatally. The calvarium is absent with a thickened and flattened skull base. Cerebral material is disorganized, leaving a flattened cerebral remnant only. (B) The Arnold-Chiari malformation describes elongation of the cerebellar tonsils and extension into the fourth ventricle. This is a temping question for those who know the association with myelomeningocele, but this is not confirmed yet, and is not the primary diagnosis in this child. (D) Spina bifida occulta tends to be a more subtle presentation of spina bifida variations.

 23 A 3-year-old child presents to her physician for a well-child visit. Her immunizations are up to date, and her mother reports that she has been healthy and has demonstrated normal milestones. Growth charts are appropriate for a child of this age. Physical examination of the heart, lungs, and abdomen is within normal limits. Fundoscopy reveals no papilledema. She has a right-sided eye droop, and her left pupil appears dilated relative to the right. Which of the following is the most likely diagnosis?

(A) Horner syndrome
(B) Left-sided acoustic neuroma
(C) Medulloblastoma
(D) Prolactinoma
(E) Right-sided facial nerve palsy

The answer is A: Horner syndrome. Horner syndrome presents with the classic triad of ptosis, miosis, and hemianhidrosis. It is a very rare condition, with no epidemiologic predilection for that reason. Commonly tested scenarios for Horner syndrome include dissection status post trauma, iatrogenic Horner syndrome (status postsurgery), and pancoast tumor invasion. Remember that it can present congenitally in the pediatric population as idiopathic Horner syndrome, as it is here.

(B) Acoustic neuromas present with tinnitus, hearing loss, and balance disturbances. Involving the eighth cranial nerve, they would not cause the symptoms seen in this patient. (C) Medulloblastoma occurs in the pediatric population (75%) and is typically located below the tentorium cerebelli, usually around the cerebellum with or without extension into the fourth ventricle. Gait abnormalities are common presentations. (D) Prolactinoma describes the condition of a prolactin-secreting adenoma. Found in the pituitary fossa, the common presentation involves visual disturbances and headache, not ptosis and miosis. (E) Right-sided facial nerve palsy describes a right-sided Bell palsy, which is a unilateral paralysis of the peripheral portion of the facial nerve. Facial droop and inability to blink are typical symptoms. It, similarly, has a wide range of etiologies.

 A 64-year-old woman presents to her physician complaining of unexplained anxiousness. Her brother has recently passed away due to autosomal dominant polycystic kidney disease (ADPKD), similar to her father and paternal grandmother. She is extremely concerned that she will suffer a similar fate. She has a benign medical history and a normal abdominal examination. Labs reveal a serum creatinine of 0.9 mg/dL. Urinalysis reveals no gross or microscopic hematuria. Renal ultrasound reveals normal-appearing, noncystic kidneys. Had she had been diagnosed with ADPKD, which of the following neurosurgical episodes is most likely to be seen in this patient?

(A) Epidural hemorrhage
(B) Subdural hemorrhage
(C) Subarachnoid hemorrhage
(D) Intraventricular hemorrhage

The answer is C: Subarachnoid hemorrhage. The question is twofold; specifically, it is asking you to recall the association between ADPKD and the presence of Berry aneurysms. Additionally, you must know that bleeding of cerebral aneurysms releases blood into the subarachnoid space. Remember that any uncontrolled hypertension predisposes to cerebral aneurysms, and there is nothing special about ADPKD's predisposition to aneurysms other than its hypertension component. Finally, patients are also prone to intracerebral hemorrhage, but note that this is not an answer choice.

(A) Epidural hematomas are commonly due to trauma and appear as convex bleeds beneath the skull as their boundaries are made by dural attachments. There is no association with ADPKD. (B) Subdural bleeds can be due to trauma or involve chronic bleeds such as those seen in the elderly. There is no association with ADPKD. (D) Intraventricular hemorrhage can occur in preterm neonates but also in patients who suffer trauma. In traumatic scenarios, it is often considered a poor prognostic indicator. The presence of blood within the ventricles is pathognomonic, typically with blood in the lateral ventricles or all ventricles.

25 An 82-year-old woman is brought to the emergency department from her assisted-living residence due to altered mental status. She has multiple chronic medical morbidities including Alzheimer dementia, hypertension, type 2 diabetes mellitus, and chronic sinusitis. Her nursing staff noticed confusion 1 day prior to admission, and somnolence starting 8 hours prior. Vitals include a temperature of 39°C, heart rate of 110 beats/min, and blood pressure of 105/80 mmHg. Physical examination reveals an elderly woman not responsive to verbal commands but moaning and withdrawing in response to nuchal flexion. A magnetic resonance imaging (MRI) demonstrates an epidural fluid collection surrounded by inflammation with some enhancement. What is the most common cause of this patient's condition?

(A) Local spread of infection from an epidural procedure
(B) Lumbar disk herniation
(C) Hematogenous spread of infection
(D) Malignant process of the spinal canal
(E) Meningococcal vaccination reaction

The answer is C: Hematogenous spread of infection. This is a classic presentation of spinal epidural abscess, where infectious signs and meningeal-like signs coincide. Spinal epidural abscesses are caused by hematogenous seeding of infection, typically with *Staph* or *Strep* bacterial species. This specific etiology of this infectious process is a commonly tested phenomenon.

(A) While infectious complications from epidural anesthesia are fairly rare, they do occur; however, we are not provided any information from the clinical history to suggest that this should be included in the differential. (B) Lumbar disk herniation commonly occurs at lower lumbar levels with pain, paresthesia, or dysthesias occurring alone the nerve roots that are compressed. The suggestion of infection and altered mental status of this patient seem to suggest a diagnosis other than disk herniation. (D) A malignant process of the spinal cord would present with a more chronic progression of disease. We are told that the signs seen in this patient began acutely. Note that epidural abscesses can present chronically, in which case they can mimic malignant processes. (E) There is no reason to believe that this is a reaction to a meningococcal vaccination, as it is not mentioned in the vignette, and a reaction of this type is atypical. The most serious reaction to the meningococcal vaccine is anaphylaxis. There is also a concern for Guillain-Barré syndrome with some meningococcal vaccine types.

Urology

1. On a routine examination, a 43-year-old woman with a history of smoking is found to have microscopic hematuria. She is otherwise asymptomatic. Repeat testing over several months shows persistent microscopic hematuria. Microscopy confirms the presence of isomorphic red blood cells. With the exception of red blood cells present in her urine, the remainder of her testing including complete blood count, urinalysis, and renal function are normal. Her physical examination is unremarkable. What is the next step in diagnosis?

   (A) Abdominal ultrasound
   (B) Cystoscopy
   (C) Observation
   (D) Renal biopsy
   (E) Repeat urinalysis

The answer is B: **Cystoscopy.** This patient has several risk factors for urothelial carcinoma (smoking and age) and should be evaluated with cystoscopy. Cystoscopy is a relatively quick and inexpensive procedure for diagnosing bladder cancer.

(A) An abdominal ultrasound is useful for identifying renal masses, hydronephrosis, and bladder masses. However, urothelial tumors of the upper urinary tract are easily missed. Thus, it is not the imaging modality of choice for working up hematuria when urothelial carcinoma is suspected. (C) This patient has risk factors for urothelial carcinoma. Observation at this point would not be appropriate. If a continued and exhaustive workup fails to identify a source of hematuria, then observation may be appropriate. (D) Renal biopsy is an invasive test and would be more appropriate if a glomerular source of bleeding was suspected. (E) At this point, several urinalyses have confirmed microscopic hematuria. Repeating urinalysis would not greatly contribute to finding the cause.

2 A 67-year-old man presents with hematuria and a 10 lb weight loss over the last 8 months. Cystoscopy reveals a large mass on the dome of the bladder. Biopsy of the mass reveals transitional cell carcinoma of the bladder. Which of the following is not a major risk factor for this type of tumor?

(A) Alcohol
(B) Dye exposure
(C) History of radiation to the pelvis
(D) Second hand smoke
(E) Smoking

The answer is A: Alcohol. Urothelial carcinoma of the bladder is the most common type of bladder cancer. There are numerous risk factors for developing urothelial carcinoma, the most important and common factor being smoking. Other known risk factors for urothelial carcinoma include (among others) chemical carcinogens (aromatic amines, dyes, occupations working with these chemicals), arsenic, chronic inflammation, human papilloma virus (although primarily associated with squamous cell carcinoma), radiation, cyclophosphamide, and phenacetin. Although there is some conflicting evidence that excessive alcohol consumption is associated with an increased risk of urothelial carcinoma, it is generally not considered an important risk factor.

(B) Dye exposure and occupations that involve exposure to dyes (hairdressers, barbers, painters) are associated with an increased risk of developing bladder cancer. Other occupations that are known to have increased risk of developing bladder cancer include metal workers, rubber industry workers, miners, cement workers, leather and textile workers, carpet manufacturers. (C) Multiple studies have shown an increased risk of developing bladder cancer in patients that have received radiation to the pelvis (previous ovarian, cervical, prostate, testicular cancers). (D) Second hand smoke has been shown to increase the risk of bladder cancer in women up to three fold. (E) Smoking is the most important risk factor for urothelial carcinoma and is the most important factor contributing to the incidence of bladder cancer in western nations. Both men and women who smoke have a significant increase in risk.

3 A 49-year-old woman presents burning during urination and mild back pain not associated with activity. She reports that she has had these symptoms off and on over the last 2 years but it has recently been getting worse. Her body temperature is 36.7°C, blood pressure 135/85 mmHg, pulse 83 beats/min, and respirations 13 breaths/min. On physical examination, there is bilateral mild costovertebral tenderness. The remainder of the physical examination including a pelvic and genitourinary examination is unremarkable. Laboratory studies and urinalysis reveal the following:

Complete Blood Count:

> Leukocytes: 6,500/mm^3
> Hemoglobin: 14.3 g/dL
> Hematocrit: 44.2%
> Platelet count: 310,000/mm^3

Urinalysis:

> pH: 7.5
> Nitrites: positive
> Protein: negative
> Glucose: negative
> Ketones: negative
> Leukocytes: moderate
> Blood: trace

Plain radiography of the kidneys–ureter–bladder (KUB) is shown in *Figure 21-1*.

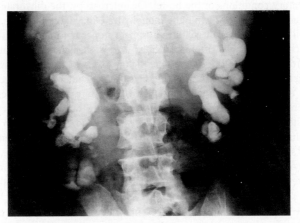

Figure 21-1

These opacities most likely represent material made up of which of the following chemical compounds?

(A) Calcium oxalate
(B) Calcium phosphate
(C) Cystine
(D) Magnesium ammonium phosphate
(E) Uric acid

The answer is D: Magnesium ammonium phosphate. This patient most likely is suffering from bilateral staghorn calculi as shown on the KUB. The most common component of staghorn calculi stones is struvite (magnesium ammonium phosphate) and calcium carbonate apatite. The pathogenesis involves infection with urease producing organisms such as *Proteus* or *Klebsiella*. Infection causes alkalization of the urine and an environment in which struvite crystals precipitate. On microscopy, these crystals appear shaped like a coffin-lid. Since women are more likely to have upper urinary tract infections (UTIs), they are also more likely to form staghorn calculi than men. Patients most frequently present with symptoms of a UTI with mild flank pain and/or hematuria. If left untreated, staghorn calculi may result sepsis and kidney failure. Medical therapy alone is usually not effective; thus, surgery is usually recommended. Percutaneous nephrolithotomy is usually the first-line method of surgical management.

(A) Calcium oxalate is the most common stone composition. They come in two forms, calcium oxylate monohydrate and calcium oxylate dihydrate. Risk factors for formation of this type of stone include dehydration, hypercalciuria, hyperoxaluria, hypernatriuria, hyperuricosuria, hypocitraturia, excessive ingestion of vitamin D or calcium, sarcoidosis, intestinal bypass surgery, and chronic inflammatory conditions of the bowel. On microscopy, the dihydrate crystals appear "envelope" shaped while the monohydrate may have a spindle, oval, or dumbbell appearance. (B) Calcium phosphate stones tend to form in alkaline urine such as in patients with renal tubular acidosis. Calcium phosphate stones also share some of the risk factors for calcium oxalate including dehydration, hypercalciuria, and hypocitraturia. Other causes include chronic ingestion of antacids. (C) Cystine stones are associated with the rare genetic disorder cystinuria where patients have a problem with renal cystine transport. On microscopy, cystine stones appear hexagonal shaped. (E) Uric acid stones tend to form in conditions with concentrated acidic urine. Medical conditions associated with uric acid stones include diabetes mellitus, gout, Lesch-Nyhan syndrome, chronic diarrhea or dehydration, high protein diet, and others. On microscopy, uric acid stones are negatively birefringent with polarization and appear needle shaped.

4 A 39-year-old white woman presents with chronic complaints of nighttime frequency, urgency, and pelvic pain with intercourse. She has a history of depression and fibromyalgia. Multiple workups including several urinalysis and urine cultures in the past have failed to find a cause for her symptoms. On cystoscopy, several ulcerative patches surrounded by mucosal edema are seen on the dome of the bladder. A biopsy of the patches reveals mucosal ulceration, chronic inflammatory cells, fibrinous exudate, and necrotic debris. Which of the following is the most likely diagnosis?

(A) Bladder carcinoma
(B) Chronic bacterial cystitis
(C) Interstitial cystitis
(D) Radiation cystitis
(E) Somatization disorder

The answer is C: Interstitial cystitis. This patient's presentation is most consistent with a diagnosis of interstitial cystitis, also called painful bladder syndrome. This diagnosis is one of exclusion. There are both ulcerative and nonulcerative subtypes of interstitial cystitis. Biopsy and cystoscopy are often normal. In many cases, interstitial cystitis is associated with other conditions such as depression, anxiety, irritable bowel syndrome, fibromyalgia, and Sjogren syndrome. Typically, patients present with suprapubic pain related to bladder filling accompanied by increased frequency. There must be no urinary infection or other obvious pathology for the diagnosis to be established. On biopsy, the ulcerative type will classically have Hunner ulcers, which are characterized on cystoscopy as reddened mucosal areas with small vessels radiating toward a central scar accompanied by fibrin deposition, rupture, and/or oozing. Nonulcerative types may have normal appearing epithelium or multiple glomerulations.

(A) On cystoscopy, bladder carcinoma will appear as a solid mass or delicate fronds on the bladder mucosa. Patients with bladder cancer frequently have hematuria. However, patients with bladder lesions on cystoscopy are almost always biopsied to rule out cancer. Microscopically, bladder cancer usually consists of neoplastic and atypical cells. This patient's cystoscopy and pathologic findings are not consistent with bladder cancer. (B) Chronic bacterial cystitis can have similar symptoms. However, there are often white blood cells and blood in the urine and urine culture will usually identify bacteria. Biopsy may have similar findings with bacteria present. (D) Radiation cystitis can occur in patients with a history of radiation to the pelvis, such as patients with a history of pelvic tumors. Cystoscopy findings in radiation cystitis include telengectasias, diffuse erythema, prominent submucosal vascularity, and mucosal edema. Biopsy of radiation cystitis will show hemorrhage and hemosiderin, fibrin deposition, acute and chronic inflammation, edema, thickened mucosal folds, vascular ectasias, and other changes. (E) Although chronic pelvic pain can be a feature of somatization disorder, this patient does not meet the criteria for somatization disorder. Additionally, the cystoscopy is abnormal. Somatization disorder is characterized by the following:

1. A history of somatic complaints starting prior to age 30.
2. At least four different sites of pain on the body. At least two sites must be gastrointestinal. One must be sexual in nature and another must be a pseudoneurologic symptom.
3. The complaints or symptoms above must not be fully explained by general medical condition or substance abuse.
4. Complaints must not be feigned.

5 A 67-year-old man presents with significant frequency, excessive dribbling after urination, hesitancy, and nocturia. He reports that these symptoms have been progressively getting worse over the last year and are causing him stress. A digital rectal examination (DRE) reveals a diffusely enlarged but soft prostate without nodules or irregularity. Laboratory studies including a urinalysis are unremarkable and a serum prostate-specific antigen is 1.4 ng/mL. Which of the following is the best management for this patient?

(A) Diphenhydramine
(B) Observation
(C) Prostatectomy
(D) Tamulosin
(E) Transuretheral resection of the prostate

The answer is D: Tamulosin. This patient is presenting with signs and symptoms of moderate benign prostatic hyperplasia (BPH). This is a common condition in elderly men (over 50) caused by prostate enlargement and progressive slowing or blocking of the urine stream. Men often present with gradual onset of symptoms such as frequency, weak urine stream, leaking/dribbling, and nocturia. Medications and lifestyle change are typically the initial management. There are currently two classes of medications that are used for treating BPH: α-blockers and α-reductase inhibitors. α-Blockers include medications such as tamulosin and work by relaxing the muscle of the bladder neck. α-Reductase medications include drugs like finasteride. These medications prevent growth or may even shrink the prostate gland and work best in men with large prostates. Both classes of drugs may be used in combination.

(A) Diphenhydramine is an antihistamine that can actually worsen symptoms of BPH. Medications such as antihistamines and decongestants should be discontinued if possible in men with BPH. (B) This man is symptomatic with stress from his symptoms. Observation is not indicated at this time. Observation may be appropriate in asymptomatic men with BPH. (C) Prostatectomy is too invasive to perform on this patient. Prostatectomies are generally reserved for patients with prostate cancer. (E) Transurethral resection of the prostate is a surgical treatment that can help with BPH. It is generally used after medical therapy and lifestyle changes have failed to improve symptoms.

---

6 A 69-year-old man presents with worsening urinary symptoms over the last several years. He reports that he sometimes has difficulty starting urination. On further questioning, he admits to frequency, dribbling, and nocturia. He denies dysuria or hematuria. His past medical history is remarkable for hypertension, for which he takes metoprolol. He smokes 1 pack per day for the last 50 years. He says that his father had prostate cancer, but died shortly after a stroke at age 80. His body temperature is 37.1°C, blood pressure 135/85 mmHg, pulse 85 beats/min, and respirations 16 breaths/min. An abdominal and genitourinary examination is unremarkable. Which of the following is the next best step in diagnosis?

(A) Cystoscopy
(B) Digital rectal exam (DRE)
(C) Prostate-specific antigen
(D) Ultrasound
(E) Urinalysis

The answer is B: **Digital rectal exam (DRE).** This patient is presenting with signs and symptoms of benign prostatic hyperplasia (BPH). However, considering his other risk factors, prostate cancer should be ruled out. The initial step in any suspected diagnosis of prostate pathology should be a DRE. In BPH, the prostate will be diffusely enlarged. In prostate cancer, it will be nodular, firm, and irregular.

(A) Cystoscopy is generally not required in the workup of BPH. (C) Although prostate-specific antigen (PSA) measurement would most likely be part of this patient's workup, a DRE should be the initial step in diagnosis. (D) Ultrasonography is useful for determining bladder and prostate size, along with the presence of hydronephrosis if present. However, it is generally not considered an essential part of the workup. Other tests such as a DRE, serum PSA, and urinalysis are usually higher yield in the initial workup. (E) Urinalysis is also part of the initial workup for BPH. However, DRE is the initial clinical test that should be performed on any patient with symptoms of BPH.

7　A 55-year-old man with a long history of smoking presents for evaluation of a right renal mass found incidentally on imaging after a car accident. He was discharged from the hospital after the accident without any major injuries. He is currently asymptomatic. Magnetic resonance imaging (MRI) is shown in *Figures 21-2A and B*.

Laboratory studies show normal renal function. Which of the following is the next best step in management?

(A) Bone scan
(B) Computed tomography–guided percutaneous biopsy
(C) Nephrectomy
(D) Nephrectomy with lymph node dissection
(E) Observation

The answer is C: **Nephrectomy.** This patient is presenting with a solid renal mass concerning for malignancy as shown on MRI. Based on the tumor size (greater than 1.5 cm), this tumor has a high probability of being renal cell carcinoma. Renal cell carcinoma is most common in men in their 50s or 60s. Smoking is a major risk factor. With the widespread use of imaging, many kidney cancers are found incidentally, and it is less common for patients to present with the classic triad of hematuria, flank pain, and a palpable mass. Currently, the best treatment for a solid renal mass is nephrectomy (partial or complete) with pathologic diagnosis after resection.

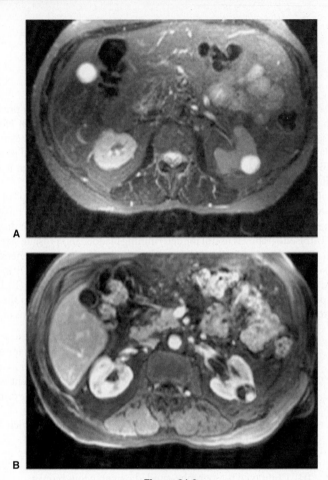

Figure 21-2

(A) Bone scans are generally recommended in patients with symptoms of bone metastasis or laboratory evidence of bone involvement such as an elevated alkaline phosphatase. (B) Percutaneous biopsy of renal cell carcinoma is not recommended due to the high level of false-negative results and high preoperative probability that this mass is renal cell carcinoma. (D) Lymph node dissection is generally not performed with localized disease. There is some recent evidence that extended lymph node dissection may be beneficial in patients with locally advanced disease and/or unfavorable clinical and pathologic characteristics. (E) Observation may be appropriate for solid renal masses found incidentally that are less than 1.5 cm.

8 A 60-year-old man presents with a 2-cm fungating mass on his right glans penis that has been growing for the last 6 months. On physical examination, there is left inguinal lymphadenopathy. Biopsy reveals a poorly differentiated squamous cell carcinoma. A partial penectomy is performed and the specimen sent for final pathologic diagnosis. Pathologic workup shows clear (greater than 2 cm) surgical margins and the tumor invading into the spongiosum. What is the next best management for this patient?

(A) Delayed lymphadenectomy
(B) Immediate bilateral inguinal lymphadenectomy
(C) Immediate left inguinal lymphadenectomy
(D) Observation and close follow-up
(E) Palliative care

The answer is B: **Immediate bilateral inguinal lymphadenectomy.** This patient has a poorly differentiated penile malignancy. Unfortunately, patients with poorly differentiated squamous cell carcinoma of the penis that invades into the penile spongiosum or cavernosum (T2) have a high rate of lymph node metastasis (approximately 20%) even with nonpalpable nodes. Since the lymphatic drainage of the penis has some crossover, contralateral metastasis can occur. Thus bilateral lymph node dissection is necessary in these patients. The dissection should be performed as soon as possible since delayed lymphadenectomy is associated with decreased survival.

(A) Delayed lymphadenectomy has been shown to have worse long-term prognosis in patients positive for nodal metastasis. (C) Although the left nodes will need to be removed, the lymphatic drainage of the penis is to both sides. (D) Surveillance has been used with low-grade disease, clear surgical margins, and clinically/radiologically negative nodal metastasis. (E) The decision to undergo palliative care is reserved for patients with advanced cancer who do not wish to undergo treatment.

9 A 72-year-old man complains of back pain and difficulty urinating. A digital rectal examination (DRE) reveals a hard and irregular-shaped prostate. Laboratory studies show a prostate-specific antigen of 19 ng/mL. A bone scan of the spine reveals multiple osteoblastic lesions. Which of the following is the next best step in management?

(A) Brachytherapy
(B) Androgen deprivation therapy
(C) Observation
(D) Radical prostatectomy
(E) Radiotherapy

The answer is B: **Androgen deprivation therapy.** This patient is suffering from metastatic prostate cancer. Since metastatic prostate cancer is not curable, the management typically focuses on relief of symptoms such as this patient's back pain and difficulty urinating. The initial step is a trial of medical orchiectomy or surgical orchiectomy. Androgen deprivation therapy is usually recommended as the initial pharmacologic step and can be accomplished with several medications that include gonadotropin-releasing hormone agonist (GnRH) agonists.

(A) Brachytherapy involves ultrasound-guided transperineal placement of radioactive seeds (iodine-125 or palladium-103). In general, brachytherapy is only recommended for local disease (less than T2a, Gleason score less than 6, and serum prostate-specific antigen [PSA] less than 10 ng/mL). (C) Observation would not be appropriate as this patient is symptomatic and can benefit from treatment. (D) Radical prostatectomy is the standard therapy for patients with localized disease and survival expectations of greater than 10 years. (E) Radiotherapy may be an option if medical or surgical orchiectomy fails to control this patient's symptoms.

 10 A 72-year-old man complains of fever, chills, dysuria, and pelvic pain that has been present for the last few days. Over the last several hours, he has also had difficulty voiding. His body temperature is 38.3°C, blood pressure 130/80 mmHg, pulse 100 beats/min, and respirations 18 breaths/min. A digital rectal exam reveals a tender and boggy prostate. Which of the following is the next best step in diagnosis?

(A) Midstream urinalysis and Gram stain
(B) Pelvic CT scan
(C) Prostate biopsy
(D) Prostatic message and secretion analysis
(E) Prostate-specific antigen measurement

The answer is A: **Midstream urinalysis and Gram stain.** This patient is most likely suffering from acute bacterial prostatitis. In elderly men, the most common pathogen is infection with *Escherichia coli*. Other pathogens in older men include *Proteus mirabilis* and *Klebsiella* species. In younger men, sexually transmitted organisms such as *Neisseria* or *Chlamydia* should be suspected. Acute prostatitis usually only occurs with predisposing risk factors such as bladder outlet obstruction or an immunosuppressed state. Workup for acute bacterial prostatitis includes a midstream urine analysis (or alternatively a urethral swab culture). This information along with the history and physical examination findings are usually sufficient to diagnose bacterial prostatitis. Treatment with antibiotics is generally indicated. Useful classes are typically directed against gram negative and include floroquinolones, trimethoprim–sulfamethoxazole, gentamicin, and ampicillin.

(B) Pelvic CT scan may be considered if the urinalysis and laboratory studies are equivocal or when no improvement is seen after medical therapy. (C) Biopsy is contraindicated in patients with acute bacterial prostatitis because of the potential to seed bacteria into the bloodstream or adjacent organs. (D) Prostatic message is contraindicated in patients with acute bacterial prostatitis. (E) Prostate-specific antigen (PSA) measurement may suggest a diagnosis of prostatitis if elevated, but is not essential to the workup.

11 A 65-year-old man is brought to the physician by his wife after she notices blood in his semen after sexual intercourse over the last 5 months. On further questioning, the man admits to occasional urinary problems including frequency and nocturia. He denies recent trauma, dysuria, fatigue, or weight loss. He has a 30-pack-year smoking history. His body temperature is 37.1°C, blood pressure 140/85 mmHg, pulse 65 beats/min, and respirations 14 breaths/min. A digital rectal examination (DRE) reveals a nodular and hard prostate. The remainder of the physical examination including a careful genital examination and urinalysis is unremarkable. Which of the following is the next best step in management?

(A) Measurement of prostate-specific antigen
(B) No further workup necessary
(C) Transrectal prostate biopsy
(D) Trimethoprim–sulfamethoxazole
(E) Total prostatectomy

The answer is A: Measurement of prostate-specific antigen. This patient has signs, symptoms, and risk factors concerning for prostate cancer. The next best step is measurement of prostate-specific antigen, especially in a man older than 50 years. Other tests that should be performed include semen analysis and culture. Based on these results, additional studies including imaging may be performed.

(B) Although the majority of hematospermia is benign, this patient has a hard and indurated prostate on digital rectal exam and needs a full workup. (C) If this patient's prostate-specific antigen (PSA) were found to be elevated, the next step would be a transrectal prostate biopsy. (D) Acute or chronic prostatitis may cause hematospermia. Urinalysis or semen culture would typically reveal evidence of infection. If this were the case in this patient, trimethoprim–sulfamethoxazole might be an appropriate next step for this patient. (E) Although total prostatectomy may be required if this patient has prostate cancer, it is not the next best step as a diagnosis should be obtained first.

12 A 42-year-old man complains of pain and excessive curvature during erections. He reports that the problem has been getting worse over the last several years and has been putting a lot of stress on his sex life.

A genitourinary examination reveals a palpable fibrous plaque on the dorsum of the penile shaft and curvature of 40 degrees. Which of the following is the best initial treatment of his condition?

(A) Biopsy
(B) Pentoxifyline
(C) Plaque excision
(D) Potassium para-aminobenzoate
(E) Vitamin E

The answer is B: **Pentoxifyline.** This patient has signs and symptoms consistent with Peyronie disease. The etiology of Peyronie disease is unknown, but most evidence points to multifactorial contributing factors including trauma, tissue ischemia, and genetics. Common symptoms include penile pain, nodularity, induration, curvature, sexual dysfunction, all of which are worse during erections. Either observation or medical management is appropriate for most patients initially, with observation often utilized in patients with less than 30-degree curvature and satisfactory erectile function. First-line medical therapy for Peyronie disease is pentoxifyline, which is thought to prevent collagen deposition. Other medical options include vitamin E, potassium para-aminobenzoate, colchicine, verapamil, and others.

(A) Biopsy is generally not required unless carcinoma is suspected. (C) Surgery is generally reserved for patients with erectile dysfunction or severe and progressive disease refractory to medical management. (D) Potassium para-aminobenzoate is an antifibrotic agent that was historically first-line treatment. However, current evidence does not support this as first-line therapy due to significant cost and difficulty ingesting the required and numerous tablets per day. (E) Vitamin E has poor efficacy in several randomized trials and is no longer recommended as a treatment option for Peyronie disease.

13 During a newborn examination, the physician notices that the baby is urinating fine. The mother requests that the child be circumcised and it is scheduled for the next day. Just before the circumcision procedure, the penis is examined, and shown in the picture in *Figure 21-3*.
    Which of the following is the next best step in management?

(A) Complete the circumcision now
(B) Halt the surgery and request a urologic evaluation
(C) Observation
(D) Start hormonal therapy
(E) Surgical correction after age 8

The answer is B: **Halt the surgery and request a urologic evaluation.** This patient has hypospadias. Since the hypospadias is severe, it may be problematic as the child grows. Treatment for hypospadias is surgical. It is usually corrected 4 to 18 months of age. The goals of repair typically include creating a

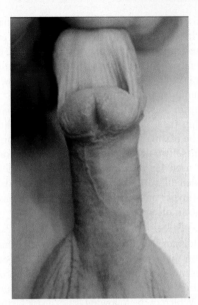

Figure 21-3

straight penis (if associated curvature is present), creating a urethra at the tip of the penis, and reforming the glans into a more natural shape. Overall, a more cosmetically acceptable penis and scrotum should be achieved. Often, foreskin can be utilized in the reconstruction. Thus, in this case the circumcision should be halted and a urologic evaluation completed.

(A) Completing the circumcision would remove valuable skin that could be used in reconstruction. (C) Observation alone is not the correct treatment in severe cases of hypospadias. It is sometimes used in cases of mild hypospadias. (D) Hormonal therapy is only sometimes used in hypospadias if the penis is small. (E) Surgical correction after age 8 is not appropriate as it is associated with an increased risk of complications such as urethrocutaneous fisultas.

 A 73-year-old man complains of poor erections. He says that he has difficulty obtaining an erection when he wants to and that the quality of his erections is poor. He reports no morning erections. He is prescribed sildenafil and asked to return in several weeks for follow-up. Which of the following medications should be avoided while taking sildenafil?

(A) Azythromycin
(B) Dapoxetine
(C) Isosorbide dinitrate
(D) Metoprolol
(E) Metformin

The answer is C: Isosorbide dinitrate. In most situations, phosphodiesterase 5 (PDE5) inhibitors are safe to use to help with erections. However, there are certain medications that should be avoided while using PDE5 inhibitors. These include nitrate medications such as isosorbide dinitrate, isosorbide mononitrate, and nitroglycerin. Taking PDE5 inhibitors with these drugs can result in life-threatening hypotension.

(A) Azythromycin does not affect the metabolism of sildenafil. However, erythromycin inhibits the CYP3A4 pathway involved in sildenafil metabolism and may increase the plasma levels of the drug. Thus, caution should be used when combining these two drugs. (B) Dapoxetine is a short-acting serotonin reuptake inhibitor used for premature ejaculation in men. It is sometimes combined with sildenafil. (D) Although sildenafil should be used with caution with other antihypertensive medications (such as metopralol), they are not necessarily contraindicated when used together.

 A 43-year-old man presents with a "weird growth" that has been increasing in size on his penis. He reports that it has been there for several years but has more recently started to bleed and become painful. Physical examination reveals a 2 cm × 1 cm exophytic and hard mass on the glans penis. Which of the following is not a risk factor for this problem?

(A) Chronic balantitis
(B) Cigarette smoking
(C) Human papilloma virus (HPV)
(D) Phimosis
(E) Presence of foreskin

The answer is E: Presence of foreskin. The presence of foreskin is not necessarily a risk factor for penile cancer. Current research suggests that the presence of foreskin itself is not a risk factor if proper hygiene is maintained, rather that the buildup of smegma and/or failure to clean underneath the foreskin are responsible for the increase in incidence in penile cancer in uncircumcised male population.

(A) Chronic balantitis and other conditions associated with inflammation are associated with an increased risk of penile cancer. (B) Cigarette smoking has been shown to increase the risk of penile cancer in men. (C) Infection with certain types of HPV may significantly increase the risk of penile cancer in men. Similar to cervical cancer, HPV subtypes 6 and 11 are generally benign but may cause genital warts. High-risk subtypes include HPV 16, 18, 31, and others. (D) Studies show that phimosis is one of the strongest risk factors for penile cancer.

 A 32-year-old man with a history of type 1 diabetes presents to the emergency department with an acute onset of pain in his genitalia. He has since developed fever and chills and says his scrotum has become itchy. He rates his pain as "10/10." He denies trauma to the area. A genitourinary examination reveals mild edema and erythema of the scrotum. Computed tomography imaging of his pelvis reveals several small empty spaces in the soft tissue near his scrotum. Which of the following is the next best step in management?

(A) Emergent surgery
(B) Hyperbaric oxygen
(C) Intravenous antibiotics and observation
(D) Intravenous crystalloids and insulin
(E) Oral antibiotics and follow-up

The answer is A: Emergent surgery. This patient is presenting with signs, symptoms, and imaging concerning for developing Fournier gangrene. Fournier gangrene is a rapidly progressing necrotizing fasciitis of the male genitalia and perineum. The most common pathogen is *E. coli*, but other organisms commonly occur as well. The infection travels along fascial planes (dartos fascia, Colles fascia, and Scarpa fascia) and primarily involves the subcutaneous tissue. Common sources of infection include the lower genitourinary tract and cutaneous infections of the genitals, perineum, or anus. Risk factors include alcohol, diabetes, and other immunocompromised states. Patients often present with painful swelling and induration of the genital tissue. The pain may be significantly out of proportion to the physical examination findings. As the infection progresses, fever, necrosis, crepitus, and other signs may ensue. The diagnosis is clinical, but CT imaging may show subcutaneous gas collection as in this patient. Treatment is emergent and aggressive surgical debridement.

(B) Hyperbaric oxygen may be useful in postoperative management but is not part of the initial treatment. (C) Although broad-spectrum intravenous antibiotics are indicated as an initial treatment, these patients will need emergent surgery. Observation is not appropriate. (D) Intravenous crystalloids should be provided aggressively with presentation. However, insulin is not part of the initial treatment and may be more appropriate if the patient was presenting with diabetic ketoacidosis. (E) Patients will need broad-spectrum intravenous antibiotics. Oral antibiotics would most likely not be potent enough for treatment.

17 A recently married 29-year-old man presents with a "swollen" scrotum that his wife "wanted me to see a doctor" for. He says that he first noticed the swelling when he was a teenager. He states that he "really isn't that concerned" because it does not cause him discomfort. He reports that the swelling is worse when he is standing. His body temperature is 37.2°C, blood pressure 128/72 mmHg, pulse 65 beats/min, and respirations 15 breaths/min. On examination, the left scrotum has grossly visible dilated vessels that are more pronounced during Valsalva.

The remainder of his genitourinary examination is unremarkable. Which of the following should be part of the initial workup for this patient?

(A) Computed tomography scan of the abdomen
(B) Magnetic resonance imaging (MRI) of the scrotum
(C) Semen analysis
(D) Surgical correction
(E) Urethral swab and culture

The answer is C: Semen analysis. This patient is most likely presenting with a varicocele, which are dilated veins in the pampiniform plexus. They are most common on the left side and occur in approximately 15% of the population. Although not all varicoceles cause infertility, they are present in a significant proportion of subfertile men. With this recently married young man, semen analysis should be part of the initial workup. Semen analysis may show decreased motility (most common finding), low sperm count, and increased abnormal forms.

(A) Right-sided varicoceles or varicoceles that have a rapid/recent onset may indicate a possible renal mass. In these patients, abdominal imaging such as computed tomography should be considered. (B) MRI may be considered for abdominal imaging when a renal mass is suspected as the cause of a varicocele, although it is usually more expensive and less preferred than other imaging modalities. This patient has a long-standing varicocele on the left side, which is unlikely caused by a renal tumor. (D) Surgical correction may be considered in patients with symptomatic varicoceles, abnormal semen analysis, or in adolescents with ipsilateral testicular atrophy. (E) This patient does not have features of a sexually transmitted disease and is an unlikely cause of this patient's symptoms.

  A 28-year-old man presents with a left scrotal mass he felt during a self-examination in the shower. His past medical history is unremarkable and he does not take any medications. He denies pain or discomfort. On examination, there is a 2-cm palpable but painless soft mass protruding from the lateral left testicle. A radical orchiectomy is performed and the pathology returns as a nonseminomatous germ cell tumor. Which of the following tumor markers may assist in the management of this patient?

(A) α-Fetoprotein (AFP) and CA-125
(B) β-Human chorionic gonadotropin (β-HCG) and AFP
(C) β-HCG, AFP, and lactate dehydrogenase (LDH)
(D) β-HCG and CA-125
(E) CA-125 and LDH

The answer is C: β-HCG, AFP, and lactate dehydrogenase (LDH). Tumor markers may assist in the diagnosis and management of testicular tumors. For nonseminomatous tumors, serum levels of AFP and/or β-HCG are elevated in approximately 80% to 85% of patients. In addition, LDH has independent prognostic significance, which indicates tumor burden, growth rate, and proliferation. LDH is elevated in 60% of patients with nonseminomatous tumors. However, LDH is not useful in posttreatment surveillance because it lacks sensitivity and specificity.

(A) Although AFP is helpful in the management of nonseminomatous germ cell tumors, CA-125 is a tumor marker for epithelial ovarian cancer and is not helpful for testicular cancer. (B) Although β-hCG and AFP will both assist in the diagnosis of nonseminomatous testicular cancers, LDH should be performed along with these tumor markers for independent prognostic significance. (D) Although β-hCG would assist in the management, CA-125 would not. (E) Out of these tumor markers, only LDH would assist in the management of this patient.

---

 19 A 60-year-old man with a long history of smoking is referred by his primary care physician for persistent gross hematuria and irritation while voiding. A cystoscopy is performed which shows diffuse velvety patches of erythematous urothelium. Random bladder biopsy shows urothelial carcinoma in situ (CIS) in 80% of the samples. Treatment for this patient involves which of the following?

(A) Intravesicle bacillus Calmette-Guérin (BCG)
(B) Methotrexate, vinblastine, adriamycin, and cisplatin
(C) Radical cystectomy
(D) Single intravesical dose of mytomycin
(E) Transurethral resection of bladder tumors followed by intravesical BCG

The answer is A: Intravesicle bacillus Calmette-Guérin (BCG). This patient has urothelial CIS. CIS is defined as urothelial cancer that is flat, high grade but noninvasive. Unfortunately when it is this diffuse, it is nonresectable by a transurethral approach. The current standard of treatment for diffuse CIS is intravesical BCG. BCG is an attenuated live vaccine of *Mycobacterium bovis* that has been shown to be effective in eradication of CIS. It works by stimulating the body's own immune system to destroy tumor cells. Multiple BCG instillations are required in the treatment over a 6-week period. Up to 70% of patients have a complete initial response to BCG. Of these patients, 52% to 71% are disease free at 5 years.

(B) Methotrexate, vinblastine, adriamycin (doxorubicin), and cisplatin is the chemotherapy regimen recommended for advanced bladder cancer. It is not used for CIS. (C) Radical cystectomy is the treatment of choice for T2–T4a bladder cancer. (D) A single dose of mytomycin is often used after transurethral resection of bladder tumors prior to BCG therapy. (E) Transurethral resection of bladder tumors followed by intravesical BCG is the standard of treatment for Ta and T1 disease.

20 A 69-year-old woman with a history of colon cancer, diabetes mellitus, and chronic obstructive pulmonary disease secondary to smoking receives cystoscopy as part of a workup for irritative voiding symptoms. During the cystoscopy, a bladder mass is found and transurethral resection of the bladder tumor is performed. Part of her treatment after resection involves intravesical instillation of Bacillus Calmette-Guérin (BCG). Which of the following is not a contraindication to BCG therapy?

(A) Active urinary tract infection (UTI)
(B) Microscopic hematuria
(C) Patient taking steroids
(D) Recent traumatic catheterization
(E) Within 2 weeks of transurethral resection of bladder tumor (TURBT)

The answer is B: Microscopic hematuria. BCG therapy is an effective treatment for early bladder cancers. However, it is not without side effects and potential complications. Common side effects include cystitis, dysuria, hematuria, malaise, fatigue, and low-grade fevers that usually resolve. A more serious but rare complication is BCG sepsis. Many of the contraindications to BCG therapy are to decrease this risk. Contraindications include gross hematuria, instillation of BCG within 2 weeks of the TURBT procedure, active UTIs, sepsis, high fever, immunosuppressed states, or previous BCG sepsis. Microscopic hematuria is not a contraindication for BCG therapy.

(A) Active UTIs increase the risk for BCG introduction into the blood and BCG sepsis. (C) Patients taking steroids are immunosuppressed and have an increased risk of BCG sepsis. (D) A recent traumatic catheterization increases the risk of introducing BCG into the bloodstream, which could cause BCG sepsis. (E) BCG therapy within 2 weeks of a TURBT procedure increases the risk of introducing BCG into the bloodstream through the resected tumor bed.

21 A 45-year-old man presents with acute episodes of left flank pain that radiate to the groin. He reports this has happened once before but resolved after a few hours and passage of the stone. His records indicate the stone was calcium oxalate. Today, his body temperature is 36.7°C, blood pressure 130/85 mmHg, pulse 100 beats/min, and respirations 18 breaths/min. On examination, there is left costovertebral tenderness. A computed tomography scan reveals a 9 mm stone in the distal ureter. Which of the following is the next best step in management?

(A) Alkalization of the urine, increased hydration, and pain management
(B) Extracorporeal shock wave lithotripsy (ESWL) and placement of ureteral stent
(C) Percutaneous nephrolithotomy
(D) Surveillance, increased fluid intake, and pain management
(E) Ureteroscopy with stone removal and placement of ureteral stent

The answer is E: Ureteroscopy with stone removal and placement of ureteral stent. This patient has an obstructing stone in the distal ureter that is unlikely to pass on its own due to its size. The treatment of choice for distal ureteral stones is ureteroscopy with stone removal. Since ureteral edema is a common complication of stone removal, a stent is often placed after the procedure.

(A) Alkalization of the urine can assist with the dissolution of uric acid stones. This is an unlikely composition of stone for this patient. (B) ESWL does not work well with stones in the distal ureter or those that are composed of calcium oxylate. (C) Percutaneous nephrolithotomy is a surgical procedure reserved for large renal or proximal ureter stone burdens, stones in calyceal diverticulum, ureteropelvic junction obstructions, and staghorn calculi. (D) Surveillance, increased fluid intake, and pain management are a conservative management that works best for stones likely to pass on their own (small distal ureter stones).

 22 A 39-year-old business executive complaining of severe penile pain is brought to the emergency department by a scantily dressed woman. He says that he is currently on a business trip and was just "partying with some friends" when he "fell" onto his penis. At that time, he reports he heard a "pop." His body temperature is 36.7°C, blood pressure 140/90 mmHg, pulse 105 beats/min, and respirations 20 breaths/min. On examination, there is a large hematoma with echymosis on the shaft of his penis. Which of the following is the next best step in management?

(A) Cavernosography
(B) Close observation and fluid resuscitation
(C) Immediate surgical repair
(D) Penile magnetic resonance imaging
(E) Penile ultrasound

The answer is C: Immediate surgical repair. This patient is presenting with a history and physical strongly suggestive of a penile fracture. When the clinical suspicion is high as in this case and there are no signs of urethral trauma, the initial step is immediate surgical repair. Imaging studies are generally not performed with the exception of a retrograde urethrography to assess for urethral trauma.

(A) Cavernosography can help reveal extravasation of contrast to confirm penile fracture. However, it is generally only performed when the diagnosis is in doubt. When used, it should not delay surgical treatment. (B) Although fluid resuscitation is important in the treatment of penile fracture, observation would be a huge mistake. (D) Penile MRI has the advantage of providing excellent imaging of the anatomy including tears or urethral injury. However, it is slow and is generally not recommended. (E) Although ultrasound has been suggested as a useful imaging modality in penile fractures, it is generally not used and would only serve to delay surgical treatment in this case.

23 A 76-year-old obese woman presents to her primary care physician because of a 1-year history of urinary incontinence. She has had five children. She says that she has to wear pads to avoid embarrassment. She admits that she leaks a small amount of urine each time she coughs, sneezes, and laughs. She denies irritative or obstructive urinary symptoms. Female pelvic examination reveals a hypermobile urethra and urine loss with cough. What is the most appropriate initial treatment for this patient?

(A) Intermittent self-urinary catheterization every 6 hours
(B) Oxybutynin
(C) Pelvic floor exercise, weight loss, and bladder training
(D) Transcutaneous or sacral nerve stimulation
(E) Vaginal sling and cystocele repair

The answer is C: Pelvic floor exercise, weight loss, and bladder training. This patient is presenting with pure stress incontinence, which should always be managed conservatively if possible. Conservative treatments include weight loss, diet modification (avoiding coffee, alcohol, carbonated beverages, etc.), bladder training, and pelvic floor (kegal) exercises. If these interventions do not work, then more aggressive measures such as surgery may be considered.

(A) Although diet modification may help with stress incontinence, intermittent catheterization generally does not. (B) Oxybutynin is an anticholinergic agent used to treat urge incontinence. It is generally not helpful for stress incontinence. (D) Sacral nerve stimulation involves implantation of a programmable stimulator that delivers low-amplitude electrical signals to sacral nerves to treat urinary incontinence, retention, and other issues. Since it is noninvasive and effective, it is gaining popularity for treating neurogenic bladder. However, it is not useful for stress incontinence since the problem is not neural in nature. (E) Vaginal slings are an option for treating stress incontinence in select patients when more conservative therapy has failed. This patient has no evidence of cystocele on examination.

24 A 31-year-old man presents to the walk-in clinic of the local emergency department with a painless right testicular mass. He reports that it has been growing over the last several months. On examination, there is small but palpable a hard nonmobile mass on the inferior right testicle. His serum placental alkaline phosphatase is increased. The tumor is excised and sent for pathologic examination. Gross examination of the tissue reveals a yellow uniform and well-circumscribed bulging mass.

Histologic examination reveals sheets of uniform large cells with abundant cytoplasm and minimal mitotic figures. What is the most likely diagnosis?

(A) Gonadoblastoma
(B) Leydig tumor
(C) Seminoma
(D) Sertoli cell tumor
(E) Teratoma

The answer is C: Seminoma. This patient is most likely suffering from a seminoma, a type of germ cell tumor. Germ cell tumors are the most common malignancy of men aged 15 to 35. Of these, seminomas account for approximately 1/3 of the diagnosis. The most common clinical presentation is a painless testicular lump. They are usually found at stage 1 and the prognosis for such patients is excellent. Seminomas appear grossly yellow and histologically as uniform populations of large cells that form sheets and nests. Serum placental alkaline phosphatase is elevated in a majority of patients.

(A) Gonadoblastomas grossly appear lobulated and histologically as complex mixture of different gonadal cells. It occurs almost exclusively in patients with disorders of sex development. (B) Leydig tumors are tumors of the gonadal interstitium. Since the tumors are typically hormonally active, feminizing or virilizing symptoms are common complaints. Grossly they appear as a solid and well-circumscribed nodule with a gold-brown cut surface. Microscopically the tumor will appear as sheets of round/polygonal cells with eosinophilic cytoplasm. Occasionally, Reinke crystals may be present. (D) Sertoli cell tumors are a type of sex cord stromal tumor derived from Sertoli cells, which are located in the seminiferous tubules. These cells normally function to support spermatogenesis. The tumors grossly appear as well-circumscribed yellow, white, or gray masses. Histologically they are composed of solid tubules containing Sertoli cells arranged in cords, nests, or sheets. Since these cells secrete testosterone, female candidates may have masculinization. (E) Teratomas are germ cell tumors composed of multiple cell types from three or more germ cell layers. Testicular teratomas usually present as a painless firm scrotal mass without accompanying symptoms. Histologically, there are multiple cell types, which may include skin, hair, sebaceous glands, sweat glands, and many other tissue types.

 25 A 26-year-old man presents to the emergency department with severe right scrotal pain. The pain started when he was playing basketball an hour earlier and has been progressing since. He admits that he was recently on a business trip where he had a new sexual partner. His body temperature is 102.5°F, blood pressure 130/85 mmHg, pulse 100 beats/min, and respirations 20 breaths/min. On examination, his left testicle appears swollen and erythematous. It is also tender to palpation. Urinalysis reveals increased leukocytes. Which of the following is the next best step in management?

(A) Ceftriaxone
(B) Repeat examination in 1 week with primary care physician
(C) Scrotal biopsy
(D) Testicular ultrasound
(E) Urine analysis and culture

The answer is D: Testicular ultrasound. This patient's presentation could be explained by several conditions including acute epididymitis and testicular torsion. This patient will need a testicular ultrasound to rule out testicular torsion since it is the most damaging possibility. If the testicle is found to be torsed, the patient will need immediate exploration and detorsion in the operating room.

(A) Ceftriaxone might be appropriate if the patient has acute epididymitis. However, testicular torsions should be ruled out first. (B) Observation would be inappropriate as this patient is in severe pain and testicular torsion must be ruled out. (C) Scrotal biopsy is unnecessary at this point. If continued workup fails to identify the problem, biopsy may be considered. (E) Although this patient's urine should be sent for culture, testicular torsion is the most damaging possibility and should be ruled out first.

26 A 23-year-old man presents with fever and testicular pain that has been progressing over the last several days. His body temperature is 38.1°C, blood pressure 120/80 mmHg, pulse 89 beats/min, and respirations 18 breaths/min. On examination, his right testicle appears swollen and is tender to palpation. He is subsequently diagnosed with viral orchitis. Which of the following is the best management for this patient?

(A) Bed rest, hot/cold packs, and scrotal elevation
(B) Ceftriaxone
(C) Doxycycline
(D) Acyclovir
(E) Gancyclovir

The answer is A: Bed rest, hot/cold packs, and scrotal elevation. Viral orchitis is an acute inflammatory condition of the testicles secondary to a viral infection. There are many viruses that can cause orchitis including coxsackievirus, Epstein-Barr virus, varicella, echovirus, paramyxovirus (mumps), and many others. The diagnosis of viral orchitis can generally be made without an extensive workup. Treatment for viral orchitis is supportive with bed rest, hot and/or cold packs, and scrotal elevation.

(B) Ceftriaxone would help treat orchitis caused by *Neisseria gonorrhea*. (C) Doxycycline would help treat orchitis caused by *Neisseria gonorrhea*.

(D) Although acyclovir may help with some viral infections such as herpes, most cases of orchitis are self-limited and are not helped by antiviral drugs. (E) Gancyclovir is an antiviral commonly used to treat cytomegalovirus infections. It is not useful for viral orchitis.

 27 A newborn neonate presents for checkup with his pediatrician after a nurse at delivery noticed an abnormal appearing penis on the newborn examination. He was found to have a short phallus with the urethral meatus located on the dorsal penile shaft. There is no obvious defect on the abdominal wall. Which of the following conditions is associated with the same embryologic defect?

    (A) Bladder exstrophy
    (B) Cryptochordism
    (C) Ectopic scrotum
    (D) Hypospadius
    (E) Penile agenesis

The answer is A: Bladder exstrophy. This patient had epispadias as indicated by the short phallus and urethral meatus located on the dorsal penile shaft. Both epispadias and bladder exstrophy are most likely caused by the same congenital defect of cloacal membrane instability. Failure of mesenchyme to migrate between the ectodermal and endodermal layers of the lower abdominal wall results in this instability and potential cloacal rupture.

    (B) Cryptochordism is caused by a blunted testosterone embryologic response and other hormone disturbances. It is not caused by the same defect in the cloaca as epispadias. (C) Ectopic scrotal tissue is uncommon congenital abnormality where there is an abnormally positioned hemiscrotum. It usually occurs near the inguinal ring. It is not generally associated with bladder exstrophy. (D) Hypospadias is caused by incomplete fusion of the urethral groove, which results in a urethra on the ventral surface of the penis. It is not caused by the same embryologic defect as epispadias. (E) Penile agenesis is a rare disorder caused by developmental failure of the genital tubercle. It is associated with cryptochordism but is rarely associated with bladder exstrophy.

 28 A 49-year-old woman has had four documented UTIs in a 6-month time period. All of the infections were cultured and revealed *E. coli* which was pansensitive to all antibiotics. Physical examination reveals a well-developed woman who looks to be her stated age. Pelvic examination reveals mild urethral hypermobility, a grade 1 cystocele, and no evidence of stress urinary incontinence with couth or straining in the lithotomy position. Regarding these repeated infections, which of the following likely contribute to this process?

(A) Bacteriostasis
(B) Eosin
(C) Hematolyxin
(D) P-fimbriae
(E) Telomerase

The answer is D: P-fimbriae. *E. coli* is the most common cause of urinary tract infection (UTI), including cystitis and pyelonephritis. Women are particularly at risk for infection. Uncomplicated cystitis (the most commonly encountered UTI) is caused by uropathogenic strains of *E. coli*, characterized by P-fimbriae (an adherence factor) and, commonly, hemolysin, colicin V, and resistance to the bactericidal activity of serum complement. Complicated UTI (pyelonephritis) may occur in settings of obstructed urinary flow, which may be caused by nonuropathogenic strains.

(A) The mechanism of resistance may relate to the presence of colicin V. (B) The mechanism of resistance may relate to hemolysin. (C) The mechanism of resistance may relate to resistance of the bactericidal activity of serum complement. (E) Telomerase relates to the mechanism of neoplasia, not infection.

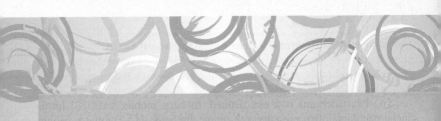

1 A 27-year-old man who weighs 70 kg presents for a body fat analysis prior to enrolling in a vigorous exercise program. Regarding the physiologic parameters in this healthy individual, which of the following statements are true?

(A) Body is 70% water by weight
(B) Estimated to have approximately 35 L of water in his body
(C) Total body water is predominantly extracellular
(D) Total body water is higher in women than in men

The answer is B: Estimated to have approximately 35 L of water in his body. The human body is 45% to 60% water by weight. In a 70-kg adult, 31.5 to 42 L of water is found throughout the body. Body mass and habitus play roles in percentage of water, as does gender with women having a slightly lower water percentage than men.

(A) The human body is 45% to 60% water by weight. (C) Total body water is predominantly intracellular comprising 60% of total body water.

2 A 54-year-old postmenopausal woman undergoes a breast biopsy for a suspected left breast lump. Physical examination reveals a 1.5-cm indurated mass lesion. The pathology report returns and indicates dilation of the subareolar ducts. Periductal inflammation, fibrosis, and ductal dilation are present. The tissue sample was 2 cm in diameter. What is the most likely diagnosis?

(A) Fibroadenoma
(B) Intraductal papilloma
(C) Lipoma
(D) Mammary duct ectasia
(E) Pseudoangiomatous hyperplasia

The answer is D: Mammary duct ectasia. This patient likely has mammary duct ectasia. This condition is characterized by dilation of the subareolar ducts with periductal inflammation and ductal dilation. It is common in perimenopausal and postmenopausal women.

(A) Fibroadenoma is a well-defined, rubbery, mobile mass. (B) Intraductal papilloma often presents with nipple discharge. (C) Lipoma is benign encapsulated adipose tissue. (E) Pseudoangiomatous hyperplasia is a benign stromal proliferation that simulates a vascular lesion.

3. In the anatomy of the femoral canal, the most lateral femoral structure in the anatomic position of the groin is:

   (A) Artery
   (B) Empty space
   (C) Lymphatics
   (D) Nerve
   (E) Vein

The answer is D: Nerve. One can use the mnemonic NAVEL (nerve, artery, veil, empty space, lymphatic) to remember the position of groin structures from lateral to medial. Nerve is the most lateral structure in the femoral canal.

(A) Artery is next most medial to the femoral nerve. (B) Empty space is not part of the mnemonic illustrated in this question. (C) Lymphatics are the most medial structure in the femoral canal. (E) The femoral vein is in the middle of the femoral canal structures between the femoral nerve and the lymphatics.

4. A 35-year-old woman with a history of multiple hamartomas scattered throughout the gastrointestinal tract presents to her primary care physician for follow-up. Physical examination reveals pigmented spots on her face and palmar surfaces of her hands. This patient is at risk for which of the following medical problems?

   (A) Brain cancer
   (B) Breast cancer
   (C) Skin cancer
   (D) Thyroid cancer
   (E) Uterine cancer

The answer is B: Breast cancer. This patient has Peutz-Jeghers syndrome. This condition is characterized by single or multiple hamartomas that can be scattered throughout the gastrointestinal (GI) tract in small bowel, colon, and stomach. Pigmented spots around the lips, oral mucosa, face, and palmar surfaces are also common. There is a slightly increased risk of various carcinomas such as stomach, ovary, breast, cervix, and lung.

(A) Peutz-Jeghers syndrome does not have an increased risk of brain cancer. (C) Peutz-Jeghers syndrome does not have an increased risk of skin cancer. (D) Peutz-Jeghers syndrome does not have an increased risk of thyroid cancer. (E) Peutz-Jeghers syndrome does not have an increased risk of uterine cancer.

 5 A 60-year-old woman presents with worsening abdominal pain of one-day duration. She also complains of nausea and two episodes of vomiting, which occurred after the pain started. While she reported that the pain was initially intermittent and diffuse, she now says that it hurts primarily in her left lower quadrant. Her temperature is 36.8°C, blood pressure 130/75 mmHg, pulse 110 beats/min, and respirations 20 breaths/min. On examination, there is tenderness in both the right and left lower quadrants. Which of the following causes of acute abdominal pain does not occur more frequently as patients age than those in younger patients?

(A) Acute appendicitis
(B) Cholecystitis
(C) Diverticulitits
(D) Intestinal obstruction
(E) Mesenteric ischemia

The answer is A: Acute appendicitis. Out of the causes of acute abdominal pain listed above, only acute appendicitis occurs more commonly in younger individuals than those that age. The incidence of appendicitis peaks in the late teens, and gradually declines with age. Interestingly, the classic picture of appendicitis is rarely seen in elderly patients as they often present more subtly.

(B) Gallstones are two to three times more frequent in female individuals than male individuals, and incidence increases with age. (C) Diverticulitis is a classic cause of abdominal pain in the elderly and increases in frequency with age. The incidence is less than 5% in patients less than 40 years old and greater than 65% in patients older than 85 years. (D) Bowel obstruction (both small and large) occurs with increasing frequency in elderly patients. (E) Mesenteric ischemia is classically caused by atherosclerotic disease associated with advancing age.

 6 A 32-year-old woman complains of frequent bruising. She reports that this bruising has been worsening over the last several months. Her physical examination is remarkable for several large areas of ecchymosis. After an exhaustive workup, the patient is diagnosed with immune thrombocytopenic purpura (ITP) and started on corticosteroids, intravenous immunoglobulin, and rituximab for 4 weeks. After several months of therapy with these medications and several others, her platelets fail to respond. Which of the following is the next best treatment for this patient?

(A) Aspirin, low dose, daily
(B) Cyclophosphamide
(C) Platelet transfusion
(D) Rho
(E) Splenectomy

The answer is E: Splenectomy. Assuming that this patient is a good surgical candidate, splenectomy is the next best step in management of this patient's ITP since it is refractory to glucocorticoid therapy. The reason for this is a higher long-term success rate with splenectomy when compared to alternative therapy options such as Rituximab.

(A) Aspirin is contraindicated in patients with ITP since it further reduces platelet function. (B) Cyclophosphamide is sometimes used in ITP that no longer have a response to other splenectomy and other medications. (C) Since the underlying autoimmune dysfunction will also destroy donor platelets, platelet transfusions are normally not recommended in patients with ITP unless there is an emergency. (D) Rho(D) immunoglobulin has been effective in some cases of ITP. However, the treatment is costly and only produces short-term improvement.

---

7 A 30-year-old man with a history of intravenous drug use and endocarditis is brought to the emergency department with fever and worsening abdominal pain. The patient localizes the pain to the upper left
quadrant. On physical examination, there is mild splenomegaly and
tenderness with guarding on the upper left abdomen. There is also mild
dullness to percussion on the left lung base. A chest radiograph shows
a left pleural effusion and elevated left hemidiaphragm. A computed
tomography (CT) scan reveals several low-density, nonenhancing,
and multiloculated lesions located within the spleen. Blood cultures
grow multiple organisms. Out of the options below, which is the best
treatment option for this patient?

(A) Broad-spectrum antibiotics and percutaneous drainage
(B) CT-guided diagnostic percutaneous aspiration
(C) Intravenous support and broad-spectrum antibiotics
(D) Splenectomy and broad-spectrum antibiotics
(E) Splenic artery embolization

The answer is D: Splenectomy and broad-spectrum antibiotics. This patient is presenting with signs and symptoms of splenic abscess. Splenic abscess typically occurs secondary to septic emboli from endocarditis or other sites of infection. Typical manifestations include fever and left upper quadrant pain. Occasionally patients may present with left-sided pleural effusion and shoulder pain related to inflammation of the left hemidiaphragm. The best way to diagnose splenic abscess is with CT imaging. The gold standard for treating splenic abscess is broad-spectrum antibiotics and splenectomy. Although percutaneous drainage may be attempted with certain abscesses (uncomplicated), it would not be recommended in this patient.

(A) Although broad-spectrum antibiotics would be important to start in this patient, percutaneous drainage would most likely not be successful with multiple lesions. (B) Although diagnostic percutaneous aspiration would be helpful in confirming the diagnosis and providing a specimen for culture, it is not necessary in this patient since he already has positive blood cultures. (C) Although intravenous support and broad-spectrum antibiotics are appropriate for this patient, they do not provide definitive treatment for splenic abscess. (E) Splenic artery embolization is sometimes used for splenic lacerations. It would not be an appropriate treatment for splenic abscess.

---

 8 A 58-year-old man presents to his physician with back pain, intermittent fevers, and anemia. He says his back pain started approximately 8 months ago and has not been getting better despite treatment with over-the-counter acetaminophen and vitamins. Radiographs of the spine reveal a lytic lesion in his thoracic vertebrae. A biopsy of the lesion reveals sheets of plasma cells. Which of the following is likely found on laboratory workup of this patient?

(A) Hypocalcemia
(B) Increased monoclonal heavy chain immunoglobulin in urine
(C) Increased monoclonal light chain immunoglobulin in urine
(D) Normal erythrocyte sedimentation rate
(E) Normal serum creatinine

The answer is C: **Increased monoclonal light chain immunoglobulin in urine.** This patient is most likely suffering from multiple myeloma, a neoplastic process involving proliferating monoclonal plasma cells. Multiple myeloma is associated with chronic pain, fevers, and anemia. There may be lytic lesions identified on radiography. The proliferating plasma cells produce nonfunctional monoclonal antibodies that may include both light and heavy chains. Urinalysis will show an increased amount of paraprotein (also called Bence Jones protein), which is composed of only monoclonal light chains.

(A) Hypercalcemia rather than hypocalcemia is characteristic of multiple myeloma. (B) Increased heavy chains are not found in the urine of patients with multiple myeloma. (D) The erythrocyte sedimentation rate is typically elevated in patients with multiple myeloma. (E) The serum creatinine is typically elevated in patients with multiple myeloma.

---

 9 A 65-year-old man presents to the emergency department with sudden onset of chest pain. His past medical history is remarkable for hyperlipidemia and hypertension. He has a history of smoking and his brother died of a heart attack at age 49. The initial electrocardiogram (ECG) shows ST elevations in leads V2 through V5. Morphine, oxygen, nitroglycerin, and aspirin are administered. Which of the following is the next best step in management?

(A) Admit to the intensive care unit for observation
(B) Cardiac catheterization
(C) Transesophageal echocardiography
(D) Transfer to the operating room
(E) Transthoracic echocardiography

The answer is B: Cardiac catheterization. This patient is most likely suffering from an anterior myocardial infarct, as indicated by ST elevations in leads V2 through V5. The next best step is cardiac catheterization, for potential removal of coronary vessel blockage and placement of stents if indicated.

(A) Admitting the patient to the intensive care unit for observation should only be done if necessary after cardiac catheterization. (C) Transesophageal echocardiography is not acutely indicated for an anterior myocardial infarction. (D) The patient does not need operative intervention for a suspected anterior myocardial infarct unless traumatic rupture of the coronary vessels is suspected. (E) Transthoracic echocardiography is not indicated for an acute anterior myocardial infarction.

 10 A 65-year-old former professional athlete and current farmer presents to his primary care physician with urinary urgency, frequency, and dysuria as well as two episodes of gross hematuria over the last 2 months. His past medical history is significant for osteoarthritis of the knees for which he takes acetaminophen and aspirin powder. Physical examination is significant for crepitus upon extension of the knees bilaterally but is otherwise without finding. What is the most likely explanation of these findings?

(A) Arteriovenous malformation
(B) Bladder carcinoma
(C) Glomerular injury
(D) Nephrolithiasis
(E) Sloughing of the renal papilla

The answer is E: Sloughing of the renal papilla. The patient described in this vignette is suffering from analgesic nephropathy brought on by overuse of over-the-counter pain relievers for his osteoarthritis. Analgesic nephropathy is more likely to occur in patients using more than one pain reliever as well as those who are dehydrated, both of which are exhibited by this patient. The disease develops via two different mechanisms operating independently to cause a compound effect on the renal papilla. Acetaminophen acts by depleting glutathione reserves and causing oxidative damage to the renal papilla, while aspirin prevents the production of prostaglandins which prevents vasodilation of the renal vasculature and produces ischemia of the renal papilla. These effects compound to cause necrosis and sloughing of the renal papilla which leads to unilateral urinary obstruction and hematuria. Patients present with hyposthenuria, gross hematuria, and renal tubular acidosis leading to stone formation. Treatment is to discontinue the use of the analgesics and treat the underlying cause of the pain which will halt progression of the disease and allow for some recovery of renal function in a select few.

(A) Arteriovenous malformation is an unlikely cause of two incidents of hematuria this late in the patient's life. Arteriovenous malformations are not associated with chronic analgesic usage. (B) Bladder carcinoma is not associated with chronic analgesic use. Transitional papillary carcinoma of the renal pelvis is, however, associated with chronic use of analgesics and papillary necrosis. (C) Chronic use of analgesics does not affect the glomerulus. (D) Although nephrolithiasis is associated with chronic analgesic usage as described above, a presentation of two episodes of hematuria in 2 months without other symptoms would be unlikely.

 A nasogastric tube is placed in a 39-year-old man with a history of peptic ulcer disease who has had a bout of intractable vomiting. If electrolyte composition were measured over a 24-hour period from the stomach in the setting of low acid, what relative volume would be expected?

   (A) 500 cm^3
   (B) 1,500 cm^3
   (C) 3,000 cm^3
   (D) 5,000 cm^3
   (E) 10,000 cm^3

The answer is B: 1,500 cm^3. In terms of volume in mL per 24 hours, the colon in the setting of diarrhea can produce up to 17,000 L of fluid. This would be seen in the situation of intractable diarrhea. The stomach in the setting of low acid would produce a volume of 1,000 to 2,500 mL/24 hours.

(A) 500 mL/24 hours of volume would be expected for pancreatic secretions. (C) 3,000 mL/24 hours would be expected for proximal and distal small bowel. (D) 5,000 mL/24 hours would be expected for stomach in the setting of high acid or colon in the setting of diarrhea. (E) In terms of volume in mL per 24 hours, the colon in the setting of diarrhea can produce up to 17,000 L of fluid.

 A 56-year-old old man who is undergoing a surgical procedure for a hernia repair is found to have incarceration of the antimesenteric portion of the bowel wall. What is the most likely explanation for this finding?

(A) Epigastric hernia
(B) Hiatal hernia
(C) Indirect inguinal hernia
(D) Richter hernia
(E) Umbilical hernia

The answer is D: Richter hernia. Richter hernia is a hernia at any site that involves only a portion of the antimesenteric wall of the bowel. Because the lumen is only partially involved, obstruction rarely occurs. However, strangulation of the involved segment is common.

(A) Epigastric hernias occur in because of a defect in the linea alba. (B) Hiatal hernia occurs because of hernia of the esophagus through the diaphragm. (C) Indirect hernias proceed directly through the inguinal canal. (E) Umbilical hernias occur because of a facial defect in the rectus muscle and fascia.

---

13 Approximately 12 hours following elective repair of an inguinal hernia in a 6-month-old male infant, he is noted to be edematous and anuric. Physical examination reveals edema of the abdominal wall. What is the most likely diagnosis?

(A) Iatrogenic ureteral injury
(B) Iatrogenic urinary bladder injury
(C) Ischemic bowel
(D) Synergistic bacterial infection
(E) Synergistic fungal infection

The answer is B: Iatrogenic urinary bladder injury. This child has a complication following inguinal hernia repair. In male infants, the bladder is the organ most frequently involved in sliding inguinal hernia, whereas in female infants, the fallopian tube and ovary are typically injured.

(A) Iatrogenic ureteral injury is common in gynecologic surgical misadventures. (C) Ischemic bowel is extremely uncommon, especially after inguinal surgery. (D) Bacterial infection is unlikely 12 hours after inguinal surgery. (E) Fungal infection is unlikely 12 hours after inguinal surgery.

---

14 A 9-year-old girl presents with swelling and pain on the left side of her neck while recovering from a common cold, which was managed symptomatically. On physical examination, she has significant swelling in her left lateral neck at the level of the hyoid bone and is audibly stridorous. White blood cell count is in the normal range. What is most appropriate next step in the management of this patient?

(A) Antibiotics, single oral dose
(B) Corticosteroids
(C) Computed tomography (CT) scan of the neck
(D) Ultrasound of the neck
(E) Watchful waiting

The answer is C: CT scan of the neck. The patient probably has a branchial cleft cyst. To confirm the diagnosis, imaging of the neck should be performed. Ultrasound is a very good modality for this, but because of the patient's symptoms (stridor), a CT or magnetic resonance imaging (MRI) should be ordered to evaluate the proximity to her airway. She should be treated with antibiotics and taken to the operating room for excision of the cyst.

(A) Antibiotics as a single oral dose are not recommended. (B) Corticosteroids will not help this patient. (D) Ultrasound will not further distinguish the type of mass in this patient. (E) Watchful waiting may be offered in the asymptomatic patient.

---

15 A 39-year-old woman undergoes a breast biopsy for a suspected right breast lump. The pathology report returns and indicates the presence of benign stromal proliferation with vascular involvement. The tissue sample was 2 cm in diameter. What is the most likely diagnosis?

(A) Cystic breast disease
(B) Fibroadenoma
(C) Lipoma
(D) Mammary duct ectasia
(E) Pseudoangiomatous hyperplasia

The answer is E: Pseudoangiomatous hyperplasia. This patient likely has pseudoangiomatous hyperplasia. This is benign stromal proliferation that simulates a vascular lesion. It is necessary to rule out angiosarcoma by obtaining a larger tissue sample.

(A) Cystic breast masses are fluid filled and do not have vascular involvement. (B) Fibroadenoma is a well-defined, rubbery, mobile mass. (C) Lipoma is benign encapsulated adipose tissue. (D) Mammary duct ectasia is characterized by dilation of the subareolar ducts with periductal inflammation and ductal dilation.

---

16 A 67-year-old retired businessman presents to his physician with a painful nodule on his lower lip that has not gone away despite home care with naturopathic remedies. He has a 50-pack-year history of smoking (2 PPD for 25 years) and reports that he enjoys golfing and drinking one to two beers/day. Physical examination reveals a 0.7 cm × 0.5 cm lesion with central ulceration on his outer lower lip. What is the next best step in management?

(A) Punch biopsy
(B) Application of topical 5-flourouracil
(C) Shave biopsy
(D) Observation, with 3-month follow-up examination
(E) Topical clindamycin antibiotic therapy

The answer is A: Punch biopsy. This patient is most likely suffering from squamous cell carcinoma on his lower lip. This occurs in greater frequency in sun-exposed areas. Smoking and alcohol are both risk factors, although more so for oral lesions. The first step in diagnosis is a punch biopsy on the edge of the lesion for histologic diagnosis. Smaller lesions may be diagnosed with excisional biopsy. Once the diagnosis is confirmed, treatment involves excision with clear and wide (greater than 1 cm) margins.

(B) Although 5-flourouracil may be an option for precancerous skin lesions including carcinoma in situ and actinic keratosis, it is not appropriate for the initial management of invasive squamous cell carcinoma. (C) A shave biopsy may not obtain enough information for pathologic diagnosis and is not recommended as an initial biopsy method. (D) Observation when localized malignancy is suspected is not appropriate. (E) Although they may be appropriate for infectious lesions, topical antibiotics are ineffective for treating squamous cell carcinoma.

---

 17 A 55-year-old woman presents with pain and swelling over her right leg. On physical examination, there is a palpable cord. She is subsequently diagnosed with superficial thrombophlebitis. Which of the following is the next best step in management?

(A) Antibiotics
(B) Aspirin and compression stockings
(C) Excision and ligation of the thrombophlebotic vein
(D) Heparin bridging followed by warfarin therapy for 6 months
(E) Warfarin therapy for 6 months

The answer B: Aspirin and compression stockings. Superficial thrombophlebitis does not require anticoagulation. Management of superficial thrombophlebitis involves the use of pain relievers (nonsteroidal anti-inflammatory drugs [NSAIDs]), compression stockings, localized heat, elevation, and education on lifestyle changes.

(A) This patient is most likely suffering from superficial thrombophlebitis. Antibiotics are not indicated for treatment of superficial thrombophlebitis. However, if signs of infection develop, intravenous antibiotics are indicated. (C) Excision and ligation of the thrombophlebotic vein is an option for persistent superficial thrombophlebitis, septic thrombophlebitis, or disease localized to the saphenous vein. (D) Although low molecular weight heparin has been shown to be useful in preventing progression of superficial thrombophlebitis to deep vein thrombosis, anticoagulation is generally not needed. (E) Anticoagulation with warfarin is not indicated for superficial thrombophlebitis.

---

18 A 69-year-old man presents with unilateral nasal obstruction and intermittent nasal bleeding that started about a month ago. He has a history of smoking and allergic rhinitis, and is employed sanding cabinets. His temperature is 37.3°C, blood pressure 130/80 mmHg, pulse 65 beats/min, and respirations 14 breaths/min. On examination, there is a polypoid mass blocking the left nasal cavity that bleeds easily when touched with the examination instruments. A CT scan shows a papillomatous lesion with some evidence of bone destruction. Biopsy of the lesion shows a thick layer of squamous epithelium with mucocytes arranged in papillary fronds. Which of the following is the treatment of choice for the most likely lesion?

(A) Medical management of sinusitis
(B) Observation
(C) Radiotherapy
(D) Surgery
(E) Surgery and radiotherapy

The answer is D: Surgery. This patient is most likely suffering from a sinonasal papilloma, an uncommon and benign tumor distinct from inflammatory nasal polyps. The tumor arises from the mucosal surface of the sinonasal tract and is almost always unilateral. Although the cause is unknown, proposed etiologies include allergic, secondary to chronic sinusitis, viral infection with human papilloma virus, and air pollution. CT is the preferred imaging modality and biopsy will establish the diagnosis. Histologically there are three subtypes, including inverted, fungiform, and cylindrical. Treatment is surgical excision with endoscopic procedures becoming more common, although recurrence rate is highly variable.

(A) Although medical management of this patient's sinusitis, if present, would be important, it would not fix the patient's complaint. (B) Observation would not be appropriate as this patient's problem is unlikely to resolve by itself. (C) Radiotherapy is generally not indicated for sinonasal papillomas, as it increases the risk for malignant transformation. (E) Although surgery is an effective way to manage sinonasal papillomas, radiotherapy, for reasons described above, is not.

---

19 A 34-year-old woman with Crohn disease returns for follow-up. CT scan reveals 15 cm of full-thickness ileal thickening and luminal construction. She is currently taking 5-aminosalicyclic acid.

Her treating physician places her on a short course of infliximab. The most appropriate indication for this medication in this patient is to heal which of the following?

(A) Colonic disease
(B) Fistulas
(C) Ileal disease
(D) Mouth ulcers
(E) Stomatitis

The answer is B: Fistulas. Antitumor necrosis factor (infliximab) is a monoclonal antibody used in the treatment of Crohn disease. Its primary indication is healing of perirectal fistulas which are common with this disease. Long-term use is not advisable.

(A) Antitumor necrosis factor (infliximab) does not improve colonic disease. (C) This medication may slightly improve ileal Crohn disease. (D) Mouth ulcer healing will be unaffected by this medication. (E) Stomatitis will be unchanged with administration of infliximab.

 20 A 19-year-old man is brought to the emergency department after failing to successfully jump over a fence in an attempt to evade law enforcement. He got to the top of the fence and then fell approximately 20 feet and hit the concrete. He lost consciousness for 2 minutes according to law enforcement. He is brought to the emergency department for evaluation. Which of the following steps in the primary evaluation of this patient are correct?

(A) A = airway maintenance with intubation
(B) B = breathing and ventilation
(C) C = immediate placement of central venous line
(D) D = drug screen
(E) E = prevent hyperthermia with cooling blanket

The answer is B: B = breathing and ventilation. The ABCDE of trauma is important to commit to memory. B represents breathing and ventilation.

(A) A represents airway maintenance with cervical spine immobilization. Intubation may not be immediately necessary in this patient. (C) C represents circulation with hemorrhage control. Placement of two peripheral lines should be undertaken. (D) D represents assessment of disability with a complete neurologic examination. (E) E represents exposure and environmental control with undressing of the patient and prevention of hypothermia. Cooling blanket is not appropriate for this patient.

 21 An 18-year-old man presents to the emergency department after suffering from a gunshot wound to the abdomen 2 hours previously.

His blood pressure is 70/50 mmHg. He is brought emergently to the operating room and was found to have an injury to his inferior vena cava which is successfully repaired. On day 2 of his hospital stay, his blood pressure remains low and his blood urea nitrogen (BUN) and K concentrations begin to rise along with decreasing urine output and the patient is placed on dialysis for several days. As his urine output begins to increase, which of the following is he at risk of developing?

(A) Hematuria
(B) Hypernatremia
(C) Hypokalemia
(D) Proteinuria
(E) Volume overload

The answer is C: Hypokalemia. The patient in this vignette is undergoing acute kidney injury (AKI) due to renal ischemia which has developed as a result of hypoperfusion. Patients suffering from AKI usually undergo three stages before the return of normal renal function. The first stage of AKI is the initiation phase which lasts for about 1 to 2 days and is characterized by only a slight increase in serum BUN and a slight decrease in urine output. The second phase, the maintenance phase, is categorized by urine output less than 400 mL/day, salt and water overload, further increases in BUN, hyperkalemia, and metabolic acidosis which usually requires dialysis for treatment. The third and final stage is the recovery stage which is heralded by an increase in urine output which can reach amounts up to 3 L/day. During this stage, the renal tubules have not yet recovered their concentrating abilities and large amounts of electrolytes, including potassium, are lost in the urine, making the patients susceptible to the effects of hypokalemia. With proper medical treatment, up to 95% of patients undergoing AKI will recover normal renal function.

(A) Although there is diffuse damage to the renal tubules, hematuria does not occur with AKI. (B) Hypernatremia occurs when there is a loss of free water in the urine. During the recovery phase of AKI the concentrating ability of the kidney is lost so hypernatremia does not occur. (D) Proteinuria does not occur during the recovery phase of AKI since the filtration portion of the glomerulus is not damaged. (E) Volume is significantly decreased, not increased, during the recovery phase of AKI since the concentrating ability of the kidney is lost.

---

22) A 28-year-old man is stabbed in the abdomen several times by an assailant who was attempting to steal his car. The patient is brought to the emergency department by rescue squad. His mental status is normal. His blood pressure is 130/90 mmHg and his pulse rate is 92 beats/min. His abdomen is soft and nontender. Three small midline stab wounds are identified. What is the most appropriate classification of hypovolemic chock in this individual?

(A) Class I
(B) Class II
(C) Class III
(D) Class IV

The answer is A: Class I. This individual appears to be clinically stable. His pulse rate is <100 beats/min and his blood pressure is normal. His blood loss is likely to be less than 750 cm³ and represents less than 15% of his blood volume. He would be classified as class I hypovolemic shock.

(B) Class II hypovolemic shock implies blood loss of 750 to 1,500 cm³. Patients are often tachycardic with normal blood pressure. (C) Class III hypovolemic shock implies blood less of 1,500 to 2,000 cm³. Patients are tachycardic and hypotensive. (D) Class IV hypovolemic shock implies blood loss of greater than 2,000 cm³. Patients have lost greater than 40% of their blood volume and are tachycardic and hypotensive.

---

23 A 75-year-old man is referred by his cardiologist to be evaluated for aortic valve replacement. The patient reports dyspnea on exertion over the last month along with two episodes of chest pain while walking his dog. A recent workup by his cardiologist shows that the patient has aortic stenosis. An abnormal value in which of the following studies is most important in determining whether the patient needs his valve replaced?

(A) Ejection fraction
(B) Left ventricular diastolic pressures
(C) Mean pressure gradient across the aortic valve on echocardiography
(D) Pulmonary artery pressures
(E) Valve area

The answer is C: Mean pressure gradient across the aortic valve on echocardiography. In a patient with aortic stenosis, the mean gradient (a measure of the pressure differences across the aortic valve) as measured during Doppler echocardiography is the best test. According to the 2006 ACC/AHH guidelines, a mean gradient of less than 25 mmHg is classified as mild aortic stenosis, between 25 and 40 mmHg moderate aortic stenosis, and greater than 40mmHg severe aortic stenosis.

(A) Ejection fraction is an unreliable measurement for determining the degree of aortic stenosis as it may be normal in patients with known stenosis. (B) While abnormal left ventricular diastolic pressures may indicate left ventricular dysfunction, they are not specific for valvular disease. (D) Similar to the ejection fraction, pulmonary artery pressures may be normal in patients suffering from aortic stenosis and are thus not a reliable value for measuring the degree of aortic stenosis. (E) While valve area is often used along with the valve gradient to determine the degree of aortic stenosis, it varies with the person's size and is less important than the mean pressure gradient.

A 29-year-old graduate student complains of inguinal pain. He presents to the student health clinic for examination. Physical examination reveals a hernia that arises lateral to the inferior epigastric vessels. What is the most likely diagnosis?

(A) Direct inguinal hernia
(B) Femoral hernia
(C) Indirect inguinal hernia
(D) Obturator hernia
(E) Sliding hernia

The answer is C: **Indirect inguinal hernia.** An indirect inguinal hernia arises lateral to the epigastric vessels, a direct hernia arises medial to the vessels, a femoral hernia is found through the femoral canal, an obturator hernia protrudes through the obturator canal, and a sliding hernia is any hernia where a portion of the sac is made up of the wall of an intraabdominal organ.

(A) Direct inguinal hernias occur within Hesselbach's triangle and occur in 1% of men. (B) Femoral hernias occur under the inguinal ligament. (D) Obturator hernias occur in the obturator canal. (E) Sliding hernia is any hernia where a portion of the sac is made up of the wall of an intraabdominal organ.

 A 37-year-old woman undergoes a laparoscopic cholecystectomy for recurrent symptomatic cholelithiasis. The procedure is uneventful. Which of the following statements regarding bile formation and secretion are correct in this patient?

(A) Bile formation and secretion occur in the liver
(B) Bile secretion is initiated in the interstitial cells
(C) Driving force of bile filtration is via hydrostatic pressure
(D) Primary bile salts include lithocolic acid
(E) Secretory IgG in bile prevents enteric infections

The answer is A: **Bile formation and secretion occur in the liver.** The formation and secretion of bile are major functions of the liver. Bile secretion is initiated at the hepatocytes, by the driving force of osmotic filtration across the sinusoids.

(B) Bile secretion is initiated by the hepatocytes. (C) The driving force of bile formation is osmotic filtration across the sinusoids. (D) Primary bile salts include chenodeoxycholic acid and cholic acid. (E) Secretory IgA prevents the systemic manifestation of enteric infections.

 A 64-year-old man with a history of vague left lower quadrant pain, bloating and alternating constipation, and diarrhea presents to his primary care physician for follow-up. Physical examination is noncontributory. Barium enema reveals multiple sigmoid diverticuli. What is the most likely explanation for these findings?

(A) Aperistaltic segment
(B) High fiber diet
(C) Increased intraluminal pressure
(D) Mass lesion in the rectum
(E) Polyposis coli

The answer is C: Increased intraluminal pressure. This patient likely has diverticulosis. This is caused by increased intraluminal pressure which causes the inner layer of the colon to bulge through this area of weakness in the colon wall. Low fiber diet, positive family history, and increase in age are considered to be risk factors.

(A) Aperistaltic segment is not thought to be an etiologic factor in development of diverticulosis. (B) Low fiber diet can cause constipation which can increase intraluminal pressures. (D) The barium enema did not reveal evidence of a mass lesion. (E) The barium enema did not reveal evidence of colon polyps.

 27 A 29-year-old man is in the operating room after being shot in the abdomen three times. He is found to have a through and through ileal gunshot wound approximately 20 cm from the ileocecal valve. Resection and bowel anastomosis are undertaken. Which of the following statements is true regarding the submucosal layer of the small intestine?

(A) Contains nerves
(B) Covers the intestinal villi
(C) Derived from the peritoneum
(D) Innermost layer
(E) Outermost layer

The answer is A: Contains nerves. The submucosa is the strongest layer and provided strength to an intestinal anastomosis. It contains nerves, Meissner plexus, blood vessels, and fibrous and elastic tissue.

(B) The intestinal villi are contained in the mucosal layer of the intestinal wall. (C) The serosa is the outermost layer and derives embryologically from the peritoneum. (D) The serosa is the outermost layer. The mucosa is the innermost layer. (E) The serosa is the outermost layer.

 28 Repair of an inguinal hernia that approximates the conjoined tendon and transversalis fascia to the inguinal ligament is known as which of the following?

(A) Bassinni repair
(B) Laparoscopic preperitoneal repair
(C) Lichtenstein repair
(D) McVay repair
(E) Shouldice repair

The answer is A: Bassinni repair. A Bassini repair joins the conjoined tendon and transversalis fascia to the inguinal ligament. A McVay repair sews the transverses aponeurosis to the Cooper ligament, a Shouldice repair combines the McVay and Bassini repairs, the preperitoneal repair involves placing a piece of mesh over the defect in the preperitoneal space, and the Lichtenstein repair uses a piece of mesh in an open repair.

(B) The preperitoneal repair involves placing a piece of mesh over the defect in the preperitoneal space. (C) Lichtenstein repair uses a piece of mesh in an open repair. (D) Shouldice repair combines the McVay and Bassini repairs. (E) Shouldice repair combines the McVay and Bassini repairs.

 (29) A 54-year-old man presents with 2 months of headaches that have become more frequent and have been associated with nausea and vomiting in the past couple of weeks. Two days ago, he suffered a seizure. He was previously healthy and has no personal or family history of cancer of any type. An magnetic resonance imaging (MRI) shows a single 5 cm × 4 cm × 3 cm tumor in the left cerebral hemisphere. Which of the following is a feature of the most likely tumor this patient has?

(A) Arising in cerebral hemispheres is rare
(B) Composed of oligodendrocytes
(C) Generally benign
(D) High recurrence rate
(E) Well-delineated

The answer is D: High recurrence rate. Although the most common brain tumors overall are metastases, this man's tumor is likely a primary tumor because he has no known cancer anywhere that could metastasize and a solitary tumor was seen on MRI (multiple tumors are more likely metastatic than primary). The most common primary central nervous system (CNS) neoplasms are astrocytomas. Astrocytomas, unfortunately, have a poor prognosis. They occur almost exclusively in the cerebral hemispheres, spread along tracts and may cross the corpus callosum, are poorly delineated, and treatments are not very effective. The recurrence rate of treated astrocytomas is high.

(A) Astrocytomas occur almost exclusively in the cerebral hemispheres. (B) The most common primary brain tumors are astrocytomas. Oligodendrogliomas are less common. (C) Meningiomas are benign primary brain tumors, but are less common than gliomas such as astrocytomas. Astrocytomas are malignant and have a poor prognosis. (E) Meningiomas are well-delineated primary brain tumors but are less common than gliomas such as astrocytomas. Astrocytomas are poorly delineated with ill-defined boundaries.

---

30 A 39-year-old man with a short bowel following multiple surgeries from Crohn disease is considering a small bowel transplantation. Which of the following is of particular concern in a small bowel transplantation?

(A) Acute rejection
(B) Chronic rejection
(C) Graft-versus-host disease
(D) Hyperacute rejection
(E) These complications occur at similar rates in all solid organ transplants.

The answer is C: Graft-versus-host disease. Small bowel transplants are less commonly performed than other types of transplants. Most are performed because of shortened bowel as occurs in congenital atresia, necrotizing enterocolitis, gastroschisis, volvulus, vascular accidents, and complications from Crohn disease as in the question stem. Because the small bowel has so much lymphoid tissue (gut-associated lymphoid tissue, GALT) that graft-versus-host disease is a more common problem in small bowel transplants than in transplants of other solid organs.

(A) Acute rejection is no more a problem with small bowel transplantations than it is with other solid organ transplantations. The large amount of lymphoid tissue within the small bowel makes graft-versus-host disease possible with small bowel transplants. Graft-versus-host disease is not a major concern with other solid organ transplantations. (B) Chronic rejection is no more a problem with small bowel transplantations than it is with other solid organ transplantations. The large amount of lymphoid tissue within the small bowel makes graft-versus-host disease possible with small bowel transplants. Graft-versus-host disease is not a major concern with other solid organ transplantations. (D) Hyperacute rejections occur when donor-recipient ABO blood groups have not been appropriately matched resulting in graft destruction by preformed antibodies in the recipient's blood. The large amount of lymphoid tissue within the small bowel makes graft-versus-host disease possible with small bowel transplants. Graft-versus-host disease is not a major concern with other solid organ transplantations. (E) The large amount of lymphoid tissue within the small bowel makes graft-versus-host disease possible with small bowel transplants. Graft-versus-host disease is not a major concern with other solid organ transplantations.

---

31 A 25-year-old medical resident is playing football with his friends when he "rolls" his ankle. He says that he was jumping to catch the ball and came down on his toes with his ankle slightly plantar flexed. He present to the emergency department for evaluation. On examination, his lateral ankle appears swollen and erythematous with prominent bruising.

There is no point tenderness, but a positive anterior drawer test of the ankle. The anterior drawer test is used to evaluate the stability of which of the following ligaments?

(A) Anterior talofibular ligament
(B) Calcaneofibular ligament
(C) Deep deltoid ligament
(D) Posterior talofibular ligament
(E) Talonavicular ligament

The answer is A: **Anterior talofibular ligament.** This patient has most likely injured his anterior talofibular ligament (ATFL). This ligament is the most commonly injured with ankle sprains and often occurs when the ankle is slightly plantar flexed. The anterior drawer test evaluates the ATFL and can be performed by securing the distal leg with one hand and applying an anterior pull to the heel with the ankle slightly planar flexed. Treatment depends on the degree of sprain, with physical rehabilitation almost always required. Surgical intervention is sometimes needed for severe ligament tears or serious athletes.

(B) Injury to the calcaneofibular ligament does not increase the amount of displacement with the anterior drawer test. (C) The deep deltoid ligament functions to prevent lateral displacement and external rotation of the talus. The anterior drawer test does not test the deep deltoid ligament. (D) The posterior talofibular ligament prevents posterior and rotary subluxation of the talus. It is not tested by the anterior drawer test. (E) The talonavicular ligament is a wide sheet-like band that stabilizes the talocalcaneonavicular joint. It is not tested by the anterior drawer test.

---

32 A 25-year-old man presents with bilaterally aching jaw that is worsened with chewing. He also has nonspecific neck, shoulder, and back pain that is worse in the morning. On examination, there is a "popping" sound of the temporal mandibular joint when moving side to side. No laboratory abnormalities are present. Which of the following is the best treatment option at this time?

(A) Arthroscopic washout of the temporomandibular joint (TMJ)
(B) Avoid soft foods
(C) Narcotics
(D) Nonsteroidal anti-inflammatory drugs and behavioral modification
(E) Ultrasonic therapy

The answer is D: **Nonsteroidal anti-inflammatory drugs and behavioral modification.** This patient is suffering from TMJ syndrome, a common syndrome that most likely has multifactorial causes, one of which is bruxism (nocturnal jaw clenching and teeth grinding) suggested by the timing of the patient's symptoms. Additional symptoms that patients may complain of include a locking jaw, headache, and an uncomfortable bite. Examination findings suggestive of TMJ syndrome include limitations of jaw opening, palpable spasms, facial swelling, crepitus over the joint, clicking or popping, and a tender TMJ joint. Treatment is almost always conservative and includes nonsteroidal anti-inflammatory drugs, muscle relaxants for any muscle spasms, and heat. Additional management should include behavioral modification including avoiding jaw clenching and teeth grinding and soft diets.

(A) Surgical management, including arthroscopic washout of the TMJ joint, may be an option for those patients who fail more conservative therapy. (B) Soft foods should be encouraged in patients suffering from TMJ syndrome. (C) Anti-inflammatory drugs should be used for pain, not narcotics due to the addiction potential. (E) Some patients who fail more conservative therapy may benefit from ultrasonic therapy.

---

33 An 8-year-old boy was noted by his school teacher to be eating chunks of hair. Computed tomography (CT) scan of the abdomen reveals a 1.5-cm trichobezoar in the stomach. What is the most appropriate treatment for this patient?

(A) Endoscopic therapy
(B) Gastrectomy
(C) Proton pump inhibitors and two antibiotic therapies for 3 weeks
(D) Splenectomy
(E) Vagotomy and pyloroplasty

The answer is A: Endoscopic therapy. Trichobezoars are accumulations of swallowed hair in the stomach and are usually treated with endoscopic therapy. However, larger lesions may require open or laparoscopic removal.

(B) Gastrectomy should not be required for this condition. Gastrotomy to remove the lesion may be required. (C) Proton pump inhibitors will not remove the lesion. (D) The spleen would be expected to be normal in this patient. (E) Vagotomy and pyloroplasty would not remove the foreign body lesion. Endoscopic or surgical removal will be the treatment of choice.

---

34 A 31-year-old obese man presents to his primary care physician for an annual examination. His blood pressure is 190/100 mmHg. Examination of the abdomen reveals purple abdominal striae on both sides of the umbilicus. What is the next most appropriate step in the management of this patient?

(A) Baseline plasma cortisol levels
(B) Computed tomograph (CT) of the abdomen
(C) Iodocholesterol adrenal scan
(D) Urinary free cortisol level
(E) X-ray of the sella turcica

The answer is D: Urinary free cortisol level. This patient may have Cushing syndrome. One must document excess cortisol production. This may be done by looking for excess urinary free cortisol excretion. One can also detect high plasma cortisol levels by drawing blood in the morning and evening. Normally, levels are high in the morning and low in the evening. In Cushing syndrome, levels are high all of the time.

(A) Cortisol levels need to be drawn in the morning and evening. (B) CT scan can detect bilateral adrenal enlargement, adrenal tumors, or pituitary neoplasms as a cause of Cushing disease. (C) Adrenal scan can detect bilateral adrenal enlargement, adrenal tumors, or pituitary neoplasms as a cause of Cushing disease. (E) X-ray of the sella turcica can detect pituitary calcifications.

---

35 A 50-year-old man from Arizona who spends a great deal of time outside presents with a lesion over the left forehead. The patient reports that it has been growing slowly over the last several years. On examination, there is a raised and waxy 1.3-cm skin mass over the left forehead. There is no lymphadenopathy and the remainder of the examination is unremarkable. What is the most likely diagnosis?

(A) Basal cell carcinoma
(B) Congenital melanocytic nevus
(C) Melanoma
(D) Sarcoma
(E) Squamous cell carcinoma

The answer is A: Basal cell carcinoma. This patient's history and examination are most consistent with a diagnosis of basal cell carcinoma. Basal cell carcinomas are the most common skin malignancy. They usually develop in sun-exposed areas in fair-skinned individuals. Although slow growing and rarely metastatic, they are locally invasive. These patients are at a much greater risk for developing new lesions, especially in areas exposed to sunlight. Histologically, basal cell carcinomas are composed of nests of malignant and basophilic cells. Treatment involves surgical resection. If the margins are tumor free, then no additional treatment is necessary. Other treatment options include topical 5-flourouricil or radiation.

(B) Congenital melanocytic nevi are benign lesions usually discovered at birth. They are often located on the head and neck and are characterized by a well-circumscribed patch of light brown to black pigmentation with a heterogeneous consistency. Microscopically, congenital melanocytic nevi appear similar to acquired nevi with the exception that cells are often found deeper within the dermis. Surgery is sometimes used for treatment as large lesions have an increased malignant potential. (C) Malignant melanoma is clinically characterized by asymmetry, irregular borders, variation in color, diameter greater than 6 mm, and an evolving appearance. This patient's presentation is not consistent with melanoma. (D) Sarcomas are malignant soft tissue tumors that rarely occur on the face. Although they may erode into the skin, this patient's presentation is highly inconsistent with this diagnosis. (E) Squamous cell carcinoma is the second most common form of skin cancer. It often occurs on the lower lip or below. It typically grows faster than basal cell carcinoma and is also locally invasive.

36 A 38-year-old woman with Crohn disease returns for follow-up. Computed tomography (CT) scan reveals 15 cm of ileocolonic disease. She is currently taking 5-aminosalicyclic acid and 6-mercaptopurine without improvement in symptoms. She is scheduled for an iliocolic resection. Which of the following surgical principles should be adhered to?

(A) Bypass disease involved segments
(B) Long side-to-side anastomosis is preferred
(C) Look for normal bowel to use for the anastamosis
(D) Use frozen section to look for uninvolved bowel
(E) Use intraoperative steroids to decrease inflammation

The answer is B: **Long side-to-side anastomosis is preferred.** This patient should have a long side-to-side anastomosis as opposed to an end-to-end anastomosis. Laparoscopic approaches can also be considered in this patient depending on the skill and expertise of the surgeon.

(A) Avoid bypass of involved segments because this leaves active disease in place. (C) Do not look for normal bowel to use for anastamoses. (D) Do not use frozen section to look for uninvolved margins; microscopic disease is nearly always present. (E) Avoid intraoperative steroids as this can impair wound healing and create undue physiologic stress.

37 A 37-year-old woman with a history of cholecystectomy for biliary colic with stones runs a half marathon 1 year after her surgical procedure. She has no other pertinent medical history. Which of the following statements are correct regarding carbohydrate metabolism?

(A) After 24 hours of fasting, glycogen is converted to glycerol
(B) After meals, absorbed carbohydrates are converted to glycogen
(C) Fatty acids are synthesized in states of glucose deprivation during the race
(D) Gluconeogenesis from amino acids comprise phenylalanine

The answer is B: **After meals, absorbed carbohydrates are converted to glycogen.** After meals, the absorbed carbohydrates are circulated systemically and reach the liver, where most of them are converted to the storage form of glycogen. This mechanism is unaffected after cholecystectomy and is also unaffected by exercise.

(A) After 48 to 72 hours of fasting, the glycogen is converted to glucose and provides a source of energy. (C) Fatty acids are synthesized in states of glucose excess. (D) Gluconeogenesis from amino acids comprise mainly alanine.

 38 A 55-year-old man with a history of alcoholism presents with an acute onset of abdominal pain. He describes the pain as worse with food. He localizes the pain to the epigastric area with radiation to his back. He has also been vomiting. His temperature today is 37.3°C, blood pressure 130/75 mmHg, pulse 105 beats/min, and respirations 20 breaths/min. On examination, the patient's mouth is dry and the abdomen is diffusely tender. Laboratory studies reveal:

Leukocytes: 13,000/mm^3
Serum alkaline phosphatase: normal
Serum bilirubin: normal
Serum amylase: 220 U/L
Serum lipase: 1,010 U/L

The patient is diagnosed with acute pancreatitis and is expected to stay at least a week in the hospital. After the initial 48 hours, which of the following will nutritionally optimize the patient's recovery?

(A) Clear liquid diet only with advancement as tolerated
(B) Maintenance fluids only and continued nothing by mouth
(C) Enteral nutrition delivered by a Dubbhoff jejunal tube
(D) Normal diet with maintenance fluids as needed
(E) Total parenteral nutrition

The answer is C: Enteral nutritional delivered by a Dubbhoff jejunal tube. This patient is most likely suffering from an acute pancreatitis. In patients with prolonged stays with nothing by mouth status, studies have shown that failure to use the gastrointestinal tract in those with acute pancreatitis may exacerbate the stress response and disease severity, leading to more complications and possibly prolonged hospitalizations. Studies have shown that patients do best when feeding is initiated early. Although total parenteral nutrition has been used historically, several trials have shown improved outcomes with enteral nutrition. The placement of a Dubbhoff jejunal tube allows food entry distal to the pancreatic ducts in this patient and thus avoids pancreatic stimulation while providing the needed nutritional support.

(A) Clear liquid diet would possibly stimulate the pancreas and worsen the patient's symptoms. (B) While the continued maintenance fluids might be appropriate, the patient's prolonged stay will require some sort of nutritional support. (D) This patient will not tolerate a normal diet, as it will stimulate the pancreas. (E) While total parenteral nutrition is an option, studies have shown that enteral nutrition has better outcomes in patients with acute pancreatitis. Parenteral nutrition should be reserved for patients who do not tolerate enteral feeds or in patients with difficult or inadequate infusions.

---

39 A 60-year-old man with a long history of smoking presents with dysphagia, fatigue, and an unintentional weight loss of 15 kg over the last 2 months. His past medical history is remarkable for Barrett esophagus, achalasia, alcohol abuse, and peptic ulcer disease secondary to infection with *Helicobactor pylori*. Esophagogastroduodenoscopy reveals a mass in the distal esophagus. Biopsy of the mass reveals glandular-like cells that appear similar to intestinal mucosa. The cells appear dysplastic, they have irregular nuclear features, and there are numerous mitotic figures appreciated. Which of the following is the greatest risk factor for this patient's condition?

(A) Achalasia
(B) Alcohol abuse
(C) Cigarette smoking
(D) History of Barrett esophagus
(E) History of infection with *H. pylori*

The answer is D: History of Barrett esophagus. Adenocarcinoma of the esophagus makes up about 40% to 50% of primary esophageal cancers, although the incidence has been increasing over the last 20 years. They primarily occur in the lower one-third of the esophagus and are most common in elderly men. Approximately 95% of cases evolve from Barrett esophagus. Indeed, having the diagnosis of Barrett esophagus increases the risk of developing esophageal adenocarcinoma by an estimated 30 to 60 times normal. Other risk factors include acid peptic disorders, motor disorders of the esophagus, other malignancies, certain medications, certain environmental exposures, diet, and nutrition.

(A) Achalasia is a risk factor for squamous cell carcinoma of the esophagus. (B) Alcohol is a risk factor for squamous cell carcinoma of the esophagus. (C) While cigarette smoking may slightly increase the risk of adenocarcinoma of the esophagus, it is a greater risk factor for squamous cell carcinoma of the esophagus. (E) Infection with *H. pylori* has not been shown to increase the risk of esophageal cancers.

---

 40 A 73-year-old woman presents with an acute onset of left-sided facial paralysis. She also complains of left ear pain over the last 48 hours and says that when she woke up this morning she could not close her left eye. She has a history of shingles. On examination, there is paralysis of the left upper and lower face. Her left eye conjunctiva appears injected and has decreased tearing. After the patient's workup, she is diagnosed with Bell palsy. The patient requests treatment. Which of the following treatment options should be initiated?

(A) Aciclovir
(B) Aciclovir and prednisone
(C) Facial nerve decompression
(D) Observation
(E) Topical ocular lubrication and ganciclovir

The answer is B: Aciclovir and prednisone. Although treatment of Bell palsy is controversial, research suggests steroids are most likely effective. The recommended dose is 1 mg/kg or 60 mg/day for 6 days, followed by a 10-day taper. Additionally, evidence suggests a viral etiology in many cases (including this patient); thus antivirals such as acyclovir or valaciclovir would be a reasonable treatment option. In addition, topical ocular lubrication is important to prevent damage to the eye.

(A) Current guidelines suggest that use of antivirals such as aciclovir alone is not an effective therapy for Bell palsy. (C) While facial nerve decompression may be an appropriate surgical option for patients with complete Bell palsy unresponsive to medical therapy, it is invasive and would not be a good initial treatment option. (D) Spontaneous recovery is fairly common in patients with Bell palsy, and observation alone may be appropriate in certain cases. However, this patient is requesting treatment, which is not unreasonable. (E) While topical ocular lubrication is an important component of the treatment, treatment with ganciclovir in a patient with suspected varicella-induced Bell palsy would not be effective.

41 A 55-year-old homeless man with a long history of alcoholism presents to the ambulatory care clinic with poor sleep, decreased appetite, loss of interest in hobbies, poor concentration, and lack of pleasure in activities he normally enjoys for the last 3 months. He is depressed and is currently taking a selective serotonin reuptake inhibitor. At the current visit he reports no improvement with his symptoms. He also complains of a new remitting and recurring painful swelling over the veins in his arms and legs. The patient's physical examination reveals a 10-lb weight loss since his last visit along with mildly yellow skin. Which of the following is the most likely diagnosis?

(A) Depression
(B) Hypothyroidism
(C) Paget disease
(D) Pancreatic cancer
(E) Substance-induced depression

The answer is D: Pancreatic cancer. This patient is presenting with weight loss, depression, jaundice, and migratory thrombophlebitis, all potential indicators of pancreatic cancer. Pancreatic cancer is the fourth leading cause of cancer deaths among both men and women. Since it is very difficult to diagnose during its early stages, patients more often present late in the disease.

(A) Although this patient does present with signs of clinical depression, studies have shown that depression may be an early sign of pancreatic malignancy. Additionally, depression would not explain the other symptoms the patient is experiencing. (B) Although hypothyroidism could account for the signs of depression, the patient would be expected to experience weight gain. Additionally jaundice and migratory thrombophlebitis are not features of hypothyroidism. (C) This patient's symptoms are not consistent with Paget disease. (E) Although this patient does have a history of alcoholism and depression, this patient's symptoms are better explained by pancreatic malignancy.

 A 43-year-old man is brought to the emergency department after suffering a rollover on his ATV. His eyes open to painful stimuli and he withdraws from painful stimuli. His only vocalizations are incomprehensible sounds. Which represents this man's Glasgow coma score (GCS)?

(A) 3
(B) 8
(C) 14
(D) 20
(E) More information is needed to assess

The correct answer is B: 8. Coma is defined as a state of depressed consciousness in which a person does not respond normally (or at all) to stimuli. There are many causes of coma; treatment depends on the cause. Often the cause is not immediately apparent, so initial management of a comatose patient involves assessing the ABCs (airway, breathing, and circulation), monitoring vital signs, and stabilizing the patient while the underlying cause can be determined. The Glasgow coma scale is a tool used to give a numerical value to a patient with depressed consciousness. This scale evaluates three types of response (eye opening, motor response, and verbal response) and ranges from a minimum of 3 in a completely unresponsive patient to a 15 in a patient who is entirely alert and oriented. The patient in the question stem would be given 8 total points: 2 points for his eye opening to painful stimulus, 4 points for withdrawing from pain, and 2 points for producing some sounds but no words.

(A) The patient in the question stem would be given 8 total points: 2 points for his eye opening to painful stimulus, 4 points for withdrawing from pain, and 2 points for producing some sounds but no words. (C) The patient in the question stem would be given 8 total points: 2 points for his eye opening to painful stimulus, 4 points for withdrawing from pain, and 2 points for producing some sounds but no words. (D) The patient in the question stem would be given 8 total points: 2 points for his eye opening to painful stimulus, 4 points for withdrawing from pain, and 2 points for producing some sounds but no words. Remember, the maximum score on the GCS is 15. (E) The patient in the question stem would be given 8 total points: 2 points for his eye opening to painful stimulus, 4 points for withdrawing from pain, and 2 points for producing some sounds but no words.

43 An obese 42-year-old woman presents to her primary care physician with complaints of frequent urination and recurrent urinary tract infection (UTI) symptoms. Her past medical history is significant for type II diabetes mellitus diagnosed 7 years ago and her last hemoglobin A1c was 11.0%. Type II diabetes has the greatest effect on disease progression in which portion of the nephron?

 (A) Ascending loop of Henle
 (B) Collecting tubule
 (C) Distal convoluted tubule
 (D) Glomerulus
 (E) Proximal convoluted tubule

The answer is D: Glomerulus. Diabetic nephropathy is one of the leading causes of chronic kidney disease in the United States and end-stage renal disease occurs in up to 40% of diabetics. Although it affects multiple portions of the nephron, most of the pathology associated with diabetic nephropathy is associated with glomerular damage. Increased serum glucose levels as well as hemodynamic changes within the glomerulus lead to capillary basement membrane thickening, diffuse mesangial sclerosis, and nodular glomerulosclerosis. These changes contribute to the development and progression of microalbuminuria, nephrotic syndrome, and end-stage renal disease. Treatment with an ACE inhibitor or an angiotensin receptor blocker will slow the progression of hemodynamically induced changes within the glomerulus.

(A) Type II diabetes does not cause significant changes within the ascending loop of Henle. (B) Diabetes insipidus and not diabetes mellitus affects the renal collecting tubule. (C) The distal convoluted tubule is not significantly affected by type II diabetes mellitus. (E) The proximal convoluted tubule is responsible for the reabsorption of glucose within the filtrate but does not undergo any pathologic change as a result of elevated glucosuria levels.

44 A 40-year-old man is found to have a relatively weak area in Killian triangle located between the inferior pharyngeal constrictors superiorly and the cricopharyngeus muscle inferiorly. This is a description of which of the following?

 (A) Esophageal leiomyoma
 (B) Meckel diverticulum
 (C) Traction mid-esophageal diverticulum
 (D) True diverticulum
 (E) Zenker diverticulum

The answer is E: Zenker Diverticulum. A Zenker diverticulum is a pulsion, or false diverticulum. This is located in a relatively weak area in Killian triangle located between the inferior pharyngeal constrictors superiorly and the cricopharyngeous muscle inferiorly.

(A) An esophageal leiomyoma is a benign tumor, not a diverticulum. (B) Meckel diverticulum is a true diverticulum containing all layers of the visceral wall. (C) Traction diverticulum is formed when inflammatory or scar tissue adheres to the esophagus, pulling away from its natural course. (D) A true diverticulum contains all layers of the visceral wall.

---

45 A 54-year-old woman with a history of chest trauma from a motor vehicle accident 10 years ago complains of intermittent significant left breast pain. In the accident, her chest and abdomen were thrust against the car door. She was not wearing a seat belt. Physical examination of the left breast reveals a tender subcutaneous cord. There is no skin or nipple retraction. Mammography reveals no evidence of abnormalities in either breast. What is the most appropriate treatment for this patient?

(A) Amoxicillin
(B) Corticosteroids
(C) Ibuprofen
(D) Stereotactic excisional biopsy
(E) Watchful waiting

The answer is C: Ibuprofen. This patient has evidence of Mondor disease. This is associated with a tender, subcutaneous cord in the lateral breast. Skin retraction may or may not be present. Treatment usually involves anti-inflammatory agents such as ibuprofen.

(A) There is no evidence of infection to suggest the need for antibiotics. (B) Corticosteroids would not be considered a first-line treatment for this condition. (D) Excisional biopsy is unwarranted. (E) Watchful waiting may be suggested if the patient did not have pain. However, this patient does have significant breast pain.

---

46 A 9-year-old girl is brought to the emergency department by her parents because of genital bleeding for 4 days. She states that she can urinate without difficulty. The child appears well and offers no complaints. She has no prior medical or surgical history. Physical examination of the heart, lungs, and abdomen is unremarkable. Pelvic examination reveals a cherry red donut of tissue at the side of the urethral meatus. An image of the lesion is shown below.

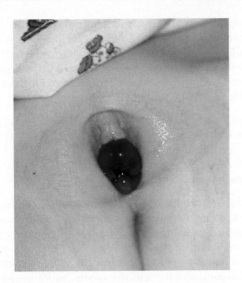

What is the most appropriate course of action for the physician to recommend?

(A) Daily baths and topical estrogen cream
(B) Metronidazole and topical estrogen cream
(C) Suprapubic urinary diversion
(D) Surgical excision
(E) Urethral catheterization

The answer is A: Daily baths and topical estrogen cream. This patient has evidence of urethral prolapse. The image shows complete prolapse of the urethral tissue which is cherry red in color. Treatment can be conservative in patients who are asymptomatic or presenting with some mild genital bleeding. The conservative approach consists of daily baths and application of topical estrogen cream for 2 weeks. Surgical therapy is warranted only in recurrent or persistent cases.

(B) Antibiotic therapy is important in cases of infection and a quinolone-type antibiotic is preferred. (C) This child can void well; therefore urinary diversion is unnecessary. (D) Surgical excision is warranted in recurrent or persistent cases. (E) Urethral catheterization is warranted in cases of urinary retention.

47 A 52-year-old man presents to his primary care physician for an annual physical. He has a new complaint of profound watery diarrhea, which started 2 months ago. He denies any blood or mucous in the stool.

He also complains of skin flushing during bouts of diarrhea, which he never had before. He denies fevers, weight loss, has some nausea with no vomiting, with no abdominal pain. Physical examination reveals no abdominal tenderness. A rectal examination is performed, which yields a normal prostate and nontender rectum. His stool is negative for occult blood. What is the most likely diagnosis?

(A) Carcinoid tumor
(B) Tropical sprue
(C) Bacterial gastroenteritis
(D) VIPoma
(E) Surreptitious laxative abuse

The answer is D: VIPoma. This patient's history of chronic watery diarrhea with skin flushing indicates he has a VIPoma. Other clues of a VIPoma are hypokalemia, achlorhydria, and dehydration. VIPomas are tumors which secrete vasoactive intestinal peptide (VIP). 90% of VIPomas originate in the pancreas from a non-β islet cell. The excess VIP secreted increases intestinal motility and secretion of water and electrolytes, which causes the diarrhea. The medical treatment of choice is octreotide, which blocks the action of VIP to decrease the intestinal motility and quell the diarrhea. Surgical excision of the tumor is the next step.

(A) Carcinoid tumors are neuroendocrine tumors which secrete serotonin. Patients usually are asymptomatic until the tumor metastasizes to the liver, which causes carcinoid syndrome (patients experience flushing, diarrhea, wheezing, abdominal cramps). (B) Tropical sprue is a malabsorption syndrome seen typically in the tropical regions. It can become a chronic steatorrhea, leading to weight loss and malnutrition. (C) Bacterial gastroenteritis can present with diarrhea, but patients typically present more acutely with fever and vomiting. The 2-month duration of the diarrhea makes this diagnosis unlikely. (E) Laxatives are used to treat constipation, and act through a variety of mechanisms to soften stool. Abuse of laxatives can cause watery diarrhea, but there is nothing in the history that indicates that this patient is abusing laxatives.

 48 A 28-year-old man is stabbed in the abdomen several times by an assailant who was attempting to steal his car. The patient is brought to the emergency department by rescue squad. His mental status is normal. His blood pressure is 130/90 mmHg and his pulse rate is 92 beats/min. His abdomen is soft and nontender. Three small midline stab wounds are identified. Two large-bore 14-gauge intravenous lines are started. Which of the following fluid replacement should be given at this time?

(A) Blood
(B) Crystalloids
(C) Crystalloids and blood
(D) No intravenous fluids are necessary in this patient

The answer is B: Crystalloids. This individual appears to be clinically stable. His pulse rate is <100 beats/min and his blood pressure is normal. His blood loss is likely to be less than 750 cm³ and represents less than 15% of his blood volume. He would be classified as class I hypovolemic shock. Given the above information, the best fluid replacement for this patient would be crystalloids.

(A) Blood is given as fluid replacement with crystalloids for classes III and IV hypovolemic shock. (C) Blood and crystalloids are given to replace fluids in patients with significant blood loss such as seen in class III or IV hypovolemic shock. (D) This patient should be managed with crystalloids.

 A cadaver kidney becomes available for transplantation into a 39-year-old man with end-stage renal disease. This patient has the following medical problems: diabetes mellitus, hypertension, history of IV drug abuse, alcoholic cirrhosis, and sleep apnea. Which of the following is an absolute contraindication to use of this organ for transplantation?

(A) ABO incompatibility
(B) Cold ischemia lasting more than 36 hours
(C) HLA tissue typing with a poor match
(D) Positive T-cell cross-match
(E) Prior positive T-cell cross-match but currently negative

The answer is D: Positive T-Cell Cross-Match. A current positive T-cell cross-match indicates the presence of circulating antibodies against class I antigens, and the certainty of a hyperacute rejection reaction. This represents an absolute contraindication to transplantation.

(A) ABO incompatibility is an absolute contraindication to use of this organ for transplantation. (B) Good renal function can be expected from kidneys that have been ischemic for 48 hours. (C) Differences in human leukocyte antigen (HLA) matching are relatively small regarding cadaver kidney matches. (E) The fact that the current cross-match is negative does not preclude transplantation.

 A 68-year-old man with a history of vague left lower quadrant pain, bloating, and alternating constipation and diarrhea presents to his primary care physician for follow-up. He has a known history of diverticulosis. Most recently, he complains of passing air through his penis as well as fecal matter. Further, he has had four urinary tract infections in the last 6 months. What is the most appropriate next step in the management of this patient?

(A) Anoscopy
(B) Digital rectal examination
(C) Computed tomography (CT) scan of the abdomen and pelvis
(D) Sigmoidoscopy
(E) Ultrasound

The answer is C: CT scan of the abdomen and pelvis. This patient with known diverticulosis now has diverticulitis with evidence of a colovesical fistula. Typical features include passage of air with urination, passage of fecal matter with urination, and recurrent urinary tract infections. The best test to diagnose this is CT scan of the abdomen and pelvis.

(A) Anoscopy will not evaluate the sigmoid colon and will miss identification of the fistula. (B) Digital rectal examination, while important in the general physical examination, will miss this lesion. (D) Sigmoidoscopy may only show erythema but not the fistula tract unless it is large. (E) Ultrasound will not identify a colovesical fistula.

---

51 A 1-month-old female infant with a history of bronchopulmonary dysplasia presents with new onset of fevers. Her current medications include furosemide and ranitidine. A workup reveals an infection and antibiotics are initiated. If furosemide is continued during the hospital stay, which of the following antibiotics should be avoided in treating this patient's infection?

(A) Amoxicillin
(B) Azithromycin
(C) Cefotaxime
(D) Erythromycin
(E) Gentamicin

The answer is E: Gentamicin. Both furosemide and gentamicin are ototoxic by themselves. Using together, the action may be synergistic and greatly increase the risk of hearing loss. Thus, in general, in pediatric patients that are maintained on furosemide, alternative antibiotic choices are appropriate. If absolutely necessary, patients may require serial vestibular, audiometric, and renal function testing to monitor for hearing loss.

(A) Amoxicillin is generally safe to use in combination with furosemide. (B) Macrolide antibiotics such as azithromycin are generally safe to use in combination with furosemide. (C) Cefotaxime is generally safe to administer in a patient taking furosemide. (D) Erythromycin, also a macrolide antibiotic, is generally safe to take in combination with furosemide.

---

52 A 50-year-old obese man presents to his primary care physician with painless jaundice and unexplained weight loss. His social history is remarkable for chronic alcoholism and a 40-pack-year smoking history. His other medical problems include diabetes mellitus. He has a family history of multiple endocrine neoplasia type I. Which of the following is the least significant risk factor for pancreatic cancer?

(A) Alcohol
(B) Diabetes mellitus
(C) Multiple endocrine neoplasia type I
(D) Obesity
(E) Smoking

The answer is A: Alcohol. This patient has multiple risk factors for pancreatic cancer. However, multiple studies have shown that alcohol is most likely not a risk factor for pancreatic cancer.

(B) Diabetes mellitus has been linked to pancreatic cancer. Studies also suggest that late-onset diabetes may be an early sign of pancreatic cancer. (C) Patients with multiple endocrine neoplasia type I have an increased risk for certain types of pancreatic malignancies including gastrinomas and insulinomas. (D) Obesity has been noted to be a risk factor for pancreatic cancer in multiple studies. In particular, central obesity patterns have the highest risk. (E) Smoking is the most common environmental risk factor for pancreatic cancer. Studies have shown that smoking may be responsible for up to 30% of cases.

 53 A 44-year-old obese woman who is gravida 3 para 3 complains of chronic intermittent right upper quadrant pain. This was made worse after eating a fried chicken meal. She has severe right upper quadrant pain. Physical examination reveals mild right upper quadrant pain to palpation without evidence of guarding or rebound tenderness. Right upper quadrant ultrasound is performed. The rationale for ordering this test includes which of the following?

(A) Detailed anatomy of benign tumors can be characterized
(B) Focal liver disease can be imaged
(C) Hepatic tumors are visualized
(D) Involves radiation
(E) Reconstruction of the biliary tree with great detail is possible

The answer is B: Focal liver disease can be imaged. Ultrasound is a quick and easy test to perform. It is noninvasive and requires no radiation. It is the primary modality to identify cholelithiasis. Focal and diffuse liver disease can be identified.

(A) Detailed anatomy of benign tumors may be accomplished with computed tomography (CT) scan. (C) Hepatic tumors can be visualized with magnetic resonance imaging (MRI). (D) Ultrasound requires no radiation. (E) Reconstruction of the biliary tree with great detail is possible with MRI.

54 A 4-year-old girl presents to the emergency department with a 2-day history of fever, drooling, and severe odynophagia. When you go to see the patient, she is sitting up in bed with her neck extended and supported with both her arms. A lateral neck x-ray is read as a possible "thumb sign." What is the most likely diagnosis?

(A) Allergic reaction
(B) Branchial cleft cyst
(C) Epiglottitis
(D) Gastroesophageal reflux
(E) Sinusitis

The answer is C: Epiglottis. This patient is showing signs of epiglottitis. You should avoid doing anything with the patient that may cause her to become upset, which can trigger respiratory compromise. The patient should be taken immediately to the operating room by the otolaryngologist and anesthesiologist. Once epiglottitis is confirmed by physical examination, the patient can be treated with antibiotics alone or may need intubation depending on the severity of the illness.

(A) Allergic reaction is possible but no history is given to suggest this, such as an environmental exposure or a injection that triggered symptoms. (B) Branchial cleft cysts are in the lateral neck and do not move with swallowing. (D) Gastroesophageal reflux should not present with signs of respiratory compromise. (E) Sinusitis should not present with signs of odynophagia and respiratory compromise.

55 A 61-year-old woman undergoes a radical cystectomy for stage T3 bladder cancer. On the third postoperative day, she complains of shortness of breath. Her temperature is 37.2°C, blood pressure is 137/85 mmHg, pulse 120 beats/min, and respirations 23 breaths/min. On examination, there is mild discomfort in her right calf with palpation. Her lungs are clear bilaterally and her heart has a regular rhythm. Her abdominal incision is clean, dry, and intact. An electrocardiogram and chest x-ray return as normal. An arterial blood gas returns with decreased PCO_2. Which of the following is the next best step in management?

(A) Immediate warfarin
(B) Send a complete blood count (CBC) and monitor the patient closely
(C) Start intravenous heparin and order a spiral computed tomography (CT) scan
(D) Venodynes (SCD)
(E) Ventilation perfusion scan

The answer is C: Start intravenous heparin and order a spiral CT scan. This patient has a high likelihood of pulmonary embolism and should be immediately started on heparin. A spiral CT scan should also be performed as soon as possible, as this will establish the diagnosis. Pulmonary emboli should be on the differential diagnosis for any patient presenting with postoperative shortness of breath.

(A) Although warfarin will be needed for anticoagulation, the patient should be bridged with heparin. Warfarin without heparin may result in initial increase in thrombosis. (B) Although this patient should be monitored closely, a CBC is unlikely to aid in the diagnosis when pulmonary emboli are suspected. (D) Venodynes (sequential compression device) are useful in the postoperative period to prevent deep vein thrombosis. However, they have no role in the acute management of suspected pulmonary emboli. (E) Although ventilation perfusion scans are still utilized for diagnosis of pulmonary emboli, spiral CT imaging is faster and more readily available in most institutions. Spiral CT imaging is currently the first-line test for diagnosis of pulmonary embolism. Additionally, in patients with a high suspicion of pulmonary emboli, heparin should be initiated as soon as possible. In a patient with pulmonary emboli, ventilation-perfusion scanning will show impaired areas of perfusion with normal ventilation.

---

 56 A 59-year-old man with chronic intermittent abdominal pain presents to his primary care physician for a follow-up examination. Physical examination reveals no evidence of guarding or rebound tenderness. Computed tomography (CT) scan of the abdomen is performed and reveals tortuous, dilated veins in the submucosa of the proximal colon wall. What is the most problematic complication that can occur in this patient?

(A) Colorectal carcinoma
(B) Colon pseudopolyposis coli
(C) Hemorrhage
(D) Herniation
(E) Inflammation

The answer is C: Hemorrhage. This patient has angiodysplasia of the colon. This condition is characterized by tortuous dilated veins in the submucosa of the colon, usually the proximal wall. This is a common cause of lower gastrointestinal (GI) bleeding in patients over the age of 60. In 15% of patients, massive hemorrhage is possible.

(A) Angiodysplasia does not predispose to colon carcinoma. (B) Angiodysplasia does not predispose to colon polyposis. (D) Herniation is not a possible complication of angiodysplasia. However, herniation of the mucosa of the bowel wall is implicated in the pathogenesis of diverticulosis. (E) Angiodysplasia is not associated with inflammation. Crohn disease and ulcerative colitis are inflammatory bowel diseases.

57 A 49-year-old woman is undergoing a right modified radical mastectomy. During the surgery, the lateral thoracic artery, as it enters the breast tissue, is transected. This vessel supplies which of the following areas of the breast?

(A) Central breast
(B) Medial breast
(C) Nipple area
(D) Posterior breast
(E) Upper outer quadrant

The answer is E: Upper outer quadrant. The blood supply to the breast comes from the internal mammary artery and the lateral thoracic artery. The lateral thoracic artery supplies the upper outer quadrant of the breast.
   (A) The central breast is supplied by the internal mammary artery. (B) The medial breast is supplied by the internal mammary artery. (C) The nipple area is supplied by the internal mammary artery. (D) The posterior breast tissue is supplied by the lateral thoracic artery and branches of the internal mammary artery.

58 A 10-month-old girl is brought to the clinic with a 4-cm bright red lesion with sharp borders that involves most of her right cheek and auricle. You note no other lesions anywhere on the child. It feels rubbery on palpation, and is nontender. Further physical examination reveals clear lung fields and no heart murmur that is readily appreciated. The mother is very worried that this might be cancer because it has grown so quickly over the past few months. What is the next most appropriate step in the management of this patient?

(A) Antibiotics
(B) Aspiration
(C) Corticosteroids
(D) Surgical excision
(E) Watchful waiting

The answer is E: Watchful waiting. Watchful waiting is the most appropriate step in the management of this patient. This lesion is most likely an infantile hemangioma. After 1 year of life, this lesion should slowly regress. The mother should be instructed, however, to take note of any stridorous breathing that may suggest subglottic involvement.
   (A) This is not an infectious condition, and as such, antibiotics are not recommended. (B) Aspiration will not remove this lesion. Bleeding will result from such a maneuver. (C) Corticosteroids will not change the size of this lesion. (D) Surgical excision could be required if this lesion does not regress.

59 If the electrolyte composition and volume of gastrointestinal fluid were measured in terms of output per 24 hours in five patients, which structure would have the highest concentration of sodium in mEq/L?

(A) Bile
(B) Colon
(C) Distal small bowel
(D) Proximal small bowel
(E) Stomach

The answer is A: Bile. Bile has the highest sodium concentration of the structures represented in this question. Bile contains approximately 150 mEq/L of sodium. Stomach, in the setting of high acid, has the lowest concentration of sodium and is measured at 20 mEq/L.

(B) Colon contains 120 mEq/L of sodium. (C) Distal small bowel contains 80 mEq/L of sodium. (D) Proximal small bowel contains 110 mEq/L of sodium. (E) Stomach in the setting of low acid contains 80 mEq/L of sodium and 20 mEq/L when in the setting of high acid.

60 An 18-year-old woman presents to the emergency department after being injured when falling off of a bike that she was riding over a patch of ice. Her knee hit a tree as she fell from the bike. She appears anxious and is complaining of right knee pain. On examination, she has an easily identifiable posterior dislocation of her right knee. The skin distal to the injury is warm and pulses are palpable. Which of the following is the next best step in management?

(A) Administer an anxiolytic
(B) Administer nonsteroidal anti-inflammatory drugs (NSAIDs)
(C) Immediate knee reduction
(D) Perform ankle-brachial or arterial indices
(E) Plain radiography

The answer is D: Perform ankle-brachial or arterial indices. Posterior knee dislocations should always be evaluated for vascular injury due to the high rate of popliteal artery injury. Patients with obvious signs of decreased perfusion (absent peripheral pulses, expanding hematomas, palpable thrills, audible bruits, pulsating hemorrhage) should receive surgical revascularization immediately. Indexes less than 0.9 indicate an abnormal result and further workup, often with duplex ultrasonography or computed tomography (CT) angiography, is required. Additionally, serial perfusion checks should be performed.

(A) Although anxiolytics may be administered, vascular evaluation should take precedence. (B) While NSAIDs may be important for pain control, this patient's vascular status should be evaluated. (C) Patients without hard evidence of arterial compromise should receive radiographs and arterial evaluation prior to reduction. (E) While plain radiography is important in this patient's evaluation, the vascular status of the limb should be evaluated first.

---

61 A 43-year-old woman presents with abdominal pain for the last 2 days. The pain is localized in the epigastric area and radiates to the right upper quadrant. She recalls a history of similar pain after eating food in the past, but reports that it has never been this severe. Her past medical history is remarkable for hypertension and hyperlipidemia. She denies smoking, drinking alcohol or other drugs. Her temperature is 37.2°C, blood pressure 150/90 mmHg, pulse 105 beats/min, respirations 20 breaths/min, and she is saturated at 98% SpO_2 on room air. On examination, there is significant tenderness in the right upper quadrant without guarding or rebound. An abdominal ultrasound is ordered which shows thickening of the gall bladder wall and pericholecystic fluid. Which of the following is the next best step in management?

(A) Antibiotics, fluid resuscitation, and surgical consultation
(B) CT scan
(C) Endoscopic retrograde cholangiopancreatography (ERCP)
(D) Percutaneous transhepatic cholecystostomy
(E) Ursodeoxycholic acid and close observation

The answer is A: Antibiotics, fluid resuscitation, and surgical consultation. This patient is suffering from acute cholecystitis, strongly suggested by her history of cholelithiasis, physical examination, and imaging. Initial treatment for acute cholecystitis includes nothing by mouth, broad-spectrum antibiotics, and fluid resuscitation. Additionally, the surgical team should be consulted for evaluation. Patients with uncomplicated cholecystitis may be treated conservatively with surgery once the acute episode resolves. This includes patients with stable vital signs, no evidence of obstruction by laboratory values or ultrasonography, no underlying medical problems or advanced age, and reliable follow-up. However, cholecystectomy is the standard of care in patients who do not fit these criteria.

(B) Although the sensitivity of computed tomography (CT) imaging is high for diagnosis of acute cholecystitis, it is not necessary unless the diagnosis is uncertain. (C) ERCP may be useful if there is a gallstone in the common bile duct. (D) For patients that are not candidates for surgery or are high risk for surgery, placement of a transhepatic cholecystostomy drainage tube is indicated. (E) Treatment with ursodeoxycholic acid is used for prevention of gallstones in patients with a history of cholelithiasis. It is not used in the management of acute cholecystitis.

---

62 A 29-year-old man who has been an alcoholic for 15 years is brought to the emergency department because of hematemesis after forceful wrenching and vomiting. He has a chronic cough from smoking

2 packs of cigarettes per day for the last 10 years. Upper gastrointestinal (GI) endoscopy confirms a distal esophageal mucosal tear. Which of the following statements are true about this condition?

(A) Is usually fatal.
(B) Is best treated with surgery.
(C) Requires computed tomography (CT) scanning for diagnosis.
(D) Can usually be treated endoscopically.
(E) Mandates *H. pylori* testing.

The answer is D: Can usually be treated endoscopically. Mallory–Weiss syndrome, a condition of bleeding from a mucosal rent at the gastroesophageal junction, has a fairly benign course and can almost always be diagnosed and treated with endoscopic hemostatic maneuvers.

(A) Bleeding stops spontaneously in greater than 90% of cases. (B) Endoscopic therapy is often effective for most patients. (C) Diagnosis can be made endoscopically as shown in this case. (E) It is not associated with *H. pylori* infection.

---

63 A 16-year-old boy is brought to the emergency department by ambulance after sustaining a gunshot to the chest during a gang fight. On arrival his temperature is 37.3°C, pulse 120 beats/min, respirations 20 breaths/min, and blood pressure 90/55 mmHg. On examination, there is a narrow pulse pressure, jugular venous distention, and muffled heart sounds. There is a larger than normal decrease in systolic pressure during inspiration. There is also hepatomegaly on the abdominal examination. Which of the following is the most likely diagnosis?

(A) Cardiac tamponade
(B) Cardiogenic shock
(C) Left ventricular rupture
(D) Pneumothorax
(E) Ruptured aorta

The answer is A: Cardiac tamponade. This patient is most likely suffering from cardiac tamponade. This is indicated by the findings of hypotension, a narrow pulse pressure, jugular venous distention, muffled heart sounds, hepatomegaly, and a larger than normal decrease in systolic pressure during inspiration (termed pulsus paradoxus). The initial management should include volume expansion, oxygen, and pericardiocentesis to remove the fluid, while leaving a closed drainage system in place.

(B) Although cardiogenic shock is possibly responsible for this patient's symptoms, the examination findings of muffled heart sounds suggest cardiac tamponade. (C) Although traumatic rupture of the left ventricle is possible in this patient, it is not the most likely diagnosis with these examination findings. (D) While a pneumothorax could explain some of the examination findings, a narrow pulse pressure and pulsus paradoxus are not typically observed in patients with a pneumothorax. (E) This patient's findings of a narrow pulse pressure, muffled heart sounds, jugular venous distention, and pulsus paradoxus are more consistent with cardiac tamponade than aortic rupture.

64 A 40-year-old man recently seen for an upper respiratory tract infection presents with "ear pain." He has a history of poorly controlled diabetes mellitus. He reports that recently he has had discharge from his ear and that it has become even more painful. Although originally the pain was only present at night, the pain is now persistent. His temperature is 38.1°C, blood pressure 135/80 mmHg, pulse 100 beats/min, and respirations 19 breaths/min. On examination, there is swelling and erythema in the left periauricular soft tissue. The external ear is exquisitely tender to palpation and the tympanic membrane is only partially visible because of swelling. There is no lymphadenopathy. Which of the following organisms is most commonly cultured from patients with this condition?

(A) *Aspergillus* species
(B) *Candida albicans*
(C) *Proteus* species
(D) *Pseudomonas aeruginosa*
(E) *Staphylococcus aureus*

The answer is D: *Pseudomonas aeruginosa*. This patient is most likely suffering from malignant otitis externa, an infection of the outer ear and ear canal. This disease is most common in diabetic patients, although it may be found in other patients with immunodeficiencies. The infection usually starts as external otitis and may eventually progress into osteomyelitis of the temporal bone. The most common organism responsible for the infection is *P. aeruginosa*, a gram-negative aerobic coccobacillus bacterium abundant in humid or moisture environments. Indeed, the infection may arise in patients from swimming or showering. Initial antibiotic coverage should be targeted toward this organism and other possible pathogens. Third-generation cephalosporins are a popular choice, although other antibiotics including fluoroquinolones are efficacious. Other treatments employed along with antibiotics include meticulous glucose control, hyperbaric oxygen therapy, and local debridement if necessary.

(A) *Aspergillus* species, a type of fungal organism, is also a less common cause of malignant otitis externa. (B) *C. albicans*, a type of fungal organism, is also a less common cause of malignant otitis externa. (C) *Proteus* species, such as *P. mirabilis*, is a potential but less common cause of malignant otitis externa. (E) *S. aureus* is the second most common cause of malignant otitis media in diabetic patients.

65 A 55-year-old man with a history of diabetes mellitus and obesity presents to the emergency department complaining of moderate pain in his chest with radiation to his back. His blood pressure is 180/100 mmHg, pulse 115 beats/min, and respirations 19 breaths/min. On examination, he appears diaphoretic. A transesophageal echocardiogram reveals a type III aortic dissection. Which of the following is the best management?

(A) Aspirin
(B) Heparin
(C) Immediate surgical repair
(D) Intravenous β-blocker
(E) Intravenous antibiotics

The answer is D: Intravenous β-blocker. This patient has a type III aortic dissection (descending aorta). Medical management is appropriate. The initial goal is to lower his blood pressure. Intravenous β-blockers and other potent hypertensives are effective for acute management.

(A) Aspirin would not be appropriate in this patient, as it would increase the risk of bleeding. (B) Heparin would not be appropriate in this patient, as it would increase the risk of bleeding. (C) Surgical repair would be required if the dissection was visualized in the ascending aorta. (E) This patient is not presenting with signs of infection thus treatment with antibiotics is not warranted.

66 A 25-year-old woman comes to her physician because she is concerned about one of her "freckles" on her shoulder. She says that she has many freckles, but that this one in particular has changed over the last several months with increased size and color changes. On examination, there are multiple small, pigmented lesions over her torso. On her left shoulder, there is a larger 1.8 cm in diameter, pigmented lesion that is asymmetrically shaped and has irregular borders. Which of the following is the next best step in management?

(A) Application of topical 5-fluorouracil cream
(B) Excisional biopsy
(C) Observation
(D) Punch biopsy
(E) Shave biopsy

The answer is D: Punch biopsy. This patient's presentation is concerning for melanoma. Melanoma risk factors include fair skin, ultraviolet light exposure, history of precursor lesions, history of peeling or blistering sunburns, family history of melanoma, and immunosuppression. Diagnosis is clinically made with the ABCDE rule where A stands for asymmetry, B for border irregularity, C for color variation, D for diameter greater than 6 mm, and E for evolution. The next best step for patients with lesions greater than 1.5 cm in diameter is a full thickness punch biopsy of the thickest part of the lesion as this will allow for adequate histologic characterization as well as depth. If the diagnosis of melanoma is established, then surgical excision is the primary treatment.

(A) 5-Flourouracil is uncommonly used for treating advanced melanoma. (B) Excisional biopsy is appropriate for lesions less than 1.5 cm in the diameter. (C) Observation is not appropriate when melanoma is suspected in a young individual such as this. (E) Shave biopsies should be avoided in patients with suspected melanoma as the prognosis is highly dependent on the depth of the malignancy. Shave biopsy will make it very difficult to determine the depth in the future.

67 A 59-year-old man with a history of chronic gastroesophageal reflux disease is found by endoscopy to have esophageal varices. His blood pressure is 80/40 mmHg and pulse is 140 beats/min. Hematocrit is 24%. In the setting of active bleeding, which of the following is the most efficacious form of treatment?

(A) Blakemore tube
(B) Somatostatin
(C) Surgical resection
(D) Transjugular intrahepatic portosystemic shunting
(E) Watchful waiting

The answer is D: Transjugular intrahepatic portosystemic shunting. Transjugular intrahepatic portosystemic shunting has largely replaced emergency surgical shunting as the standard of treatment for esophageal bleeding. This is useful in patients who are unresponsive to endoscopic and pharmacologic treatment.

(A) Blakemore tune is successful in 50% of cases. (B) Somatostatin decreased bleeding by 50% through vasoconstriction. (C) TIPS has replaced surgical shunting as the treatment of choice for patients with esophageal bleeding. (E) Watchful waiting is not recommended for this hemodynamically unstable patient.

68 A 78-year-old man presents with a hand tremor at rest, shuffling gait, and difficulty getting started walking. He also exhibits ratcheting rigidity with passive motion of his upper extremities. Which test could be used to confirm the diagnosis?

(A) EEG
(B) Functional magnetic resonance imaging (fMRI)
(C) Nerve conduction study
(D) No further testing is necessary
(E) Peripheral nerve biopsy

The answer is D: No further testing is necessary. The symptoms and signs described for this patient are consistent with Parkinson disease. Diagnosis is clinical; there are currently no tests or studies useful for diagnosing Parkinson disease. The findings include a "pill rolling" resting tremor (disappears with voluntary movement), shuffling and stooping, difficulty initiating the first step, and "cogwheel rigidity," meaning a jerking, ratcheting motion with passive movement of the limbs. These movement abnormalities are the result of depletion of dopaminergic neurons in the substantia nigra and locus ceruleus in the midbrain.

(A) An EEG might be useful in evaluating seizure disorders if an EEG can be performed during a seizure, but would have no role in evaluating Parkinson disease. Parkinson disease is a clinical diagnosis. (B) fMRI scans are used largely in research to visualize changes in blood flow related to neural activity. It has no use in evaluating Parkinson disease, which is a clinical diagnosis. (C) Nerve conduction studies may be used to evaluate suspected carpal tunnel syndrome, ulnar neuropathy, or other causes of paresthesias. It has no use in evaluating Parkinson disease, which is a clinical diagnosis. (E) Nerve biopsies may reveal demyelinating diseases, but the neural changes in Parkinson disease are in the central nervous system and are not biopsied. Parkinson disease is a clinical diagnosis.

 69 A 57-year-old man with advanced colorectal carcinoma is treated with 6 weeks of external beam radiation in an effort to reduce tumor bulk. He presents to his physician for a follow-up examination. Which of the following symptoms, if present in this patient, would be most worrisome to the treating physician?

(A) Bleeding
(B) Diarrhea, transient
(C) Malaise
(D) Nausea
(E) Vomiting

The answer is A: Bleeding. Acute phase injury of the bowel is due to mucosal injury. Common symptoms include nausea, vomiting, and diarrhea. However, bleeding and perforation can occur which may require surgical intervention. Thus, bleeding is a worrisome symptom for the treating physician to be aware of as an underlying perforation could be present.

(B) Transient diarrhea would be expected in this patient given the radiation received. (C) Malaise is a common symptom of radiation injury. (D) Nausea is a common symptom of radiation injury. (E) Vomiting is a common symptom of radiation injury.

 70 A 29-year-old man with a history of HIV disease and intractable diarrhea is hospitalized on the medical service. He is admitted for fluid replacement. Assuming that he weighs 50 kg, which of the following statements are true about maintenance fluid resuscitation for this individual?

(A) 4 mL/kg for the first 10 kg of body weight
(B) 3 mL/kg for the second 20 kg of body weight
(C) 2 mL/kg for the third 30 kg of body weight
(D) 0.5 mL/kg for each additional measurement of body weight

The answer is A: 4 mL/kg for the first 10 kg of body weight. In the adult, fluid maintenance requirements approximate 30 mL/kg/body weight/24 hours. Maintenance fluid after resuscitation can be estimated by the 4–2–1 formula. 4 L/kg is administered for the first 10 kg of body weight.

(B) 2 mL/kg is administered for the second 10 kg of body weight. (C) 1 mL/kg is administered for all additional weight. (D) This statement is incorrect. 1 mL/kg is administered for each additional measurement of body weight.

71 A 58-year-old man with a history of respiratory acidosis is hospitalized in the medical intensive care unit. An arterial blood gas is drawn from his right femoral arterial line. The results return with a serum pH of 7.40. Given this information and assuming that there is no potassium wasting, what would his predicted serum potassium be?

(A) 2.6 mEq/L
(B) 3.8 mEq/L
(C) 4.1 mEq/L
(D) 5.1 mEq/L
(E) 5.9 mEq/L

The answer is C: 4.1 mEq/L. It is useful to know that it is possible to predict serum potassium from serum pH assuming that no potassium wasting is occurring. In this patient, his normal serum pH of 7.40 correlates with a predicted serum potassium of 4.1 mEq/L.

(A) A serum of pH of 7.70 correlated with a serum potassium of 2.6 mEq/L. (B) A serum of pH of 7.50 correlated with a serum potassium of 3.8 mEq/L. (D) A serum of pH of 7.20 correlated with a serum potassium of 5.1 mEq/L. (E) A serum of pH of 7.10 correlated with a serum potassium of 5.9 mEq/L.

72 A 48-year-old woman presents to her primary care physician with a new rash on her buttocks. She also complains of losing 20 pounds over the past 3 months, and feeling "a little off." Physical examination reveals that the rash appears as an area of erythematous blisters on her lower buttocks down into her perineal region, along with some swelling of the area. Her blood tests show an elevated blood glucose level of 1,040 mg/dL, as well as a hemoglobin level of 8.4 g/dL. Should this condition be due to neoplasm, which of the following would be the most likely origin of the lesion?

(A) Pancreatic α-cell
(B) Zona fasciculata
(C) Pancreatic acini
(D) Adrenal medulla
(E) Pancreatic δ-cell

The answer is A: Pancreatic α-cell. This patient has a glucagonoma, which is a rare tumor of the pancreas that produces excess levels of glucagon. Glucagon is a hormone produced by pancreatic α-cells which acts to increase blood levels of glucose via stimulation of glycolysis and gluconeogenesis in the liver, stimulation of lipolysis in peripheral adipose, and stimulation of protein breakdown in skeletal muscle. Excess glucagon levels causes hyperglycemia, anemia, and a dermatologic condition called necrolytic migratory erythema (NME). NME appear as erythematous blisters and swelling which occurs in areas subject to greater friction and pressure, like the buttocks and perineum in this patient. The origin of this tumor is the pancreatic α-cells in the islets of Langerhans.

(B) The zona fasciculata is the middle zone of the adrenal cortex responsible for glucocorticoid production. Tumors from this region can cause Cushing syndrome. (C) Pancreatic carcinoma originates from the pancreatic acinar cells. It classically present with painless jaundice. (D) The adrenal medulla is the main source of catecholamines into the bloodstream. Pheochromocytomas are tumors of the adrenal medulla. (E) Malignant transformation of pancreatic δ-cells can form somatostatinomas, which manifest as steatorrhea and hyperglycemia.

---

73 A 61-year-old nondiabetic woman is brought to the emergency department because of suprapubic pain and not being able to urinate for the last 24 hours. Ultrasound shows a distended bladder and a cervical mass. She has a Foley catheter placed and is admitted for observation and further treatment. As the nurse taking care of the patient places the orders into the computer, which of the following labs should she have monitored regularly over the next 24 hours?

(A) Albumin
(B) Basic metabolic panel
(C) CA-125
(D) Complete blood count (CBC)
(E) Fingerstick glucose

The answer is B: Basic metabolic panel. Postobstructive diuresis is a clinical picture that follows prolonged urinary obstruction which can result in electrolyte abnormalities. Although the pathogenesis of this phenomenon is not completely understood, it is thought that products of serum filtration are reabsorbed by the renal interstitium due to the obstruction of urine outflow causing increased pressure and stagnation of urine in the tubules. Once this outflow is reestablished, a high concentration of diuretic and natriuretic compounds in the serum causes a profound diuresis of sodium chloride rich urine which can be as much as 1,000 mL/h. This high flow rate through the tubules can cause increased potassium secretion in the collecting duct. To monitor for electrolyte disturbances, a basic metabolic panel should be performed regularly, while urine output is still high postobstructively.

(A) Albumin levels are not affected by postobstructive diuresis and do not need to be checked regularly. (C) A CA-125 test is not indicated in the presence of a cervical mass and is also not necessary to be checked regularly in the postobstructive phase of diuresis. (D) A complete blood count does not need to be checked regularly during postobstructive diuresis since a nephritic syndrome is not present and no blood loss is occurring. (E) Serum glucose levels are not indicated in asymptomatic nondiabetic patients.

---

 74 A 24-year-old man is stabbed in the abdomen several times by an assailant who was attempting to buy drugs from him. The patient is brought to the emergency department by rescue squad. He is confused. His blood pressure is 90/40 mmHg and his pulse rate is 125 beats/min. His abdomen is rigid and tender in all four quadrants. Two large midline stab wounds are identified measuring 1 cm each. Two large-bore 14-gauge intravenous lines are started. Which of the following fluid replacement should be given at this time?

(A) Blood
(B) Crystalloids
(C) Crystalloids and blood
(D) No intravenous fluids are necessary in this patient

The answer is C: Crystalloids and blood. This individual appears to be clinically unstable. His pulse rate is >120 beats/min and he is hypotensive with a blood pressure of 90/40 mmHg. His blood loss is likely to be greater than 1,500 cm³ and represents more than 30% of his blood volume. He would be classified as class III hypovolemic shock. Given the above information, the best fluid replacement for this patient would be crystalloids and blood.

(A) Blood is given as fluid replacement with crystalloids for classes III and IV hypovolemic shock. This patient would also benefit from crystalloids as well. (B) Crystalloids alone would be given to replace fluids in patients with class I or II shock. (D) This patient should be managed with crystalloids and blood.

---

 75 A 47-year-old man presents to the emergency department following contact with a high-tension electrical power line while trying to fix his satellite dish. On examination, there is an entrance wound visible on the patient's right hand and an exit wound visible on his right upper arm. The patient is stabilized in the emergency department and scheduled for surgical debridement. Which of the following medications may this patient require to avoid renal failure?

(A) Aluminum chloride
(B) Dopamine
(C) Epinephrine
(D) Mannitol
(E) Oxacillin

The answer is D: Mannitol. This patient has suffered an electrical injury to his arm. Unfortunately, electrical burn injuries are usually much more extensive than they may superficially appear. Extensive surgical debridement of the soft tissues along the path of the electrical current is often necessary. Adequate hydration is extremely important in the initial management for these patients. If severe muscle damage is expected, an osmotic diuretic such as mannitol and/or alkalinizing agent is indicated to prevent acute renal failure from myoglobinuria. In addition to mannitol administration, urine alkalization with sodium bicarbonate increases the rate of myoglobin clearance.

(A) Aluminum chloride is a medication used to acidify the urine. It would be contraindicated in the use with electrical burn injuries since acidification of the urine would increase the chance of developing acute renal failure. (B) Dopamine is a vasopressor that increases medullary oxygen demand. Withdrawal from dopinergic agents may cause rhabdomyolysis. However, this is not a medication that will help this patient avoid renal failure. (C) Epinephrine will not help avoid acute renal failure in this patient. (E) Oxacillin is a penicillinase-resistant β-lactam antibiotic and will not help this patient avoid renal failure.

 A 34-year-old woman returns for follow-up after undergoing a cadaveric renal transplant. She is now approximately 6 weeks post-op and presents for a routine scheduled follow-up examination. She has a history of diabetes and hypertension. She complains of a 2-day history of headache. Her blood pressure is 164/105 mmHg. Examination of the heart, lungs, and abdomen is unremarkable. Her serum creatinine is 2.3 mg/dL and her cyclosporine level is 300 ng/mL. Ultrasound of the abdomen reveals no evidence of fluid collections. What is the most appropriate management of this patient?

(A) Begin OKT3
(B) Biopsy of the transplant kidney
(C) Discontinue immunosuppression
(D) Increase prednisone and decrease cyclosporine
(E) Intravenous pulse steroids for 1 week

The answer is D: Increase prednisone and decrease cyclosporine.
This patient has cyclosporine nephrotoxicity. This patient should have their cyclosporine levels decreased and increase the dose of prednisone. This will guard against rejection. If there is no improvement in serum creatinine, renal biopsy is necessary.

(A) OKT3 should be administered if the renal biopsy suggests rejection.
(B) Biopsy will be necessary if there is no improvement in serum creatinine.
(C) Immunosuppression should be stopped in the face of serious infection.
(E) Pulse steroids will not lower the elevated cyclosporine levels seen in this patient.

 77 A 17-year-old boy is brought to the emergency department by his parents after being struck in the side of the head with a baseball while playing without a helmet with friends. The patient is saying he feels fine except for a mild headache, but two friends who accompanied him to the hospital say he was unconscious for a few seconds after being struck. What is the next best step in the management of this patient?

(A) Aminocaproic acid
(B) Emergent craniotomy
(C) Monitor for 24 hours
(D) Nonsteroidal anti-inflammatory drug (NSAID) for headache
(E) Order head computed tomography (CT)

The answer is E: Order head computed tomography (CT). This patient's story raises high suspicion for an epidural hematoma. Epidural hematomas generally occur following a blow to the side of the head that ruptures the middle meningeal artery which bleeds into the space between the bones of the skull and the dura mater. The classic presentation is less common, but involves a brief loss of consciousness followed by a lucid interval. As blood continues to flow into the epidural space, coma ensues. Ipsilateral mydriasis is seen in about half of cases. A head CT scan would show a lens-shaped hematoma at the trauma site.

(A) Aminocaproic acid promotes coagulation by inhibiting plasmin. It may theoretically help slow the bleeding of an epidural hematoma, but is not used for this purpose because treatment requires most importantly rapid surgical decompression. No treatment should be given until the diagnosis is made with CT scan regardless. (B) Rapid surgical decompression is the treatment for epidural hematoma, but no intervention should be pursued until the diagnosis is made with CT scan. (C) This patient may have an epidural hematoma. Witholding treatment may result in his demise. The next step would be a head CT scan to assess the injury. (D) NSAIDs would impair platelet function and are contraindicated in patients suspected of having an intracranial bleed (or any significant bleed). The next step would be a head CT scan to assess the injury.

A 93-year-old woman with a history of 36 hours of severe abdominal pain is brought to the emergency department for evaluation. She has a prior medical history of coronary artery disease and hypertension. Physical examination reveals severe pain to palpation in the lower quadrants out of proportion to the light tough of the physician. What is the most appropriate next step in the management of this patient?

(A) Chest x-ray flat and upright films
(B) Computed tomograph (CT) scan of the abdomen without contrast
(C) Flat plate film of the abdomen
(D) Magnetic resonance imaging scan of the abdomen
(E) Mesenteric angiography

The answer is E: **Mesenteric angiography.** This patient likely has acute mesenteric ischemia. This is due to a compromised blood supply to the colon via the superior mesenteric vessels. Diagnosis is by mesenteric angiography. Treatment involves fluid hydration via intravenous and broad-spectrum antibiotics. Injection of vasodilators such as papavarine may be necessary.

(A) Chest x-ray will rule out pulmonary diseases such as pneumonia and pneumothorax. However, this patient does not have any pulmonary complaints. (B) CT scan will not reveal mesenteric vascular abnormalities but can show other colon pathology. Mesenteric angiography is the test of choice for acute mesenteric ischemia. (C) KUB of the abdomen is a useful test to indicate free air from bowel perforation but will not show evidence of mesenteric ischemia. (D) Magnetic resonance imaging (MRI) scan will not reveal mesenteric vascular abnormalities.

 A 19-year-old man is brought to the emergency department complaining of left upper quadrant pain after an automobile accident. He was sitting in the passenger seat and his left side struck the dashboard on impact. Physical examination reveals ecchymosis of the left flank. Computed tomography (CT) scan of the abdomen reveals a splenic injury. What other injury should the treating physician also consider in the evaluation of this patient?

(A) Liver laceration
(B) Prostate infarction
(C) Renal contusion
(D) Rib fracture
(E) Spinal cord infarction

The answer is D: **Rib fracture.** This patient has suffered blunt trauma to the left abdomen and has findings of a splenic injury on CT scan. Fractures of the lower left rib cage are most commonly associated with splenic injury and must be considered as such.

(A) Liver laceration is less commonly associated with splenic injury. (B) Prostatic infarction can be seen on CT scan of elderly men with long-standing prostate enlargement. (C) Ipsilateral renal contusion may be associated with splenic injury due to the proximity of the organs. (E) Spinal cord infarction is unlikely to occur given the extensive blood supply to this region.

---

80 A 43-year-old woman is in the operating room undergoing a laparoscopic-assisted cholecystectomy. She is morbidly obese and weighs 310 lb. With the laparoscope in the peritoneum, the surgical procedure is now in progress. Which of the following anatomic statements is correct?

(A) The gall bladder is supplied by a branch of the left hepatic artery
(B) The gall bladder is olive shaped
(C) The gall bladder comprises four anatomic portions
(D) The medial surface of the gall bladder is covered by peritoneum
(E) The inferior surface is associated with the hepatic fossa.

The answer is C: The gall bladder comprises four anatomic portions.
The gall bladder has four anatomic portions which include the fundus, body, infundibulum, and neck. The gall bladder is pear shaped and can distend to accommodate approximately 50 cm^3 of fluid.

(A) The gall bladder is supplied by a branch of the right hepatic artery which is known as the cystic artery. (B) The gall bladder is pear shaped. (D) The inferior and lateral surface of the gall bladder is covered by peritoneum. (E) The superior surface of the gall bladder is covered by peritoneum.

---

81 A previously well 4-year-old boy measuring in the 75th percentile for height and 55th percentile for weight is brought to the physician complaining of right leg and knee pain for the last month. His mother says he has been limping around as well. The mother reports no fever, morning stiffness, or history of trauma. His vital signs are within normal limits. On examination, his right knee is nontender to palpation and has a normal range of motion. Examination of his right hip reveals limited range of motion with hip flexion, abduction, and internal rotation. There is no observable trauma, erythema, or tenderness of the hip joint. Which of the following is the most likely diagnosis?

(A) Legg-Calvé-Perthes disease
(B) Osteomyelitis of the hip
(C) Rheumatoid arthritis
(D) Septic arthritis of the knee
(E) Slipped capital femoral epiphysis

The answer is A: Legg-Calvé-Perthes disease. This patient is most likely suffering from Legg-Calvé-Perthes disease, or avascular necrosis of the femoral head. The condition is most common in boys between the ages of 3 and 12 years. It is not associated with obesity. Although the mechanism of action is not thoroughly understood, it is thought to be caused by temporary disruption of vascular supply. Symptoms include an insidious onset of intermittent knee, hip, groin, or thigh pain. Limping with a Trendelenburg gait is caused by the femoral head collapse leading to decreased abductor muscle tension. The diagnosis is made with plain radiographs of the pelvis and "frog-leg" laterals. The prognosis is excellent in children with a bone age of less than 6 years. Treatment is aimed at keeping the femoral head contained within the acetabulum and maintaining good range of motion. This can usually be accomplished with observation, activity restriction, partial weight bearing, traction, and/or physical therapy. Rarely surgery may be needed.

(B) This patient does not have a fever or history of trauma; thus osteomyelitis of the hip is less likely. (C) This patient's lack of morning stiffness makes rheumatoid arthritis less likely. (D) The physical examination of this patient's knee is unremarkable and there is no fever making septic arthritis unlikely. (E) Slipped capital femoral epiphysis is more common in obese and older (average age of 13) patients.

 82) A 18-year-old man falls from a tree while trimming branches. On arrival to the emergency department via ambulance, he is conscious and complaining of chest and abdominal pain. He has two large-bore intravenous lines in place and has already received 2 L of crystalloids. His blood pressure on arrival is 95/50 mmHg, pulse is 135 beats/min, and respirations are 27 breaths/min. He appears anxious but is not in respiratory distress. On examination, there are several superficial head and body lacerations and large bruises over the chest and abdomen, but no obvious head injuries or other bony deformities. A chest x-ray shows clear lungs and a normal cardiac silhouette, although there are several broken ribs. Initial fluid resuscitation is continued and an abdominal ultrasound prepared. Just before starting the abdominal ultrasound, the patient loses consciousness and endotracheal intubation is required. A repeat blood pressure measures 80/40 mmHg, and the patient seems to be quickly deteriorating. Which of the following is the next best step in management?

(A) Abdominal ultrasound
(B) Exploratory laparotomy
(C) CT scan
(D) Place external pressure on lacerations
(E) Plain radiography of the femur

The answer is B: **Exploratory laparotomy.** This patient is suffering from hypovolemic shock from hemorrhage. Hypovolemic shock can occur with 25% or more of blood volume loss. An average adult has 5 L of blood. Since no significant external hemorrhaging can be found in this patient, attention should be focused on finding and stopping an internal source. Only several places in the body can accommodate enough blood to account for hypovolemic shock. These include the chest, abdomen, pelvic cavity, and more rarely hematomas within the thighs. Without obvious injuries elsewhere and a negative chest x-ray, and in a patient with an insignificant response to fluid resuscitation, an immediate exploratory laparotomy is indicated.

(A) Although an abdominal ultrasound is an excellent way to look for free blood in the abdomen, this patient is quickly deteriorating and there is a high suspicion for blood in the abdomen. Immediate laparotomy is indicated, as an abdominal ultrasound would simply delay treatment. (C) Although a CT scan is an excellent way to evaluate for intraabdominal injuries in a stable patient, this patient would most likely not survive if surgery is delayed. (D) Although there are some superficial lacerations, none of these would account for enough blood loss to explain this patient's condition. (E) Although enough blood loss to cause hypotension can occur with femur fractures, an abdominal source is much more likely in this patient.

 83 A 62-year-old man presents to the ambulatory care clinic complaining of a 4-month history of intermittent diarrhea and lightheadedness. On further questioning, he reveals the symptoms are episodic in nature. He also complains of skin flushing, and occasional "asthma attacks" during these episodes. He has a 15-lb weight loss, even though he has been "eating more than ever." His physical examination shows no abnormalities. On his laboratory results, he is found to have an albumin of 2.5, and an international normalized ratio (INR) of 1.8. His 24-hour urine is negative for vanillyl mandelic acid (VMA), and is positive for the presence of 5-hydroxyindoleacetic acid (5-HIAA). In this condition, which amino acid is in highest demand?

(A) Alanine
(B) Tyrosine
(C) Tryptophan
(D) Threonine
(E) Histidine

The answer is C: **Tryptophan.** This patient's history of episodic diarrhea, flushing, and wheezing is classic for carcinoid syndrome. Carcinoid syndrome is caused by liver metastasis of a carcinoid tumor, which is a neuroendocrine tumor of the gastrointestinal (GI) tract which produces excess serotonin. In the case of a localized carcinoid tumor, this excess serotonin is removed from the bloodstream by the liver and the patient is asymptomatic. But with liver metastasis, as in our patient with a low albumin and elevated INR, the normal liver tissue is unable to remove the serotonin. It then enters the systemic circulation and patients become symptomatic. The amino acid precursor of serotonin is tryptophan, which is readily consumed by the carcinoid cells. Tryptophan is quickly depleted by this outflow of serotonin.

(A) Alanine does not play a role in the synthesis of serotonin. Its most important role is in the alanine-glucose cycle, where it travels from skeletal muscle to the liver to aid in gluconeogenesis. (B) Tyrosine is the main building block of the catecholamines dopamine, norepinephrine, and epinephrine. (D) Threonine is not used in the synthesis of neurotransmitters or hormones. (E) Histidine is the precursor of histamine, which is released by mast cells in type I hypersensitivity reactions.

84 A 22-year-old man has an exploratory laparotomy for a gunshot wound to the abdomen at which time a through-and-through injury to the infrarenal inferior vena cava is encountered. His blood pressure is 90/40 mmHg and his pulse is 105 beats/min. He has received 5 units of packed red blood cells during the procedure. His most recent blood pressure intraoperatively is 110/80 mmHg and his pulse is 90 beats/ min. What is the appropriate management of this patient?

(A) Ligation of the suprarenal inferior vena cava
(B) Primary repair of the injuries
(C) Polytetrafluoroethylene (PTFE) patch graft
(D) Saphenous artery patch graft
(E) No treatment is necessary

The answer is B: Primary repair of the injuries. Injuries to the inferior vena cava result from gunshot wounds to the abdomen. Inferior vena cava injuries are diagnosed by a thorough exploration of the retroperitoneum. Primary venorrhaphy is the simplest and quickest method of repair.

(A) In patients who are unstable, ligation of the infrarenal inferior vena cava is a possible treatment. (C) PTFE patch graft is not a primary treatment of this condition. (D) Saphenous vein graft is a possible treatment of this condition. (E) This patient will require primary repair, ligation of the vena cava, or a vein patch graft.

85 A 5-year-old girl presents to her pediatrician with a 1-day history of fever and midline neck swelling which has become red and tender. She is otherwise asymptomatic. On examination, it is noted that the mass is fluctuant and elevates when she is asked to swallow. There is no thyromegaly noted. What is the appropriate treatment for this child?

(A) Antibiotics
(B) Aspiration
(C) Corticosteroids
(D) Surgical excision
(E) Watchful waiting

The answer is A: Antibiotics. This patient has a thyroglossal duct cyst, which has become infected. This infection should be treated with appropriate antibiotics. She should then be taken for surgery to remove the cyst and center of the hyoid bone, which is involved in the migration of the thyroid gland from the tongue to the anterior neck.

(B) Aspiration will not remove this lesion. Bleeding will result from such a maneuver. (C) Corticosteroids will not change the size of this lesion. (D) Surgical excision could be required if this lesion does not regress. (E) This lesion is infected and required treatment.

 86 During a radical mastectomy in a 43-year-old woman with suspected right breast cancer, indurated lymphatic tissue is dissected and removed from the area medial to the pectoralis minor muscle against the chest wall. This implies disease in which of the following nodal levels?

(A) Level I
(B) Level II
(C) Level III
(D) Level IV

The answer is C: Level III. Nodal levels are important to understand in the relationship to metastatic spread from breast cancer. Patients with level III nodal involvement have disease that is medial to the pectoralis minor and against the chest wall.

(A) Level I lymph nodes are inferior and lateral to the pectoralis minor. (B) Level II lymph nodes to the pectoralis minor. (D) Level IV lymph nodes are not part of the metastatic spread of breast cancer.

 87 The pathologist receives an unlabeled specimen of small and large intestine from a 36-year-old woman who suffered from chronic abdominal pain, fevers, chills, and night sweats. Macroscopic examination reveals a 4-cm tumor of the bowel with perforation. The tumor is solid. Microscopic examination reveals significant infiltrate with lymphocytes. What is the most likely tissue origin of this lesion?

(A) Duodenum
(B) Jejunum
(C) Ileum
(D) Rectum
(E) Sigmoid colon

The answer is C: Ileum. Primary small bowel lymphomas usually arise in the ileum. Perforation is a frequent presentation. Lymphomas can also present with fevers of unknown origin which was also noted in this patient. Malabsorption and abdominal pain are also noted in these patients.

(A) The duodenum is an unlikely location for these tumors. (B) The jejunum is an unlikely location for primary small bowel lymphoma. (D) Adenocarcinoma is a more common tumor of the rectum than lymphoma. (E) Adenocarcinoma is a more common tumor of the sigmoid colon rather than lymphoma.

 A 35-year-old man is in a mining accident where he falls from a coal car approximately 15 feet. Witnesses note that he has lost consciousness. He is unable to be easily rescued from the mine and a hole has to be drilled for him to be pulled to safety. Initially, upon conversation with rescue personnel, it is noted that he is able to open his eyes to pain, is confused, and is able to follow commands. His Glasgow coma scale (GCS) score is estimated to be which of the following?

(A) 2
(B) 4
(C) 6
(D) 8
(E) 12

The answer is E: 12. The Glasgow coma scale grades eye opening, verbal response, and motor response. The minimum score is 3 and the maximum score is 15. This individual has a GCS of 12. He obtains 2 points for being able to open his eyes to pain, 4 points for being confused, and 6 points for being able to follow commands.

(A) GCS of 2 is unlikely to be compatible with life. (B) GCS of 4 shows essentially none to minimal responsiveness. (C) GCS of 6 may show some eye opening, verbal response, and motor responses. (D) GCS of 8 is more positive than the other GCS values above but is still quite low.

 A 13-month-old boy is brought to the clinic by his mother for ear pain and a sensation of fullness in the ear. This is the third visit in the last 3 months. The child also describes a popping-like sensation. Otoscopy examination reveals a bulging and cloudy tympanic membrane. Which of the following is the most significant modifiable risk factor for otitis media in a child?

(A) Breast feeding
(B) Mold removal
(C) Passive cigarette smoke
(D) Pneumococcal vaccination
(E) Removal of dust from the house

The answer is C: Passive cigarette smoke. This patient is most likely suffering from acute suppurative otitis media. The most significant modifiable risk factor out of the choices above is exposure to passive cigarette smoke. Another major modifiable risk factor is the use of a pacifier after the age of 11 months.

(A) Breast feeding is thought to be protective against otitis media, not a risk factor. (B) Although significant mold exposure does increase the risk for acute otitis media, it is not as significant of a risk factor as smoking or pacifier use. (D) While vaccinations are important to protect against a variety of childhood illnesses, clinical trials with the pneumococcal vaccines have not shown significant impact on rates of acute otitis media. (E) Although significant dust exposure does increase the risk for acute otitis media, it is not as significant of a risk factor as smoking or pacifier use.

 90 A 57-year-old woman presents to the emergency department with acute abdominal pain and distension. She has vomited two times since she arrived, and has not had a bowel movement in 2 days, which she says is way behind usual routine. She is diagnosed with a small bowel obstruction and is scheduled for surgery. In the operating room, the surgeon identifies a large duodenal tumor, which he sends to pathology for an intraoperative frozen section. The tumor is identified as a carcinoid tumor. What is the surgical treatment of choice for carcinoid tumor?

(A) Local excision
(B) Pancreaticoduodenectomy
(C) Segmental intestinal resection
(D) Wide excision of bowel and mesentery
(E) Local excision and mesenteric lymph node dissection

The answer is B: Pancreaticoduodenectomy. The surgical management of carcinoid tumor varies depending on the tumor size, site, and whether or not metastatic disease is present. This patient has a large duodenal tumor, which is treated with a Whipple procedure (also known as a pancreaticoduodenectomy). For tumors less than 1 cm without any metastasis, segmental intestinal resection is indicated. For tumors larger than 1 cm, or multiple tumors, or lymph node involvement, the surgery indicated is a wide excision of bowel and mesentery. For tumors of the terminal ileum, a right hemicolectomy is indicated. For small duodenal tumors, local excision is indicated. And for extensive disease which cannot be locally controlled, surgical debulking is indicated for palliation.

(A) Local excision is indicated for small duodenal tumors. (C) Segmental intestinal resection is indicated for localized tumors under 1 cm. (D) For tumor larger than 1 cm, wide resection of bowel and mesentery is indicated. (E) This surgical procedure is not indicated for any carcinoid tumors.

91 A 32-year-old African American woman has a small benign mole removed from her upper ear lobe. Six months later, she presents with a large, rubbery hypertrophic mass of tissue that appears to be invading the surrounding tissue. Biopsy shows wide bands and bundles of collagen in an unordered arrangement with brightly eosinophilic and glassy appearing fibers. The edge of the tissue appears "tongue-like" and pushing underneath the epidermis. There are horizontally arranged fibrous bands in the upper reticular dermis. What is the most likely diagnosis?

(A) Basal cell carcinoma
(B) Chronic folliculitis
(C) Dermatofibroma
(D) Hypertrophic scar
(E) Keloid scar

The answer is E: Keloid scar. This patient is most likely suffering from a keloid scar. Features that suggest a keloid scar include the initiating event (biopsy or trauma), patient's race (much more common in black patients), location (most commonly occurs on the ear lobe), and histologic features. This type of scar is composed of mainly type III or type I collagen, depending on the maturity. They are benign but can sometimes be painful or itchy.

(A) Basal cell carcinomas are the most common skin malignancy. They usually develop in sun-exposed areas in fair-skinned individuals. Although slow growing, they may erode into adjacent structures. Histologically, they are composed of nests of basophilic cells. This patient's presentation is not consistent with this diagnosis. (B) Chronic folliculitis is defined as inflammation of a hair follicle and will histologically be composed of increased inflammatory cells. This patient's history and histologic features are not consistent with chronic folliculitis. (C) Dermatofibromas are hard solitary slow-growing papules that are benign tumors. They may be related to previous insect bites or thorn pricks. They are composed of disordered collagen and are usually found on the leg. (D) Hypertrophic scars may often be confused with keloid scars. However, there are some key differences. The primary difference is that hypertrophic scars do not grow beyond the original boundaries of the wound. Additionally, they often appear as erythematous raised fibrotic lesions and may undergo spontaneous regression.

92 During a laparoscopic cholecystectomy in a 29-year-old woman with cholelithiasis, the cystic artery is identified in the triangle of Calot. This triangle is bordered by the common hepatic duct medially, the cystic duct laterally, and which of the following structures superiorly?

(A) Common bile duct
(B) Cystic artery
(C) Cystic duct
(D) Jejunum
(E) Liver

The answer is E: Liver. The triangle of Calot is an important landmark in gall bladder surgery. The cystic artery crosses the triangle of Calot. Identification of the triangle, and visualization of any structure within, is very important during a cholecystectomy to avoid injury to the right hepatic artery. The liver is the superior boundary of the triangle of Calot.

(A) The liver is the superior boundary of the triangle of Calot. (B) The cystic artery runs in the triangle of Calot. (C) The cystic duct lies outside the triangle of Calot. (D) The jejunum is nowhere near the triangle of Calot.

---

93 Which of the following statements is correct about the gastric peptide ghrelin?

(A) Inhibits acid secretion
(B) Initiates protein digestion
(C) Produced by oxyntic glands
(D) Secreted by parietal cells
(E) Stimulates starvation

The answer is C: Produced by oxyntic glands. Ghrelin is produced by oxyntic glands. It is an orexigenic hormone, and it stimulates food intake.

(A) Somatostatin inhibits acid secretion. (B) Pepsins initiate protein digestion. (D) Intrinsic factor is secreted by parietal cells. (E) Ghrelin stimulates food intake.

---

94 A 17-year-old girl who participates in competitive swimming presents with severe and intermittent right lower abdominal pain that started 1 day ago and has since been worsening. The pain is described as radiating suprapubically and into the right thigh and is associated with nausea and vomiting. On examination, there is tenderness with palpation of the lower right abdomen. There is no rebound tenderness or guarding. Which of the following is the next best step in diagnosis?

(A) Abdominal and pelvic CT
(B) Complete blood count (CBC) and measurement of interleukin-6
(C) Immediate operative management
(D) Ultrasonography and pregnancy test
(E) Urinalysis and magnetic resonance imaging

The answer is D: Ultrasonography and pregnancy test. This patient is suffering from lower abdominal and pelvic pain. While there are multiple causes of lower abdominal and pelvic pain, ovarian torsion should remain high on the differential in a patient with the described symptoms. The first step in diagnosis of ovarian torsion is abdominal or transvaginal ultrasound with Doppler flow. In patients with confirmed ovarian torsion, the most common finding on ultrasound is an enlarged heterogenous appearing ovary. Other findings suggestive of torsion include a cranial displaced adnexa, thickening of the adnexal wall, multiple peripheral follicles, and cystic hemorrhage. Doppler imaging may show decreased blood flow. In the majority of surgically confirmed cases of torsion, a cystic, solid, or complex adnexal mass as well as free fluid in the cul-de-sac was visualized on ultrasound. However, normal ovaries on ultrasound do not rule out the possibility of torsion. Also on the differential is an ectopic pregnancy, which is the reason for the pregnancy test.

(A) While CT scan may assist in the diagnosis, it typically has less diagnostic value than transvaginal ultrasound. Computed tomography (CT) findings suggestive of torsion include a large predominantly solid oval mass with low-density center and possibly other small cysts consistent with follicles. Other findings include thickened fallopian tube, ascites, and uterine deviation. (B) Although a CBC should be part of the initial workup, interleukin-6 is currently not utilized for the diagnosis of torsion as further research is needed into this marker. However, early studies show that this is elevated in patients with ovarian torsion. (C) While many cases of torsion cannot be confirmed except surgically, other less invasive procedures should be performed first in this patient. (E) While urinalysis is an important part of the initial workup, magnetic resonance imaging (MRI) is less valuable than ultrasonography for diagnosis of ovarian torsion.

---

95 A 61-year-old man returns for a follow-up appointment for medial knee joint pain and "clicking." His symptoms are worse when he plays golf. He has a prior medical history of mild arthritis and diet-controlled diabetes mellitus. He has already tried acetaminophen and physical therapy for his knee pain. At his last appointment, he received an intraarticular steroid injection and reports no improvement of his symptoms. An magnetic resonance imaging (MRI) of his knee joint reveals a medial meniscus tear and chondrosis of the underlying bone. Which of the following is the next best treatment?

(A) Arthroscopic partial meniscectomy
(B) Continued use of acetaminophen and physical therapy
(C) Intraarticular viscosupplementation
(D) Observation alone with discontinuation of physical therapy
(E) Total knee replacement

The answer is A: Arthroscopic partial meniscectomy. This patient has suffered a meniscal injury. First-line treatment for meniscal injuries includes nonsteroidal anti-inflammatory drug (NSAID) use and observation. Goals of therapy are to minimize the effusion, normalize the gait, and maintain fitness. A trial of conservative treatment should be used almost all meniscal injuries with the exception of the most severe. In this patient, his symptoms have not responded to conservative therapy; thus surgery is needed. Arthroscopic partial meniscectomy is a procedure used for treating meniscal tears nonresponsive to more conservative treatment or areas of the meniscus that are avascular.

(B) Continued NSAID use and observation would not be appropriate, as he has not responded to trials of conservative treatment. (C) Published clinical trials have failed to show a significant benefit for this treatment. (D) While observation is part of the treatment, it should be combined with pain relief, physical therapy, and other treatment modalities to maximize rehabilitation. (E) Total knee replacement is invasive and rarely necessary for meniscal tears.

 A 55-year-old man complains of muscle weakness that has been worsening over the past few months. He first noticed the weakness in his arms, finding it harder and harder to perform yard work like he used to. More recently, he has also had more difficulty climbing his stairs. Repeated use of the physical examination shows 4/5 strength in all four extremities, but his sensation is completely intact. Which of the following is the most likely cause of this man's weakness?

(A) Amyotrophic lateral sclerosis
(B) Cerebrovascular accident
(C) Guillain-Barré syndrome
(D) Multiple sclerosis (MS)
(E) Muscular dystrophy

The answer is A: Amyotrophic lateral sclerosis. Amyotrophic lateral sclerosis (ALS) is a disease of the anterior horn cells and corticospinal tracts of the spinal cord. Signs of damage to upper motor neurons (spastic paralysis) as well as to lower motor neurons (flaccid paralysis) may be present. Importantly, sensory function is not affected in ALS. Most cases present between 50 and 70 years of age. There is currently no effective treatment and the 5-year mortality is 80%.

(B) Cerebrovascular accidents (strokes) can cause muscle weakness if they affect a motor area of the brain, but the chance of multiple strokes causing weakness in multiple muscle groups bilaterally without causing any sensory deficit is vanishingly small. This patient's presentation is more consistent with ALS. (C) Guillain-Barré syndrome is an ascending demyelinating polyneuropathy due to antibodies targeted against foreign antigens that happen to cross-react with neural proteins. The pattern of weakness begins in the lower extremities (unlike in this patient, where the weakness was first noticed) and may also affect sensation. (D) MS is a demyelinating central nervous system (CNS) disease that is more common in women than men, and the most common initial presentation is transient sensory deficits. Motor symptoms may also appear, but the course of MS generally involves random symptoms that relapse and remit. The insidious onset and unrelenting course in this patient are more consistent with ALS. (E) Muscular dystrophy, both Duchenne and Becker, would present earlier in life than 55 years old. Duchenne muscular dystrophy manifests in childhood and patients have an average life expectancy of 25 years. Becker muscular dystrophy has a less severe course, with some patients surviving to a nearly normal lifespan. Even so, symptoms of Becker muscular dystrophy generally present before age 25.

 97 A 73-year-old farmer presents with a worsening cough over the last week. His past medical history is remarkable for chronic obstructive pulmonary disease and hypertension, which is managed with inhalers and hydrochlorothiazide, respectively. He has smoked 2 packs per day for the last 55 years. A chest x-ray reveals a possible mass in the lower lobe of the left lung. A previous chest x-ray shows no mass. Which of the following is the most important next step?

(A) Chest CT
(B) Initiate antibiotics
(C) Initiate radiation and chemotherapy
(D) Obtain a biopsy of the lesion
(E) Obtain serum tumor markers

The answer is A: Chest CT. This patient is presenting with a lung lesion that could potentially be cancer. The fact that the lesion is not seen on a previous x-ray makes it even more suspicious. The next step in diagnosis is to obtain advanced imaging to characterize the lesion. Computed tomography (CT) imaging can often provide extensive information about the location and provide clues about the type of cancer. It is also used in staging. CT imaging has been examined as a screening tool for lung cancer. While currently not recommended for screening, CT imaging is still an important diagnostic tool in patients with lung cancer.

(B) Although the cough could be pneumonia, the patient does not have other symptoms such as a fever that would indicate an infective process. (C) While radiation and chemotherapy may be an option for this patient depending on the type and extent of cancer, it is still too premature to begin therapy. (D) Biopsy is also a very important step in the workup of patients with suspected lung malignancy. However, it is usually obtained after or less frequently along with imaging if CT-guided biopsy is indicated. (E) Possible lung cancer markers include neuron-specific enolase (increased in small cell carcinoma), carcinoembryonic antigen (increased in adenocarcinoma), cytokeratin-19 fragments (most sensitive marker for non–small cell carcinoma of the lung), and others. Although no markers have yet been shown effective as screening tools, they are sometimes helpful in monitoring treatment response.

---

 98 A 5-year-old boy is admitted to the hospital with a 3-day history of bloody diarrhea, which began hours after a picnic. The patient has been lethargic since and has been unable to eat because of vomiting. Physical examination reveals an ill-appearing child who is difficult to arouse. Vital signs are temperature 39.2°C (102.2°F), blood pressure 89/74 mmHg, heart rate 131 beats/min, respiratory rate 23 breaths/min. Numerous petechiae are noted on his legs. The abdomen is diffusely tender, with decreased bowel sounds. Laboratory studies reveal the following: blood urea nitrogen (BUN), 72; creatinine, 8.1; WBCs, 11,000/mm³; Hgb, 5 mg/dL; platelet count, 10,000/mm³; prothrombin time (PT), normal; partial thromboplastin time (PTT), normal. The peripheral smear demonstrates numerous schistocytes. What is the most likely diagnosis?

(A) Crohn disease
(B) Disseminated intravascular coagulopathy (DIC)
(C) Hemolytic uremic syndrome (HUS)
(D) Idiopathic thrombocytopenic purpura (ITP)
(E) Ulcerative colitis

The answer is C: Hemolytic uremic syndrome (HUS). This patient has HUS, which is usually associated with *E. coli* infection and begins with bloody diarrhea and abdominal pain. The classic triad is thrombocytopenia, anemia, and renal failure.

(A) Ulcerative colitis and Crohn disease are not supported by the lab findings or peripheral smear. (B) DIC can be confused with HUS, but coagulation studies are normal with HUS and increased in DIC. (D) ITP shows isolated thrombocytopenia without anemia or renal failure. (E) Ulcerative colitis and Crohn disease are not supported by the lab findings or peripheral smear.

---

 99 A 39-year-old woman with a history or end-stage renal disease is 1-year status postcadaveric renal transplant. She is now 16 weeks' pregnant. Physical examination of the heart, lungs, and abdomen is unremarkable. A healed right iliac fossa scar is noted. The fundus is palpable 4 cm below the umbilicus. During this patient's pregnancy, the renal glomerular filtration rate (GFR) can increase by as much as

(A) 10%
(B) 25%
(C) 50%
(D) 75%
(E) 100%

The correct answer is C: 50%. The GFR increases early in pregnancy by up to 50%. This increase occurs at the beginning of the second trimester. The elevation in GFR persists until term. The mechanism of increase has not been identified.

(A) GFR during pregnancy can increase by up to 50%.
(B) GFR during pregnancy can increase by up to 50%.
(D) GFR during pregnancy can increase by up to 50%.
(E) GFR during pregnancy can increase by up to 50%.

---

 100 A 62-year-old man presents to his primary care physician complaining that he gets all flushed and has trouble breathing on occasion. Upon further questioning, he describes a 2-month history of episodic wheezing and skin flushing. He also complains of diarrhea, which did not improve even though he tried to increase his dietary fiber. His physical examination is normal, as are his complete blood count (CBC) and basic metabolic panel. On further workup, he has a 24-hour urine study, which is negative for vanillyl mandelic acid (VMA), but is positive for the presence of 5-hydroxyindoleacetic acid (5-HIAA). What is the most appropriate treatment for this patient?

(A) Labetalol
(B) Phenoxybenzamine and atenolol
(C) Diphenhydramine
(D) Diphenhydramine and atenolol
(E) Ocreotide

The answer is E: Ocreotide. The patient's episodes of flushing, wheezing, and diarrhea are consistent with carcinoid syndrome. Carcinoid syndrome is caused by a malignancy of neuroendocrine cells of the gastrointestinal (GI) tract which secrete excess amounts of serotonin. When this malignancy invades the liver, the excess serotonin is able to enter the systemic circulation causing symptoms. The medical treatment of choice for carcinoid syndrome is ocreotide. Ocreotide is a somatostatin analogue that decreases the symptoms of diarrhea and flushing caused by carcinoid syndrome. It does this by decreasing the amount of serotonin released by the carcinoid tumor cells.

(A) Labetalol is a nonselective β-blocker which has α-blocking effects as well. It can used in the treatment of pheochromocytoma. (B) For the treatment of pheochromocytoma, α- and β-blockers are used. Phenoxybenzamine and atenolol are examples of these, respectively. (C) Diphenhydramine is a first-generation antihistamine which may be used as an adjunct medication for symptomatic relief of Carcinoid syndrome. It is not very effective alone. (D) This answer choice is a distractor; atenolol can be used for treatment of pheochromocytoma after α-blockade is established. Diphenhydramine may be used for some symptomatic control of carcinoid syndrome.

Figure
Credits

Figure 2-1 Fleisher GR, Ludwig S, Baskin MN. *Atlas of Pediatric Emergency Medicine.* Philadelphia, PA: Lippincott Williams & Wilkins; 2004.

Figure 2-2 Bucholz RW, Heckman JD. *Rockwood & Green's Fractures in Adults.* 5th ed. Philadelphia, PA: Lippincott Williams & Wilkins; 2001.

Figure 2-3 Eisenberg RL. *An Atlas of Differential Diagnosis.* 4th ed. Philadelphia, PA: Lippincott Williams & Wilkins; 2003.

Figure 3-1 Leyendecker JR, Brown JJ. *Practical Guide to Abdominal Pelvic MRI.* Philadelphia, PA: Lippincott Williams & Wilkins; 2004.

Figure 3-2 Mulholland MW, Lillemoe KD, Dohery GM, Maier RV, Upchurch GR. *Greenfields Surgery: Scientific Principles and Practice.* 4th ed. Philadelphia, PA: Lippincott Williams & Wilkins; 2006.

Figure 4-1 Eisenberg RL. *An Atlas of Differential Diagnosis.* 4th ed. Philadelphia, PA: Lippincott Williams & Wilkins; 2003.

Figure 4-2 Eisenberg RL. *An Atlas of Differential Diagnosis.* 4th ed. Philadelphia, PA: Lippincott Williams & Wilkins; 2003.

Figure 5-1 Daffner RH. *Clinical Radiology: The Essentials.* 3rd ed. Philadelphia, PA: Lippincott Williams & Wilkins; 2007.

Figure 5-2 Fleisher GR, Ludwig S, Baskin MN. *Atlas of Pediatric Emergency Medicine.* Philadelphia, PA: Lippincott Williams & Wilkins; 2004.

Figure 6-1 Fleisher GR, Ludwig S, Baskin MN. *Atlas of Pediatric Emergency Medicine.* Philadelphia, PA: Lippincott Williams & Wilkins; 2004.

Figure 6-2 Mulholland MW, Maier RV, et al. *Greenfields Surgery: Scientific Principles and Practice.* 4th ed. Philadelphia, PA: Lippincott Williams & Wilkins; 2006.

Figure 7-1 Mulholland MW, Lillemoe KD, Dohery GM, Maier RV, Upchurch GR. *Greenfields Surgery: Scientific Principles and Practice.* 4th ed. Philadelphia, PA: Lippincott Williams & Wilkins; 2006.

Figure 7-2 Mulholland MW, Lillemoe KD, Dohery GM, Maier RV, Upchurch GR. *Greenfields Surgery: Scientific Principles and Practice.* 4th ed. Philadelphia, PA: Lippincott Williams & Wilkins; 2006.

Figure 8-1 Gorbach SL, Bartlett JG, Blackow NR. *Infectious Diseases.* Philadelphia, PA: Lippincott Williams & Wilkins; 2004.

Figure 8-2 Leyendecker JR, Brown JJ. *Practical Guide to Abdominal Pelvic MRI.* Philadelphia, PA: Lippincott Williams & Wilkins; 2004.

Figure 8-3 Eisenberg RL. *An Atlas of Differential Diagnosis.* 4th ed. Philadelphia, PA: Lippincott Williams & Wilkins; 2003.

Figure 8-4 Leyendecker JR, Brown JJ. *Practical Guide to Abdominal Pelvic MRI.* Philadelphia, PA: Lippincott Williams & Wilkins; 2004.

Figure 9-1 Mulholland MW, Lillemoe KD, Dohery GM, Maier RV, Upchurch GR. *Greenfields Surgery: Scientific Principles and Practice.* 4th ed. Philadelphia, PA: Lippincott Williams & Wilkins; 2006.

Figure 9-2 Harris JR, Lippman ME, Morrow M, Osborne CK. *Diseases of the Breast.* 3rd ed. Philadelphia, PA: Lippincott Williams & Wilkins; 2004.

Figure 11-1 Goodheart HP. *Goodheart's Photoguide of Common Skin Disorders.* 2nd ed. Philadelphia, PA: Lippincott Williams & Wilkins; 2003.

Figure 11-2 Eisenberg RL. *An Atlas of Differential Diagnosis.* 4th ed. Philadelphia, PA: Lippincott Williams & Wilkins; 2003.

Figure 12-1 Leyendecker JR, Brown JJ. *Practical Guide to Abdominal Pelvic MRI.* Philadelphia, PA: Lippincott Williams & Wilkins; 2004.

Figure 12-2 Leyendecker JR, Brown JJ. *Practical Guide to Abdominal Pelvic MRI.* Philadelphia, PA: Lippincott Williams & Wilkins; 2004.

Figure 13-1 Fleisher GR, Ludwig W, Baskin MN. *Atlas of Pediatric Emergency Medicine.* Philadelphia, PA: Lippincott Williams & Wilkins; 2004.

Figure 13-2 Goodheart HP. *A Photoguide of Common Skin Disorders: Diagnosis and Management.* Baltimore, MD: Lippincott Williams & Wilkins; 1999.

Figure 14-1 Leyendecker JR, Brown JJ. *Practical Guide to Abdominal Pelvic MRI.* Philadelphia, PA: Lippincott Williams & Wilkins; 2004.

Figure 14-2 Yochum TR, Rowe LJ. *Yochum and Rowe's Essentials of Skeletal Radiology.* 3rd ed. Philadelphia, PA: Lippincott Williams & Wilkins; 2004.

Figure 15-1 Crapo JD, Karlinsky JB, King TE. *Baum's Textbook of Pulmonary Diseases.* 7th ed. Philadelphia, PA: Lippincott Williams & Wilkins; 2004.

Figure 15-2 Eisenberg RL. *An Atlas of Differential Diagnosis.* 4th ed. Philadelphia, PA: Lippincott Williams & Wilkins; 2003.

Figure 16-1 Fleisher GR, Ludwig W, Baskin MN. *Atlas of Pediatric Emergency Medicine.* Philadelphia, PA: Lippincott Williams & Wilkins; 2004.

Figure 16-2 Swischuk LE. *Imaging of the Newborn, Infant, and Young Child.* 4th ed. Philadelphia, PA: Lippincott Williams & Wilkins; 1997.

Figure 17-1 Eisenberg RL. *An Atlas of Differential Diagnosis.* 4th ed. Philadelphia, PA: Lippincott Williams & Wilkins; 2003.

Figure 17-2 Mulholland MW, Lillemoe KD, Dohery GM, Maier RV, Upchurch GR. *Greenfields Surgery: Scientific Principles and Practice.* 4th ed. Philadelphia, PA: Lippincott Williams & Wilkins; 2006.

Figure 18-1 Daffner RH. *Clinical Radiology: The Essentials.* 3rd ed. Philadelphia, PA: Lippincott Williams & Wilkins; 2007.

Figure 19-1 Courtesy of William Phillips, MD.

Figure 19-2 Moore KL, Dalley AF. *Clinically Oriented Anatomy.* 4th ed. Baltimore, MD: Lippincott Williams & Wilkins; 1999.

Figure 20-1 Swischuk LE. *Emergency Imaging of the Acutely Ill or Injured Child.* 3rd ed. Philadelphia, PA: Lippincott Williams & Wilkins; 1994.

Figure 20-2 Topol EJ, Califf RM, Isner, J. *Textbook of Cardiovascular Medicine.* 3rd ed. Philadelphia, PA: Lippincott Williams & Wilkins; 2006.

Figure 20-3 Eisenberg RL. *An Atlas of Differential Diagnosis.* 4th ed. Philadelphia, PA: Lippincott Williams & Wilkins; 2003.

Figure 21-1 Daffner RH. *Clinical Radiology: The Essentials.* 3rd ed. Philadelphia, PA: Lippincott Williams & Wilkins; 2007.

Figure 21-2 Leyendecker JR, Brown JJ. *Practical Guide to Abdominal Pelvic MRI.* Philadelphia, PA: Lippincott Williams & Wilkins; 2004.

Figure 21-3 Courtesy of T. Ernesto Figueroa.

Figure Q46 Fleisher GR, Ludwig W, Baskin MN. *Atlas of Pediatric Emergency Medicine.* Philadelphia, PA: Lippincott Williams & Wilkins; 2004.

Index

Note: Page numbers followed by *f* indicate figures; those followed by *t* indicate tables.